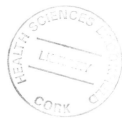

THE LOURDES HOSPITAL INQUIRY

An Inquiry into peripartum hysterectomy at Our Lady of Lourdes Hospital, Drogheda.

REPORT

Of

JUDGE MAUREEN HARDING CLARK S.C.,

January 2006

BAILE ÁTHA CLIATH
ARNA FHOILSIÚ AG OIFIG AN tSOLÁTHAIR
Le ceannach díreach ón
OIFIG DHÍOLTA FOILSEACHÁN RIALTAIS,
TEACH SUN ALLIANCE, SRÁID THEACH LAIGHEAN, BAILE ÁTHA CLIATH 2,
nó tríd an bpost ó
FOILSEACHÁIN RIALTAIS, AN RANNÓG POST-TRÁCHTA,
51 FAICHE STIABHNA, BAILE ÁTHA CLIATH 2,
(Teil: 01 - 6476834/35/36/37; Fax: 01 - 6476843)
nó trí aon díoltóir leabhar.

———

DUBLIN
PUBLISHED BY THE STATIONERY OFFICE
To be purchased directly from the
GOVERNMENT PUBLICATIONS SALE OFFICE,
SUN ALLIANCE HOUSE, MOLESWORTH STREET, DUBLIN 2,
or by mail order from
GOVERNMENT PUBLICATIONS, POSTAL TRADE SECTION,
51 ST. STEPHEN'S GREEN, DUBLIN 2,
(Tel: 01 - 6476834/35/36/37; Fax: 01 - 6476843)
or through any bookseller.

———

(Prn. A6/0246)   €10.00

Wt. —. 3,000. 2/06. Cahill. (M92291). G.Spl.

; 17026283

TABLE OF CONTENTS

INTRODUCTION AND OVERVIEW

1 HISTORICAL BACKGROUND LEADING TO THE HOLDING OF THIS INQUIRY

1.1 In September 2003 Dr. Michael Neary, a well respected, busy and popular consultant obstetrician and gynaecologist at Our Lady of Lourdes Hospital, Drogheda, was struck off the Medical Register following a lengthy hearing before the Fitness to Practise Committee of the Irish Medical Council.

1.2 This action was the culmination of a series of investigations carried out by the management of the hospital at which Dr. Neary worked, the North Eastern Health Board (the owners of the Lourdes Hospital since 1997, in succession to the Medical Missionaries of Mary (MMMs)), the Institute of Obstetricians and Gynaecologists in Ireland and finally the Fitness to Practise Committee of the Irish Medical Council. The process started in late October 1998. Two midwives working at the Maternity Unit of the Lourdes Hospital reported that it was their perception that Dr. Neary was carrying out an unusual number of caesarean hysterectomies and that some of his clinical practices were perceived as being out of date. Initial investigations confirmed that there was substance in the allegation that Dr. Neary had carried out a number of caesarean hysterectomies, some of them on very young women.

1.3 It is appropriate to explain at this time what exactly is meant by peripartum hysterectomy, which is sometimes referred to as obstetric hysterectomy or caesarean hysterectomy. A peripartum hysterectomy is an operation to remove the womb within six weeks of a delivery. It is not a common procedure. The peripartum period is the period following parturition or birth. A caesarean hysterectomy is a hysterectomy performed during the initial surgery for caesarean section after the baby has been removed or within a short period subsequent to it. Caesarean hysterectomy is more narrowly defined than peripartum hysterectomy as it excludes hysterectomy following ordinary vaginal delivery. Obstetric hysterectomy is a more general description, which includes both procedures and alerts the reader to the fact that the hysterectomy took place in the context of a pregnancy. Obstetric hysterectomy includes all hysterectomies associated with pregnancy - for instance following a late miscarriage or following evacuation of products of conception. Ordinary hysterectomies, which take place in a gynaecology theatre and which are associated with older women with gynaecological problems such as fibroids, endometriosis, or cancer, are not connected with pregnancy and are therefore excluded. Some obstetric hysterectomies are planned in advance in cases where there is known cancer or other disease. Most of the hysterectomies with which we are concerned are hysterectomies, which were carried out as emergency procedures in the same theatre in which a caesarean section had been performed and are referred to as caesarean hysterectomies. A total hysterectomy is where the cervix and uterus are removed. A sub total hysterectomy leaves the cervix behind. In both cases, unless there is a very good reason, the ovaries are conserved.

1.4 On October 28th 1998 a meeting was arranged between Health Board senior management and Dr. Neary to discuss the midwives' concerns. Dr. Neary was asked to take administrative leave for two weeks in order that the allegations could be further investigated. At the end of that period Dr. Neary sought to return to work. Dr. Ambrose McLoughlin, the Assistant Chief Executive Officer of the North-Eastern Health Board, had in the meanwhile become better informed in relation to the incidence of peripartum hysterectomies and therefore had serious misgivings concerning Dr. Neary's return to work. He sought to have Dr. Neary's suspension extended during which time his cases of caesarean hysterectomy during the period of 1996 to 1998 would be subject to peer review and audit by the Institute of Obstetricians and Gynaecologists in Ireland. At that time it was erroneously believed that the caesarean hysterectomy rate was within acceptable limits before 1996.

1.5 Dr. Neary consented to this audit, but argued through his legal representatives that it was unprecedented for a consultant Obstetrician and Gynaecologist to be suspended before the peer review had taken place, and that this action would have such negative consequences on his practice that civil damages would not be an adequate remedy. Dr. Neary's advisors then obtained copy files of the seventeen caesarean hysterectomies identified from the original search through the maternity theatre register. He sought to have these cases reviewed by three established, eminent and practising consultant colleagues attached to the major teaching hospitals in Dublin.

1.6 The three obstetricians met together with Dr. Neary and considered the files in turn. At all stages they accepted the explanations provided by Dr. Neary. Eight of the seventeen cases they were asked to review were excluded on the basis that Dr. Neary informed them that these were consent hysterectomies - necessitated because of the prohibition in the hospital of tubal ligation.

The three consultant Obstetrician/Gynaecologists did not consider these 8 files.

They produced two reports. They stated that the reason for reporting was:

"Dr. Michael Neary, a consultant Obstetrician and Gynaecologist in Drogheda has received a letter from the North Eastern Health Board detailing certain perceptions concerning his practice, with particular reference to the number of caesarean hysterectomies carried out under his care at Our Lady of Lourdes Hospital in Drogheda. He has been informed of the wishes of the Health Board to hold an inquiry into his practice and of their wish that he suspend practice during such investigation.

This report is a preliminary report following a brief examination of the case records of those patients who have had caesarean hysterectomies under the care of Dr. Michael Neary during the last three years, and a study of the caesarean hysterectomy rates at the hospital during the three years 1996 to 1998. Because of the immediacy of the situation we have had insufficient time to prepare a comprehensive report but have sought to determine whether or not there are grounds for an investigation into Dr. Neary's practice whether it is in the patients' or the Health Board's interests to suspend Dr. Neary during such investigation."

The three consultant Obstetrician/Gynaecologists reviewed Dr. Neary's last 9 cases of caesarean hysterectomy which, according to Dr. Neary's information, were hysterectomies carried out for obstetric reasons.

Two of those Obstetricians concluded:

> *"Having reviewed the case notes, we are of the opinion that all of the nine cases reviewed can be justified in the prevailing situation. We note that if female sterilisations were available in the Lourdes Hospital the incidence of caesarean hysterectomy would be reduced by 50% immediately. We find no evidence of questionable clinical judgement, poor operative ability or faulty decision making. Quite the contrary, we find that Dr. Neary, in the exercise of his clinical judgement, has under difficult circumstances probably saved the lives of several mothers. We note that some of the mothers may have been under-transfused after the operation but accept Dr. Neary's explanation that these mothers were very reluctant to receive even the volume of blood that was transfused as we have had the same experience here in our own hospital. We do not now transfuse patients for postpartum anaemia unless they are symptomatic with haemoglobin of less than 7grams/dl.*
>
> *On the evidence presented we find no grounds to suspend Dr. Neary or to place any restrictions on his practice (public or private).*
>
> *We recommend that the North Eastern Health Board take urgent steps to implement the following procedures:*
>
> - *That female sterilisation be made available where considered by the patient and her attending Obstetrician. This is the practice in the majority of obstetric units in the state, and is in accordance with Department of Health policy.*
>
> - *That Prostaglandin F2Alpha be available to treat refractory cases of postpartum haemorrhage.*

- *That appropriate surgical back-up from a surgeon trained in vascular surgery be available for consultation in cases of uncontrollable post partum or intraoperative bleeding. We do not consider it appropriate that a surgeon be called in from Navan for this purpose."*

The third Obstetrician reported as follows:

- *"I have scrutinised photocopies of the notes presented to me of the 9 patients who underwent emergency hysterectomy in the three years 1996 to 1998 at the practice of Dr. Michael Neary in Drogheda. Seven of these patients had intraoperative haemorrhage and two had a post-partum hysterectomy because of haemorrhage which had not responded to appropriate therapy. Dr. Neary was called in to a further five cases during the three years in question to help a colleague. Dr. Neary's undoubted reputation at management of postpartum haemorrhage was in my opinion life saving in these cases. From the data provided by Dr. Neary his rate of caesarean hysterectomies is not dramatically different from that of his colleagues.*

- *It is my conclusion that Dr. Neary has no case to answer concerning his management of any of the patients in question. On the contrary it would seem to me that the North Eastern Health Board has a number of situations which need to be dealt with urgently.*

- *A more enlightened attitude by management is required into the intrinsic risks of motherhood and the stresses of contemporary obstetric practice on all involved at a clinical level.*

- *Female sterilisation should be made available and this would significantly reduce the number of caesarean hysterectomy.*

- *There should be appropriate surgical backup and the provision of vascular surgery should be examined.*

- *The methods of dealing with perceived high rates of intervention should be dramatically altered. There must be some way where the practice of a senior and highly respected obstetrician can be evaluated on a mutually agreed basis without the fear of suspension, legal action and so on.*

It is my firm conclusion that Dr. Neary should continue to work in Our Lady of Lourdes Hospital pending any formal investigation. It would be wrong to put restrictions on his practice and it is my view that the mothers of the North Eastern Health Board are fortunate in having the service of such an experienced and caring obstetrician."

Dr. Neary's 9 most recent caesarean hysterectomies were thus not criticised and his practices were deemed to present no danger to patients.

1.7 The solicitor and the three consultants involved in that first report have attended for interview and explained that this limited report was prepared on a confidential basis to enable Dr. Neary to continue working, pending the outcome of the review of his practice by the Institute of Obstetricians and Gynaecologists. It is apparent that, at this time, Dr. Neary was fully confident that any review of his practice would exonerate him fully and that he would be returning to work. In those circumstances therefore it is understandable that he had very grave concerns with regard to his future practice if he were to be suspended pending the expected review.

1.8 The Inquiry accepts that permitting Dr. Neary to work pending the review by the Institute of Obstetricians and Gynaecologists may well have been the intention of his union advisors and his three colleagues in presenting their report. The report may have been prepared for limited viewing but the language, which is not qualified, is regrettable. I believe that the three obstetricians involved have had serious regrets for their part in producing these reports, which were motivated by compassion and collegiality. They ought to have been alarmed that one obstetrician carried out 17 caesarean hysterectomies in three years in a middle sized Maternity Unit notwithstanding the lack of tubal ligations, a vascular surgeon or the use of prostaglandins.

As a result of their report, Dr. Neary returned to work - subject to restrictions - and the Health Board sought the views of an independent specialist outside the jurisdiction.

1.9   The Health Board engaged Mr. Michael Maresh, an English obstetrician practicing as a consultant at St. Mary's Hospital in Manchester where he was the Lead Clinician in the labour ward. St. Mary's Hospital delivers more than 6,000 babies every year and is a tertiary referral centre. Mr. Maresh is held in high esteem there as a clinician. He is an advisor to the Royal College of Obstetrics and Gynaecology, and has published a large volume of research papers and articles.

On 8th December 1998 The Health Board received a report from Mr. Maresh. His report reviewed the same nine cases as were reviewed by the three obstetricians acting for Dr. Neary. Mr. Maresh stated in his report that he had major concerns about Dr. Neary continuing to practice currently as a consultant obstetrician. He believed Dr. Neary's clinical judgement to be significantly impaired and that women appeared to be put at risk. Dr. Maresh also indicated that he had concerns about other aspects of Dr. Neary's management of patients and in addition he expressed concerns about his skills at caesarean section currently if there were complications. He also expressed the view that Dr. Neary's perception of events appeared impaired. A copy of Mr. Maresh's report was furnished to the Health Board solicitor and the solicitors for Dr. Neary's professional union. Having taken account of Mr. Maresh's report, the CEO invoked Appendix IV of the Consultants' Contract and instructed Dr. Neary to take immediate administrative leave with effect from the 11th December 1998.

1.10   In the meantime, a more thorough search of the maternity theatre register had been conducted. This search went back to 1991 which is the date when the then current register was commenced and one year after the move to the new hospital. For the first time, it was apparent that peripartum hysterectomy had been carried out more frequently than originally thought. Although Dr. Neary carried out the vast majority of the operations, peripartum hysterectomies were attributed to all the consultants working in the unit and to some registrars. They were not confined to Dr. Neary nor did they commence in 1996 when Dr. Neary's wife was diagnosed with ovarian cancer as originally thought. In fact, the years 1993, 1994 and 1995 had some of the highest rates of caesarean hysterectomy in the unit since records were kept.

1.11 On 14th December 1998 full details of the nine cases reviewed by Mr. Maresh were published in the Irish Times. The report was leaked to the Irish Times immediately following its receipt by the Health Board and Dr. Neary's solicitors. The details caused deep hurt, anguish and upset to those patients who had no idea until then that they had possibly undergone unnecessary hysterectomies, or that there had been any doubt over Dr. Neary's competence, or that their cases had been subject to review. Each of the women was able to recognise similarities to her own circumstances, which permitted her to identify herself as a former patient of Dr. Neary. Neither the hospital nor Dr. Neary was named in the reports but their identities were thinly disguised.

We have been unable to fully determine how or why the contents of Mr Maresh's report were leaked to the Irish Times. It is very probable that journalists had access to an informed person in the Health Board who leaked this and other documents. We became aware at an early stage that there were and are deep divisions in the politics of healthcare in this region and in the hospital. The leak meant that patients were made aware of concerns regarding their procedures in an utterly inappropriate manner.

1.12 Following the media coverage which followed the leaking of the report and Dr. Neary's suspension, many supporters marched to the gates of Our Lady of Lourdes Hospital in Drogheda and demanded that he be reinstated. We understand that some of these supporters also marched to the Dáil. We have been informed, but have been unable to confirm, that the march in support of Dr. Neary's reinstatement included at least one obstetrician, midwives, nurses, nuns and other hospital staff. From questions that we put to witnesses, we are aware that some, but not many, midwives marched, but that the majority of the supporters came from Dr. Neary's patients. We have seen hundreds of letters from former patients sent to the manager of the Lourdes Hospital, which speak in very laudatory terms of the care they received from Dr. Neary. It is clear that he was a well liked consultant.

Perhaps the intention of the person leaking Mr. Maresh's report was to balance the hostility in the hospital among some consultants and medical staff to the Health Board's handling of the complaints made about Dr. Neary's practices and to redress some misinformation circulating in the hospital and outside in the wider community. The leaking of the report engaged public interest in the allegations and to some extent weakened support for Dr. Neary's reinstatement but animosity towards senior management figures continued. In the weeks and months following its publication there was intense media speculation and sensational reporting of the events that led to Dr. Neary's suspension. The pendulum seemed to swing the other way.

In the aftermath of these media reports, the Health Board set up a patient helpline so that former patients of Dr. Neary could contact the hospital and seek advice in relation to procedures which had been carried out on them. The helpline appears to have been confined to queries relating to Dr. Neary, and not to queries arising out of procedures in general carried out in the Maternity Unit.

1.13 The media coverage of the 9 cases, including a programme on RTE Prime Time, was such that the Fitness to Practise Committee of the Medical Council became involved. They sought Dr. Neary's suspension through the High Court under Section 51 of the Medical Practitioners Act, 1978, pending an inquiry into his practice. Dr. Neary was suspended from practice by Order of the High Court on the 5th day of February 1999 and resigned from the practice of medicine in June 1999. He has not practised since. For ease of reference the section of the Act is found below.

Application by Council for order suspending registration.

51.—(1) Whenever the Council is satisfied that it is in the public interest so to do, the Council may apply to the High Court for an order in relation to any person registered in any register maintained under this Act that, during the period specified in the order, registration of that person's name in that register shall not have effect.

(2) An application under this section may be made in a summary manner and shall be heard otherwise than in public.

(3) The High Court may make, in any application under this section, such interim or interlocutory order (if any) as it considers appropriate.

1.14 While the Medical Council was taking steps to seek Dr. Neary's suspension in the public interest, the Institute of Obstetricians established a Review Group to carry out a review of Dr. Neary's practice in relation to peripartum hysterectomies. They obtained the case notes of all 42 patients who were identified as having undergone peripartum caesarean hysterectomy between 1992 and 1998, including the 17 cases received by the first review group and the 9 cases examined by Mr. Maresh. This list of 42 was subsequently reduced to 39, as 3 cases were deemed to belong to Dr. Finian Lynch and the records in 3 cases were not available. The Review Group did not have sight of the first report carried out by the three Consultant Obstetrician/ Gynaecologists, nor did they know the identities of the women whose cases were reviewed by Mr. Maresh. Each case was given an identifying number, and the Review Group then examined the contents in depth. They visited the Maternity Unit at the Lourdes Hospital and spoke to pathologists, senior nurse management and anaesthetists as well as the midwives who made the complaint. They also interviewed Dr. Neary, Dr. Lynch and the other consultant obstetrician Dr. Seosamh O'Coigligh. They examined the Code of Ethics for the hospital and received submissions from Dr. Neary in relation to the ethics code.

In all, they carried out a fairly robust and comprehensive analysis of Dr. Neary's practices in the new Maternity Unit. I was much impressed with their findings, which differed little from ours which involved a very much larger group of witnesses.

1.15 In April 1999 the Institute of Obstetricians Review Group reported their findings to the Hospital and Dr. Neary. They noted that the caesarean section rate at the Lourdes Hospital was high, and made similar findings in relation to induction of labour. They found a high caesarean hysterectomy rate. Dr. Neary had a personal caesarean hysterectomy rate of 5% of his caesarean sections. Out of 39 cases reviewed, they found that 18 represented unacceptable practice, 5 were doubtful and in 16 cases his practice was acceptable. These cases included instances where hysterectomy may have been carried out because tubal ligation was unavailable. The Review Group had concerns about Dr. Neary's treatment and assessment of blood loss, which seemed to precipitate hysterectomy at a low threshold. They felt that he made a diagnosis of morbidly adherent placenta or other unusual uterine abnormalities too frequently and, when those diagnoses were not confirmed on histology, he seemed not to discuss the findings with the pathologists. The Group found little evidence that Dr. Neary consulted with colleagues before carrying out a hysterectomy.

1.16 The Review Group's report discussed at some length the hospital's position with regard to direct sterilisation and Dr. Neary's well documented difficulties with the hospital owners over this issue. Dr. Neary said that if he had been permitted to carry out tubal ligations, 8 cases of caesarean hysterectomy carried out by him in the last 3 years would not have been necessary. The 8 cases of indirect sterilisation appear to be the same 8 cases extracted from the 17 cases reviewed by the first group of 3 Dublin obstetricians. The Institute Review Group stated that -

> "In previous years, in Ireland, some patients may have had a peripartum hysterectomy as a method of sterilisation and although some of Dr. Neary's patients may have fitted the criteria for indirect sterilisation, in the opinion of the Review Group, the choice of

peripartum hysterectomy for the purposes of sterilisation is not now acceptable."

The Review Group seemed to have difficulty accepting Dr. Neary's argument that he would lose his job if he carried out a tubal ligation.

The Review Group noted that the anaesthetists who were present for the hysterectomies all thought that each hysterectomy was necessary. Dr. Neary was considered by the anaesthetists to be a safe surgeon. The Group noted that the midwives who were interviewed were concerned at the young age of the patients undergoing hysterectomy, and their low parity, rather than at the fact of the operation itself. The frequency of the operation was accepted without question as just *"one of those things"*. Dr. Neary had a strong personality with very strong views on many subjects and his demeanour and mood had a major influence on the unit. It was an open secret that he had a bad relationship with management.

The Review Group looked at the history of the unit, in particular the difficulties that arose from attempts at integration of the Maternity Unit into the general hospital. They noted that the Maternity Unit had a rigid and definite policy that only allowed clinical patient management to be reviewed if a patient complained. The Review Group found that senior midwives and medical staff had not noted the high rate of hysterectomies, nor had they asked the consultants the reasons for this high incidence. They noted that there was no audit, no regular meetings, no discussions nor any clinico-pathological conferences and no evidence of organised training programmes. In this atmosphere it was difficult for any member of staff to express clinical concerns. The Review Group made a number of recommendations in relation to:

- Audit
- Regular meetings between medical and midwifery staff
- Perinatal conferences
- Journal club and a forum for case discussions
- Regular departmental meetings to discuss protocols with involvement of midwives and trainee medical staff
- An annual clinical report similar to that produced by the Dublin hospitals

- Periodic visits by the Institute of Obstetrics and Gynaecology, RCPI and RCOG
- Rotating responsibility for meetings
- Regular attendance at national and international meetings
- Improved teaching for undergraduates and postgraduates
- Changes in the Code of Ethics to include removal of the ban on sterilisation for contraceptive purpose.

In relation to Dr. Neary, the Review Group recommended a supervised postgraduate programme of retraining for a continuous period of six months with attendance and observation of colleagues in theatre and delivery wards, hospital conferences, library and laboratories. Dr. Neary was never given the opportunity to retrain, as he had been suspended by Order of the High Court in February 1999 under S.51 of the Medical Practitioners Act 1978.

THE MEDICAL COUNCIL

1.17 The Medical Council received complaints from 15 patients who had procedures carried out by Dr. Neary during the years 1986 to 1998, including ten complaints alleging unwarranted peripartum hysterectomies. The Medical Council commenced its Inquiry on the 6th June 2000 and continued hearing evidence over the next two years. These ten complaints included the 9 cases reviewed by the Review Group and Mr. Maresh.

1.18 On 29th July 2003 the Medical Council's Fitness to Practise Committee found that the facts in relation to 10 complaints alleging unwarranted peripartum hysterectomies were proved, and that Dr. Neary was guilty of professional misconduct. The Medical Council determined that his name should be erased from the General Register of Registered Medical Practitioners. Dr. Neary did not apply for cancellation of the decision pursuant to Section 46(3) of the 1978 Medical Practitioners Act and thereafter the Medical Council applied to the President of the High Court, Mr. Justice Finnegan on the 2nd day of September 2003 to confirm the decision. The waiting period between the start of the hearings and the decision to remove Dr.Neary from the register was a difficult time for all parties affected by the Inquiry. Those who had complained were anxious to know how the Medical Council, which sets standards for the medical profession, viewed their complaints. The delay in arriving at a final decision caused great anxiety to many different parties with totally opposite views and expectations.

1.19 During this time a grey cloud hung over the Hospital in general, and the Maternity Unit in particular. Information was scarce although the midwives and obstetricians were acquainted with the findings of the report prepared by the Institute of Obstetrics Review Group and must have known that their findings included criticisms of the numbers of inductions and caesarean sections and the lack of meetings, audit and supervision of junior doctors. Few knew the facts surrounding either Dr. Neary's suspension or the Medical Council's Inquiry, which was heard in private, and there was a lot of ill-informed rumour and speculation. The leaking of Mr Maresh's report to the media did not help. Many of the patients who had called the help-line to obtain their hospital charts had sought the views of obstetricians, sourced and funded by the Health Board, on the appropriateness of those procedures. They too were concerned to hear the decision of the Medical Council.

1.20 Even more seriously, many other patients who had contacted the help-line learned that their charts were missing and not available. These patients now remain in a state of unknowingness, which must be painful. So far, they have not received any meaningful explanation as to why their charts were unavailable, and the Medical Council Inquiry did not, and could not, provide answers. They will, from this Inquiry and Report, become aware of the extent of the deliberate and malicious activity involved in the removing of their records.

1.21 The decision of the Medical Council in July 2003 and the Order of the High Court in September 2003 caused much media comment. Former patients of Dr. Neary, who had strongly defended the service they received from him and had been happy with their treatment now began to question every aspect of their care. A smaller group of patients also targeted the practices of the other practising obstetricians at the Lourdes Maternity Unit. They claimed that they had also carried out hysterectomies and were not being made accountable. A larger picture was emerging which needed to be explored. Mr. Mícheál Martin TD, the Minister for Health and Children, announced that an inquiry would be set up to look at the situation referred to by the Medical Council when they stated in their report that :

"It was clear from the statistics that Dr. Neary was by no means alone in having a high caesarean hysterectomy rate. The medical culture in Drogheda was different and, in particular, a mode of clinical management was adopted that led to this difference.

The Committee cannot accept that a substantial falling below medical standards can in any way be justified by the fact that colleagues may appear, or be alleged to have adopted a similar approach…….. What occurred in these cases in Drogheda was unacceptable both by the standards which should have prevailed in that hospital, by the standards which the patient had a right to expect and by the standards prevalent generally in this country."

They further stated that:

"There was substantial evidence of a curious internal and external culture of isolation and absence of consultation within Our Lady of Lourdes Hospital. There appears to have been little evidence of peer review, consultation with colleagues or consultation with practitioners in other disciplines, such as pathology, in order to preserve and maintain acceptable medical standards. Effective communication and case review is at the heart of the good practice of medicine. There is regrettably substantial evidence that these ingredients were absent, both within the hospital and between Our Lady of Lourdes Hospital and other units elsewhere. It is deeply regrettable that it was not until this Inquiry that the statistics referred to earlier came to light fully.

The evidence discloses a series of profound errors of judgement with very serious consequences for each of the patients, a regrettable absence of insight and objectivity and the non-existence of any mechanism either within the hospital or elsewhere to ensure that such errors as occurred might be corrected or that a pattern of adverse or unusual outcomes could be properly monitored."

1.22 As a result of these comments, and because of many submissions made by Patient Focus on behalf of women who had undergone peripartum hysterectomies, Minister Mícheál Martin asked the Government to set up an Inquiry. In November 2003 the Minister requested me to take up the position of Chairman and sole member of the Inquiry. He also committed me to gather a legal team to assist in the Inquiry. In particular, the Minister requested that I establish how the normal system of peer review and outside assessment of the Maternity Unit in the Lourdes Hospital failed to disclose the high number of peripartum hysterectomies. As a result of requests made by Patient Focus, an additional Term of Reference covering missing charts was included.

1.23 This non-statutory private Inquiry was established by a decision of the Government on the 6th of April 2004 when the following terms of reference were approved.

WE PRESENT THE TERMS OF REFERENCE TO REMIND READERS OF THE INQUIRY'S MANDATE:

TERMS OF REFERENCE

1) To examine the rate of peripartum hysterectomy at Our Lady of Lourdes Hospital, Drogheda ("the hospital") with particular reference to the period covered in the report of the Fitness to Practise Committee of the Medical Council ("the report") and the period since the publication of that report and to determine how this rate compared with the rate in other Maternity Units of similar status.

2) To ascertain what system of recording of peripartum hysterectomy took place at the Hospital; to ascertain whether all expected records are now extant; and, if not, to inquire into what has become of such records.

3) To inquire into whether Dr. Neary's practice in relation to peripartum hysterectomy was commented on or acted upon by Consultants or other

medical staff, by midwives and other nursing staff within the hospital, or by the management of the hospital.

4) To inquire into what, if any, review and consultation took place, either within the hospital, or externally following peripartum hysterectomy.

5) To ascertain whether periodical clinical reports were prepared by the Maternity Unit at the hospital and, if so, the purpose of those reports; to whom they were furnished; and the action, if any, which was taken on foot of those reports.

6) To inquire into what practices and protocols have been adopted at the Maternity Unit of the hospital since October 1998 or arising from the publication of the Report.

7) To advise the Minister for Health and Children on whether additional protocols and systems of control should now be put in place to prevent a recurrence of the events that gave rise to the findings of the Report.

8) In the event of the withholding or withdrawal of full co-operation from the Inquiry by staff or former staff of the hospital, by the North Eastern Health Board, its servants and agents, the former proprietors of the Hospital or any State authority, or any suggestion that co-operation is being withheld, to report that fact immediately to the Minister.

9) In the event that the Inquiry cannot produce a final report within 9 months of the date of appointment by the Minister, the Inquiry will submit a progress report to the Minister.

1.24 The Inquiry set out to determine how many caesarean and peripartum hysterectomies had been carried out in the Maternity Unit at the Lourdes Hospital, and to compare that rate with the rate in other similarly sized units throughout the State. This Inquiry was therefore not confined to the practices of Dr. Neary, but considered the whole unit from 1960 to the present day. We did this in the expectation of establishing how the rate of peripartum hysterectomy was as high as it was in the 1990s with so little comment or appreciation.

We set out to determine how the medical culture in this hospital was different to that in other hospitals, how the style of clinical management allowed that culture to be different, and how the standards of maternity care were allowed to fall so far below what should be expected. We set out to determine whether the obstetricians and their practices were protected by any parties who knew or ought to have known of these practices. We tried to determine the extent of missing records and how these records came to be missing.

Finally, we consulted widely to learn how such mistakes can be prevented from occurring again, to report on what systems are now in place, and to advise whether those systems are adequate.

1.25 Between the 30th June and the 3rd of July 2004 advertisements were placed in national and local newspapers, with details of the Inquiry's Terms of Reference and inviting any person with information relevant to those terms of reference to contact the Inquiry offices at Bow Street in Dublin. In addition, 30-second radio advertisements ran on LMFM between 1st and 4th July 2004. We also published the Guidelines on how the interviews, which would be held in private, would be conducted to ensure confidentiality and the highest standards of constitutional justice.

1.26 In the beginning, witnesses were very reluctant to make themselves available for interview. Many legal representatives were unhappy with the safeguards for their clients in relation to confidentiality and the procedure following any subsequent adverse findings. All witnesses were assured of the maximum confidentiality available and of fair procedures. Eventually, as the Inquiry progressed, the cooperation which we received from witnesses who were invited to attend was almost 100 percent. At the end of the Inquiry, although some witnesses clearly harboured resentment at being questioned at all and appeared to maintain strong loyalties to the MMMs or to Dr. Neary, only 2 witnesses actually refused to cooperate and 1 witness provided partial cooperation. In total we heard 268 witnesses, some of whom were heard a second or third time. We received extensive submissions and responses to written questions from Dr. Neary and Dr. Lynch.

2 STARTING UP

2.1 Before we could start work on the Inquiry it was necessary to obtain and furnish suitable premises. There are currently no permanent premises set aside for the hearing of inquiries, nor is there a body of experienced personnel to manage the conduct of such inquiries. Each inquiry is therefore obliged to start from scratch, and much time is spent on very basic preparation. It should also be understood that when premises are identified, those premises must be equipped and furnished. It is essential to engage a competent office manager so that contracts can be negotiated under Government tender regulations for the supply of furniture, phone, computer and security systems for the building.

2.2 Security was a constant worry and expense. The premises we operated from were subject to three criminal forced entries including one on a Saturday afternoon when a member of the team was working there. I am deeply indebted to Rob Walsh, the office manager who was seconded to the Inquiry from the Department of Health & Children. It was he who had to respond to the break ins and the many alarm alerts. His hard work and his familiarity with the tendering process and his general competence were an enormous help to us.

2.3 The legal team consisted of Robert Haughton, SC, Johanna Ronan Mehigan and Denise Brett as Junior Counsel, Judy O'Kane Solicitor, (seconded from Hayes Solicitors a firm which specialises in medico legal defence), one part-time Research Assistant - Rebecca Broderick BL, and Dr. James Feeney FRCOG to advise and guide on all medical matters. Finally, Kevin Feeney SC advised on a needs basis on legal issues. Ann Mulvaney was our receptionist and secretary and Anne Coyle typed the interview notes and formatted this report. I was privileged to work with such an efficient, knowledgeable, supportive and happy team.

2.4 Once the building was ready, the legal team wrote to various bodies who it was considered would be in a position to assist the Inquiry with relevant documentation. We reviewed a large number of files from the North-Eastern

Health Board, the current owners of Our Lady of Lourdes Hospital in Drogheda, as well as from the Medical Missionaries of Mary. It was with the assistance of both those institutions that we were able to make out a list of witnesses whose evidence we felt would be relevant to the Inquiry. We wrote to all General Practitioners practising in the North East area asking them to contact the Inquiry if they had any relevant information. We received 3 replies, all from doctors who never had a patient with a hysterectomy. No GP who had a patient who had undergone hysterectomy contacted us.

2.5 We took advice on the circumstances in which one would expect to see a caesarean hysterectomy. Dr. Feeney directed the Inquiry team towards a large volume of published research on caesarean and peripartum hysterectomy. Mr. Maresh advised that:

"caesarean hysterectomy is invariably performed because of uncontrollable haemorrhage from the uterus at caesarean section following delivery. It is performed when the various measures, which have been taken to control bleeding, have failed, and there is concern over the woman's life. Such a decision is taken by a consultant. In view of the rarity of the problem, and the difficult manoeuvres required to try to stop the bleeding, another consultant may sometimes be called in to assist, as the registrar helping the consultant is unlikely to have experience of the procedure.

One of the results of caesarean hysterectomy is that it prevents the woman from having any more children. Therefore, great efforts must be taken to avoid this procedure on young women who have not completed their families. However, delaying performing a hysterectomy with continued bleeding could cause its own problems. Excessive bleeding is associated with reduced clotting of the remaining blood and this may increase haemorrhage. A blood transfusion on its own will not correct this. Accordingly, it is difficult to decide at what stage it is necessary to abandon conservative measures to save the uterus and proceed to hysterectomy, another reason why today a second opinion should be considered."

2.6 Dr. Feeney has advised and counselled the Inquiry that this definition excludes a situation almost unknown in the UK in the last 30 years, but which continued in Ireland until tubal ligations became commonly available from about the mid 1980s. He explained that there are circumstances where at caesarean section the obstetrician may note that the patient's uterus has become stretched and thin and is difficult to repair. The obstetrician may well suture the uterus as well as his/her skill permits, and advise strongly against any other pregnancy because of the danger of rupture. Rupture during pregnancy almost inevitably leads to death of the baby and greatly endangers the life of the mother. The mother may have had any number of heart or kidney conditions making further pregnancy dangerous. It is therefore important to note that Mr. Maresh's above definition presupposes that a woman who has been advised not to become pregnant again because the condition of her health or her uterus will follow that advice.

2.7 In modern obstetrics, such a patient would probably be advised to have a tubal ligation to protect against further pregnancy and the couple would be fully advised to use additional barrier methods of contraception to ensure minimal risk until the effectiveness of the tubal ligation was assured. Male vasectomy might also be discussed as an option. These options were not available at The International Missionary Training Hospital of Our Lady of Lourdes in Drogheda. No forms of contraception advice, apart from the rhythm or Billings method, were countenanced by the ethos of the owners of the hospital. The obstetricians there, in common with obstetricians in other Catholic hospitals with a Catholic ethos, may have carried out hysterectomies to protect the woman's health from a further pregnancy.

Readers are reminded of the significance of this limitation with regard to the care available to the patients of the Maternity Unit. This is the background in which the events which gave rise to this Inquiry occurred. This aspect of the consequences of a Catholic ethos in a maternity hospital was referred to by the Review Group at paragraph 1.16 above. Hysterectomies were carried out in such circumstances at this Maternity Unit. They were what are described as "indirect sterilisations"

The Medical Missionaries of Mary have objected to this part of the report. Their stated position is -

"The MMM were not aware that any peripartum hysterectomies were carried out at OLLH in order to protect a woman's health in a future pregnancy nor would it make any sense. There is no evidence to support this most serious contention. There are no medical records outlining this, nor was this matter put to any member of the MMMs.

The Inquiry's failure to put these comments, insofar as they may be accurate, in context or to identify any specific case in the draft report where a patient was allegedly advised to have a tubal ligation, which was unavailable, and thereafter went on to have a peripartum hysterectomy, due to weakness of the uterus, is unbalanced and grossly unfair to the MMMs. It also now appears that the women were young and of low parity. In circumstances where no specific cases were put to the MMMs as to this having actually occurred, it is inappropriate to suggest that it was a reality. Futhermore we contend that the statement in the report that :-

> *'This aspect of the consequences of a Catholic ethos in a maternity hospital was referred to by the Review Group at paragraph 1.16 above. Hysterectomies were carried out in such circumstances at this Maternity Unit.'*

The Inquiry should take account of Paragraph 7.6.2 Introduction page 53 which states:
> *' Many of the women used modern family planning to space their families. They accepted the Catholic ethos of the MMMs, but they did not let it interfere with their personal decision about family planning' "*

The Inquiry's response to this objection was

> "Before you reach paragraph 2.7 of the Introduction it would be fair to note that there are several preceding paragraphs which quote sources recommending that female sterilisation and contraception be made available in the hospital. These recommendations were made following

a medical examination of the high rate of peripartum hysterectomy in the hospital and Dr. Neary's contention that the lack of tubal ligations contributed to this high rate. It was acknowledged by these obstetricians that hysterectomy for sterilisation purposes had been carried out.

The preceding paragraphs, 2.6 and the first part of 2.7 describe how hysterectomy was carried out in circumstances where the woman's health would be impaired if she were to become pregnant again.

I note what you say that the MMMs were not aware that hysterectomy was carried out in such circumstances and I am therefore prepared to append your clients' stated position to this particular section in an appropriate highlighted format. I think I ought to point out however that Sr. B. did say during one of her interviews that if sterilisations by tubal ligation were carried out because of medical reasons there would be no problem (page 37, interview 12th July 2004). In a later interview on 4th August 2004 at page 14 Sr. B. said, *"Let me say that I was aware that hysterectomies were done in Ireland more often than was necessary because sterilisation was ethically non- acceptable"*.

The import of the interview with Sr. B. is that she was aware that hysterectomy was more common in Ireland because of Catholic mores.

The Inquiry was not mandated to look specifically at the medical records of women who had undergone obstetric hysterectomy. We did in fact see records and read reports which were furnished to us by patients or the Health Board. Dr. James Feeney examined many records from patients who underwent peripartum hysterectomy from 1960. We did not require to put specific cases to any witnesses in the light of the clear and open acknowledgement. We nevertheless put the position presented by Dr. Neary and Dr. Lynch to other investigating bodies to several of the MMMs. We specifically put the question that the ethos of the hospital which forbade contraception or sterilisation led to a number of planned hysterectomies for sterilisation purposes. I do not believe

that you could seriously contend that such questions were not put to many of the MMMs who had occupied a position of authority in the Maternity Unit and in the general hospital.

There was an abundance of evidence from obstetricians, midwives and professionals in the hospital, theologians, articles and text books, which led me to the inescapable inference that compassionate hysterectomies and planned hysterectomies were carried out as obstetric operations in the Lourdes Hospital Maternity Unit and in other Maternity Units in the country and in other Catholic hospitals."

2.8   The first letters we wrote enclosing our Terms of Reference and our proposed guidelines for interviews were to the four consultant obstetricians and gynaecologists who worked in the Maternity Unit during the period with which we were concerned. They were Dr. Liam O'Brien now retired, Dr. Michael Neary, Dr. Finian Lynch who practises at the Maternity Unit and Dr. Seosamh O'Coigligh appointed in 1997 and practising in the unit. We invited them to come in and to answer questions.

2.9   Dr. O'Brien was more than willing to attend for interview. Dr. Neary indicated that he was unwilling to come, but was prepared to answer questions by letter. Dr. Finian Lynch's wife was terminally ill and although he was willing to cooperate, we felt that he was facing into a very difficult few months and let him know that we would defer his attendance until he felt ready to speak to us. Dr. O'Coigligh was on leave awaiting major surgery and was facing a long recovery period. The absence of these critical witnesses at the early stages of the Inquiry caused us to take a different approach to our investigations.

2.10   We considered it important to know something of the background and history of the Hospital, the people who worked in the Hospital, the nature of the complaints and how they came about, and how so many women were injured by the failures of that institution.[1] We were aware that many questions remained

---

[1] The MMMs reject this contention.

unanswered following the Fitness to Practise Committee's report, and we set out, within the Terms of Reference, to address those questions.

2.11 We learned at an early stage that many decent hardworking doctors, nurses and managers feel hurt, betrayed and aggrieved by the glare of hostile media attention on them and their workplace. They feel that all their efforts during the bad days of a weak economy and difficult work conditions have been set at nought by the continuing adverse publicity which works almost daily as a corrosive on their morale and on their commitment to patients. Many of the new consultants who have taken up their position in recent years were not even aware of who the personalities in the Maternity Unit were and are irritated by the seeming immediate connection in the minds of the public of the Lourdes Hospital with events in the past.

2.12 It became apparent that there were politics and personal agendas at work in this region, as well as many camps and divisions. It was apparent that leaks to journalists were a potent method of advancing causes. Another method of stirring knee jerk reactions was raising questions in the Dáil. At times it seemed some people preferred bizarre and fantastic explanations for human failings rather than facts.

We came across people who held simplistic reasons and explanations that demonise Dr. Neary and the personnel in the Maternity Unit. We came across others who hoped that we would prove the Medical Council wrong and find an innocent explanation for what occurred. We had tremendous difficulty in spreading the message that this was an inquiry into the practices at the Maternity Unit, and not exclusively into Dr. Neary. To this day, we note that the Inquiry is erroneously described as the "Neary Inquiry".

2.13 At the early stages of this Inquiry many perceptions were presented to us from both sides including the following statements which we heard

- Dr. Neary hated women
- Dr. Neary had a fear of uterine cancer in women
- Dr. Neary panicked when he saw blood

- Dr. Neary was protected by the nuns who thought he "walked on water"
- Dr. Neary's wife's death from ovarian cancer had caused him to carry out hysterectomies
- Dr. Neary took sadistic pleasure from mutilating women
- Dr. Neary thought he was God and could decide which women should have children
- Everyone knew what was happening in the unit
- Any one who tried to report Dr. Neary was sacked

OR

- Dr. Neary was an incredibly good and hard working doctor who has been totally misrepresented
- All the women who underwent hysterectomy are looking for compensation
- Dr. Neary did the best he could in very difficult conditions
- Dr. Neary was carrying out sterilisations on women who had requested hysterectomy
- Dr. Neary saved many women's lives
- Dr. Neary held up the whole maternity system in the Lourdes since 1974
- Dr. Neary carried most of the work load

2.14 We started the Inquiry against this background of unsubstantiated perceptions by first reading the various documents which were available. The key documents were:

- the files given to us by the Health Board
- the history of the Hospital given to us by the Medical Missionaries of Mary
- the findings of the Fitness to Practise Committee of the Medical Council and the transcript of hearings
- the report of the Institute of Obstetricians and Gynaecologists into Dr. Neary's practice between 1992 and 1998

- various reports commissioned by the Health Board into different aspects of the Maternity Unit.

2.15 When we were in a position to hear witnesses, we advertised the Terms of Reference and invited any interested parties to attend. We put details of our contact addresses and telephone numbers on a web site. The first witnesses we wanted to interview were the midwives who worked at the unit during Dr. Neary's tenure at the hospital. We wished also to speak to the original owners and managers of the hospital, being the Medical Missionaries of Mary (MMMs), and to the patients, in order to form a picture of events which exposed the unit's practices to scrutiny.

2.16 Initially, patients were very reluctant to be interviewed. The members of Patient Focus and other patients were unhappy that the Inquiry was not statutory - with full powers of compulsion. They believed that we would not obtain the cooperation of the midwives and doctors without such powers. They had also expressed the view that they wished to see the midwives, the obstetricians, theatre staff including the anaesthetists and the pathologists cross-examined in public.

2.17 The midwives were also initially reluctant to be interviewed. We were told that they felt scapegoated and were resentful and quite understandably suspicious. Most of the midwives were represented by the INO (Irish Nurses' Organisation). We are grateful for the assistance of Ms. Patsy Doyle of the INO who accompanied many of the midwives to interview. We were able to reassure them through their representatives that the interviews would be held in private and that their identities would be protected so far as possible. Eventually the cooperation that we received was good, although we can fully understand that many of the midwives believe that the personalities of other consultants played a role in their failure to realise that caesarean hysterectomy was being carried out too frequently and that there was something they could do about it. They wished the events to be seen in context.

2.18 The legal team was anxious to have input from patients who were central to the Inquiry. The legal team met with Patient Focus members and their spokesperson, Ms. Sheila O'Connor, on a number of occasions to discuss their fears and reluctance to engage with a non statutory inquiry.

2.19 Patient Focus decided not to attend and continued to lobby for a full sworn statutory inquiry. I wrote to Ms. O'Connor expressing my regret that they would not cooperate but informing the group that the Inquiry would go ahead regardless, and that our door would remain open.

2.20 The Inquiry team wrote to various proposed witnesses and discussed the conditions under which we would operate. From the outset, I was determined that we would operate on an informal basis where open discussion could take place. We conducted interviews and not interrogations. We promised the maximum confidentiality possible in exchange for cooperation. We were open in exchanging information which we had received in order to elicit informed responses. We operated an open door policy for witnesses to contact us.

2.21 Following the advertising of our Terms of Reference, more than 100 people contacted the inquiry office to arrange an interview. Almost 200 others were contacted by the Inquiry solicitor and came in for interview. The Inquiry got under way with interviews commencing in July 2004. We are very grateful to the many former patients of the Maternity Unit at the Lourdes Hospital who contacted us, and also for the very full assistance and cooperation we subsequently received from Ms. Sheila O'Connor and Patient Focus.

2.22 We conducted almost 320 interviews with 280 witnesses including patients, midwives, sisters of the Medical Missionaries of Mary, retired and practising obstetric specialists, anaesthetists and pathologists from the Maternity Unit and elsewhere, IT specialists, statisticians, nurse managers and Matrons, health board officials, risk managers, members of VHI, priests, officials from the Department of Health and Children, members of the Medical Council, GPs, administrative and secretarial assistants, Healthcare advisers, Capita Consulting, members of the Institute, members of the RCOG and many, many others. All of these witnesses made themselves available on a voluntary basis.

The interviews were mostly held at the Inquiry headquarters at 31-35 Bow Street, Smithfield, Dublin 7. Witnesses were also interviewed in London, Donegal, Castlebar, Galway, Ballinasloe, Kilkenny, Wicklow and Drogheda. National and international interviews were conducted by teleconference. The Inquiry received full and extensive assistance from The Institute of Obstetricians and Gynaecologists in Ireland, The Medical Council and The Department of Health and Children and the Royal College of Obstetricians and Gynaecologists in London.

I am immensely impressed with and grateful to the number of witnesses who travelled very great distances to make themselves available to the Inquiry for interview. I am grateful and impressed that so many witnesses travelled without any compensation for expenses incurred to assist the Inquiry. Without their assistance I would not have been able to understand fully the complexity of the issues involved nor would I have been able to arrive at what I consider to be fair and considered findings.

3 WHAT THE INQUIRY ESTABLISHED

3.1   We uncovered a complex story, and many strands remain tangled in the personalities of the participants and the difficult relationship between religious beliefs and human reproduction overlaid with a sense of intense loyalty to the Maternity Unit. It is a story set in a time of unquestioning submission to authority, whether religious or civil, when nurses and doctors were in abundant supply and permanent jobs were few and treasured. The MMMs ran a very ordered hospital in an austere and dedicated manner.

3.2   It is the story of a relatively small but very busy hospital which operated by a separate and unique set of rules, and was accountable to a religious community rather than to objective medical standards. Its owners set out to provide the best medical care to the people of Drogheda in a Catholic setting and to train doctors and nurses for the missions in Africa.

In order that this hospital and its staff, as well as the obstetric communities in all similar units, never repeat the same mistakes, we have to try and learn and understand what happened at the Lourdes Hospital.

3.3   To begin with, it must be remembered that no one died and it is highly probable that some mothers' lives were saved when hysterectomy was the only procedure to stop intractable haemorrhage. The events must be seen in the context of the position of the catholic ethos of the hospital that permitted "secondary sterilisations" where the condition of the uterus might seriously compromise the mother's health in another pregnancy. In these situations, the "offending organ could be isolated" which was another description for a peripartum hysterectomy.

3.4   Establishing the rate was difficult as key registers were missing. We are nevertheless fairly satisfied that we have established the correct number of peripartum hysterectomies carried out in the Lourdes hospital since 1974. The vast majority were caesarean hysterectomies and a smaller number were carried out in the gynaecology theatre following normal vaginal delivery and post partum haemorrhage. The numbers are truly shocking.

3.5   **188 peripartum hysterectomies were carried out in the 25 years 1974 – 1998 in the Unit as a whole.** 129 hysterectomies are attributed to Dr. Neary. 59 are attributed to either one of the other three consultants working there over the 25 year period or to registrars or locums.

3.6   The Inquiry was able to obtain the patients previous parity details in all but 5 cases. 3 of those cases were former patients of Dr. Neary. An analysis of the 129 cases attributed to Dr. Neary indicates that 53 hysterectomies were carried out in the period from the Summer of 1990 after the move to the new Maternity Unit until the end of October 1998.

3.7   Parity details were unavailable in 3 of Dr. Neary's cases. An overall analysis shows that there was a different profile for the women undergoing hysterectomy under Dr. Neary compared with the rest of the unit. This was partly explained by the fact that Dr. Neary's antenatal clinic included a higher proportion of problem pregnancies and a higher proportion of repeat sections than the other consultants. Repeat caesarean sections carry higher risks and are somewhat self-limiting in that most women who can only safely deliver by caesarean section do not have large families.

3.8   Of the 129 hysterectomies carried out by Dr. Neary over 25 years, 25 hysterectomies involve women who were having their first baby and 26 involve women who were having their second delivery including 3 sets of twins. Included in that figure were 2 women whose babies died and were thus childless. Of the remaining 75 cases, 26 mothers excluding the three sets of twins had three children, 21 mothers had 4 children and the remaining mothers had between 5 and 13 children at time of hysterectomy. **There were only two women who underwent peripartum hysterectomy who ended up childless. A crude statistic is 40% of Dr. Neary's peripartum hysterectomy patients were having their first or second baby.**

3.9   The other obstetricians carried out 59 hysterectomies. No peripartum hysterectomy was associated with a patient who ended up childless. 2 hysterectomies involved women having their first delivery and 4 involved women having their second delivery. All the rest of the hysterectomies carried out involved women with 3 children or more. Some of the women were of very high parity.

3.10   **70% of the 183 women who had hysterectomies in the Unit and for whom parity details are available had at least 3 children. This figure is lower for Dr. Neary.**

3.11   The figure that caused the most surprise was the 91 peripartum hysterectomies carried out in the period from mid 1990 to 1998 when the maternity service moved from the old hospital into a purpose built unit adjacent to the general hospital. The breakdown between the obstetricians is:

Dr. Neary 53
Dr. Lynch 29
Dr. O'Brien 1
Dr. O'Coigligh 2
Registrars 5
Locum 1

3.12 According to the consultants and midwives who attended for interview, peripartum hysterectomy was associated mainly with women of high parity, older women and women having their fourth or more caesarean section. The birth rate was falling generally during the 80s and 90s. Nevertheless the profile of Dr. Neary's patients changed considerably after the move into the new Maternity Unit. In the 8 year period that he was practising in the new unit, 12 of his patients were primigravida, 13 were having their second baby and 14 were having their third baby. This was not remarked upon until there was almost an epidemic of such operations in 1996. Even then, the concept that there was a problem with Dr. Neary's judgement, technique or tolerance of blood loss was not articulated. It was inconceivable to the doctors and most of the midwives who so often assisted him that the hysterectomies on young women were anything more than bad luck. The vast majority of witnesses believed that the patients were well managed at the time. No one who worked with Dr. Neary has suggested that he had any ulterior motive for what he did.

3.13 The several midwives who told us of their concerns from about 1996 were concerned at the younger age and lower parity of these women. The Matron was concerned with Dr. Neary's rising caesarean section rate and believed that they were connected. For the rest of the Maternity Unit staff the continuing hysterectomies involving older women or high parity passed without remark or concern. Some of these hysterectomies contributed to by the condition of the uterus may well have been anticipated and planned. These hysterectomies masked concerns relating to those which were emergency procedures and utterly unplanned and we now know medically and statistically unacceptable.

3.14 Few complained or questioned[2] -

_ not the patients, their partners nor their families;

---

[2] A patient complained about Dr. Neary through her Solicitor in 1980. She did not proceed as she had been assured in legal correspondence that an obstetric hysterectomy was extremely rare and only carried out in the presence of an intractable haemorrhage. Another patient engaged a Solicitor 1998 complaining of her treatment, including peripartum hysterectomy, carried out in January of the same year.

    –   not the obstetricians who worked in the Maternity Unit and who knew of the operations carried out;

    –   not the junior doctors nor the post membership registrars;

    –   not the anaesthetists, who received the patient, administered the anaesthesia, wrote up the operation notes and spoke to each patient in the recovery room and were always present at the operations[3];

    –   not the surgical nurses who were frequently midwives, and always women, who handed the hysterectomy clamps to the surgeons and counted the swabs[4];

    –   not the midwives who cared for the women after their operations and who recorded each day the women stayed in the post natal ward and the fact that they had had a peripartum hysterectomy;

    –   not the pathologists and technicians who received the wombs and specimens from the maternity theatre, who dissected, examined and reported[5];

    –   not the Matrons who made ward rounds and who contacted the public health nurses[6];

    –   not the sisters of the Medical Missionaries of Mary who owned the hospital and employed the obstetricians[7];

    –   not one of the various GPs whose patients attended the IMTH and underwent caesarean hysterectomy;

    –   not any of the parties who read the maternity hospital's biennial reports in the years when it was published.

No one made a formal complaint and no one questioned openly.

3.15   The Royal College of Obstetricians and Gynaecologists inspected the Maternity Unit in 1987 and 1992 and found it to be suitable for training obstetric registrars. On each occasion deficits in the training programme were noted and the approval for training was lukewarm. In 1992 the report of the visiting committee of the RCOG made 8 recommendations to the

---

[3] A junior anaesthetist who had completed 6 months training at the Coombe was very seriously concerned in early 1998.

[4] Several junior midwives were concerned from 1996 and especially when a midwife who had trained outside the Lourdes joined the staff in 1997.

[5] One of the pathologists had concerns in 1981. Another and recently appointed pathologist had serious concerns in 1998.

[6] The Matron of the Maternity Unit was concerned in 1979 and 1980 and again in the mid 1990s

[7] A temporary tutor who was also a sister in the MMMs tried to voice concerns in 1980

Maternity Unit. No return visit was planned to ensure implementation and no efforts were made to determine whether the recommended changes were effected. It was advised that tubal ligation be introduced as a choice for patients. On neither occasion were the recommendations made by the RCOG fully implemented.

3.16 The medical school at the Royal College of Surgeons in Ireland approved the Maternity Unit for undergraduate training.

3.17 An Bord Altranais carried out periodic assessments of the midwifery school at the maternity hospital for accreditation purposes. They advised as far back as 1980 that women should be offered a full choice on contraception and that midwives ought to be fully trained on these methods. Nothing happened.

3.18 No person or institution raised any issues until October 1998 when two experienced midwives, who were consulting the Health Board Solicitor on an unrelated matter, sought his advice on serious concerns which one of the midwives had about Dr. Neary's practices.

3.19 The story of Dr. Neary's fall from grace is one of enormous tragedy for the hospital at which he worked for 25 years, for the staff who worked with and supported him and especially for the women who entered the maternity hospital to face the joy of a new baby and who returned home to recuperate from a hysterectomy. It has also had a profound affect on Dr. Neary's life, and on his family. This is not a simple story of an evil man or a bad doctor, nor is it a story of wholesale suppression of facts. The facts were there for all to see. There was no attempt to hide the procedures or pretend they were something else. The operations were carried out in the presence of consultant anaesthetists, assisted at by trainee obstetricians who had all the textbooks available to them and frequently observed by spouses and partners. The operations were openly recorded.

3.20 Neither is it the story of a surgeon with poor surgical skills or a doctor deficient in academic excellence. Dr.Neary completed his professional qualification examinations on the first attempt and did well. His trainers speak very highly of him and have universally expressed amazement that he was struck off the register. It is the story of a doctor who, at critical points during his training, was inadequately supervised. He came to work in a unit which lacked leadership, peer review, audit or critical capacity. It is the story of a doctor with a deep fault line, which was recognised early but never corrected. It is a story of a committed doctor with a misplaced sense of confidence in his own ability. It is a story of deep misunderstanding and misapplication of clinical independence.

3.21   Dr. Neary's senior colleague Dr. O'Brien carried out very few caesarean or peripartum hysterectomies compared with either Dr. Neary or Dr. Lynch, or even the registrars. If he was aware of his colleagues' practices, he felt it was not his business.

3.22   Dr. Lynch carried out a significant number of hysterectomies although the number was not in the same league as Dr. Neary's. No one in the hospital, either in the past or now, expressed any concern about Dr. Lynch's rate of hysterectomies or those performed by any of the registrars.

3.23   There is the very strong suspicion that a number of hysterectomy procedures were carried out because of the ethos at the hospital. These hysterectomies - which were medically indicated sterilisations - masked unwarranted resort to hysterectomy. These issues are dealt with at the appropriate Term of Reference in the body of the report.

The medical Missionaries of Mary object to this finding and wish to state their position on this paragraph:

"At no stage were any statistics or figures put to our client in regard to specific hysterectomies carried out for the purposes of sterilisation. At no stage were the MMMs aware of a suggestion or suspicion that the ethos of the hospital in regard to sterilisation had any bearing on the necessity for a peripartum hysterectomy and in that context the MMMs are appalled at the comments outlined above. With respect we believe it incumbent for the Inquiry to draw its conclusions on more than mere suspicions. Furthermore, as the Inquiry is

aware, many hospitals in Ireland had the same ethos, yet the rate of peripartum hysterectomy was not at the same level as OLLH."

4 BRIEF HISTORY OF THE HOSPITAL

4.1   In May 1997 the North Eastern Health Board formally took over the ownership of the Lourdes Hospital, the biggest hospital in the region. It had previously been owned by the Medical Missionaries of Mary (MMMs), who were founded in 1939 by Mother Mary Martin. It was the first hospital founded by the order. The order set up the hospital, then called the "International Missionary Training Hospital", in Drogheda. It served the people of Drogheda and the surrounding regions, and it also served to train personnel for hospitals in Africa.

Nurses and patients for the most part refer to the hospital as "The Lourdes", a shortened version of its full title Our Lady of Lourdes Hospital. Many of the older consultants referred and still refer to the hospital as the IMTH, (International Missionary Training Hospital). The hospital provided services that accorded with the ethos of the Roman Catholic Church – including its teachings on human reproduction.

The hospital started from small beginnings funded first by private donations and contributions from local people and businesses followed by substantial allocations of cash from each Government Health Department. It grew into the biggest hospital in the counties of Meath, Louth, Cavan and Monaghan.

When the Lourdes Maternity Hospital was founded in 1939, it was housed in a converted 18th century mansion close to the Order's convent. Later, a school of nursing was built, followed by a school of midwifery, a nurses' home, a medical residence and a separate general hospital.

4.2   When the general hospital was built the maternity hospital enjoyed a considerable degree of autonomy and continued to operate more or less as a separate institution. The Matron of the Maternity Hospital, Miss Phelan, held her old position without involvement with the general hospital. The new general hospital was located about 300 metres from the existing maternity hospital. Getting from one building to the other involved a long and inconvenient walk braving the elements.

4.3   The distance between the two hospitals meant that anaesthetists had to travel some distance to service patients who needed general anaesthesia. In addition, the Maternity Unit was separated from blood supplies, the pathology and radiology departments and the baby special care unit. Patients were delivered on the first floor, but all surgery was carried out on the ground floor. For much of the time that the maternity hospital was in service, there was no lift. Until 1986 theatre nurses had to travel from the main hospital to assist in caesarean sections and other peripartum procedures including caesarean and peripartum hysterectomies. In 1986, a group of midwives was trained to be scrub nurses in theatre. Gynaecological hysterectomies and other gynaecological procedures and operations were carried out in the main operating theatres in the main hospital.

4.4   Many witnesses have described the premises as "primitive", "unbelievable", "run on a shoestring", and "Dickensian". Be that as it may, it was the place of choice or necessity for thousands of mothers to have their babies delivered, until the new Maternity Unit was opened in 1991. Many mothers, fathers and doctors who were familiar with the premises praised the friendly, homely atmosphere that prevailed in spite of the clear lack of comfort. It provided private obstetric care with private and semi private rooms.

4.5   The birth rate at the Maternity Unit, with all its shortcomings and economies during the 60s and 70s, exceeded the birth rate now prevailing at the new unit. This is in spite of the closure of the Maternity Units in Dundalk and Monaghan, the rising population and the refugee centre at Mosney. During most of this period there were only 2 consultant obstetricians attached to the Lourdes Hospital, a small number of junior doctors and one registrar. Many young newly graduated doctors spent six months in the Maternity Unit learning the obstetrics necessary to be accredited to practise as a General Practitioner. All describe horrendous workloads.

4.6   There was a midwifery school on the campus, and midwifery students received their practical training in the Maternity Unit. All the candidates at the midwifery school were qualified nurses, and the majority of these nurses had been trained in the nursing school attached to the General Hospital. There was a strong sense of loyalty in the nurses and midwives to their hospital. They felt privileged to train and work there.

4.7   Until the late 90s, jobs were scarce in Ireland. Many young girls who wanted to become nurses had to train and work in the UK. The Lourdes Hospital was (and still is) a major employer in the region and jobs there were eagerly sought after. If one became a staff nurse one had a job for life. For much of this period, natural wastage was the only route to a new job opening up, especially at a time when nurses continued in employment after marriage. There was very little turnover of staff during that period. Job insecurity may have influenced a climate of silence. Consultants could, and did cause nurses to be transferred. Many witnesses recounted to us that a junior paediatrician encountered Dr. Neary's displeasure causing her contract not to be renewed.

4.8   The Lourdes Maternity Hospital published periodic reports similar in style to those produced by the National Maternity Hospital at Holles Street. Sometimes it appeared as an annual report and sometimes as a biennial report. Sometimes the publication was several years late, e.g., the 1980 report might have been published in 1983. The reports contained valuable information relating to statistics on morbidity, mortality, stillbirths, eclampsia, caesarean sections and so forth. Symphysiotomies were detailed as were caesarean hysterectomies. Since 1952 there were few years when some caesarean sections did not end in hysterectomy. Similarly, high parity was associated with problems like uterine rupture leading to hysterectomy for haemorrhage. The figures were broadly in line with what one would expect from a provincial unit.

4.9   In the last three decades nationally, the treatment of post partum haemorrhage has improved to such an extent that the rate of hysterectomy following delivery or caesarean section had fallen significantly in every hospital in the State - apart from the Lourdes Hospital. The changing size of families has also decreased the obstetrical problems associated with high parity.

We have been advised that new obstetric problems have replaced the problems of unstable lie, atonic uterus and rupture associated with older mothers of high parity with the problems associated with older first time mothers and mothers having repeat caesarean sections, obesity and diabetes. We have been advised of a large body of recent literature indicating an increasing incidence of placenta previa and accreta or morbidly adherent placenta associated with repeat caesarean sections leading to caesarean hysterectomy.

4.10   In July 1990, the old maternity hospital was closed down and the hospital moved into a brand new purpose-built unit attached to the main hospital by a tube like link corridor. The cost of construction and furbishment was borne mostly by a grant from the Department of Health. The MMMs, who were still the owners and proprietors of the two hospitals, financed the balance. The religious ethos of the hospital continued.

In the new maternity hospital, mothers soon had access to routine epidural injections for the control of pain during labour. The baby care unit was immediately adjacent to the operating theatres, which were beside the labour ward delivery suites. Access to anaesthetists, blood supplies, and the pathology laboratory was much improved.

4.11   In common with the Dublin maternity hospitals, the rate of caesarean section in the Lourdes was rising steadily. Nationally the rate of peripartum hysterectomy on the other hand fell to such a low rate throughout the country that the adverse event was no longer mentioned in hospital statistics. In the mandatory form used by the RCOG for the gathering of obstetric statistics, peripartum hysterectomy was absent. The Lourdes maternity hospital entirely abandoned annual reports - the last one was for 1984 and was probably printed and disseminated in 1986/87.

4.12   From the late 70s, the rate of peripartum hysterectomy at the Lourdes Maternity Unit averaged about 7 per annum. This rate rose dramatically after the move to new modern premises. No one questioned this rate until 1998. When the patient undergoing caesarean hysterectomy was older or of high parity, there appeared to be a tacit understanding that it was a sterilisation. This belief or suspicion served to quell curiosity or concern when the mothers were young and of low parity when it was assumed to be for a good reason. No one seemed to know the actual numbers or suspect that anything was amiss or unusual

The Medical Missionaries of Mary object to this aspect of the report on the basis that :

> *"This was not put to any members of the MMM and we are not aware that any member of the MMM had a tacit understanding that it was a sterilisation. The Inquiry should specify what party had this understanding and if there is some particular reason why the Inquiry cannot name the individual or individuals who had this understanding, their occupation should be named. The draft report does not specify the basis for this "tacit understanding". The MMMs wholly reject any such suggestion. It is unclear why the MMMs would condone unnecessary peripartum hysterectomies yet disallow sterilisation. It is not logical."*

They reiterate that they are not aware of any actual evidence that peripartum hysterectomies were carried out as a form of sterilisation and reiterate that no specific cases were put to the MMM witnesses.

4.13   Hospitals appear to run in a hierarchical system based on division of tasks. There is hierarchy among the nurses, and a co-relating medical hierarchy, from the medical students to the interns, the SHOs, the registrars and the consultants. Hierarchy works well in normal life. A move up the ladder ought to be commensurate with experience and increased knowledge, with the higher echelons reserved for candidates who show leadership qualities. If there is little upward movement or if promotion automatically follows tenure, hierarchical structures can create a negative and dangerous environment.

4.14   Things were no different in the Lourdes Hospital. Nurses were more constant in their place in the hierarchy. Student nurses frequently moved on in search of permanent posts. Several midwives who had been students in the Midwifery School described being fearful of voicing any criticisms of consultants. Those former students described how they believed that they would be dismissed if they crossed a consultant. Those who stayed tended to work their way up from staff nurse to ward sister. There was very little change in the hierarchy in the Maternity Unit. There were only two Matrons in the Maternity Unit between 1954 and 1998, and between 1945 and 1997 there were only 4 consultant obstetricians. Over the years a loyalty developed between the senior nurses and those consultants. There was very little movement of staff. The same anaesthetists and pathologists were in the hospital for decades. No new consultants were appointed between 1983 and 1996.

4.15   As the hospital was owned and managed by a religious order, continuity at management level was assured. The sisters belonged to an era when nurses were efficient, ordered and respectful. They carried out orders and did not question consultants. Matron maintained a formal, distant authority over nurses. The nuns who had set the practices and protocols for training nurses and midwives in the hospital in the 50s thus produced suitable nurses who fitted their mould – hardworking, respectful, Catholic nurses who were well trained, knew their place, trusted the consultants and suspended their critical or questioning faculties. They were trained to certain tasks - and to those tasks only.

4.16   The International Missionary Training Hospital developed an extraordinary cocoon of confidence and self assurance around itself. It simply did not occur to anyone within the body of management in the hospital that practices in the Maternity Unit were different from the accepted norm. It was not until 1997 and 1998 when midwives who had trained outside the unit raised concerns which were acted upon by the North Eastern Health Board.

4.17 Training and reflection are at the heart of good medical practice. To be effective the trainers must be aware of best practice, and in touch with evidence-based recommendations. It is not enough to teach what was always taught. It is not enough to teach and demonstrate, without also applying and maintaining a critical eye to procedures and outcomes on the floor. In this hospital, training for hard work and dedication to specific tasks was not enough to create a healthy questioning environment where high standards are maintained.

5 THE ETHICAL POSITION AS PRACTISED BY THE MMM

5.1 This issue was not always easy to understand, but it gave some insight into the problems in the Maternity Unit. The Catholic ethos prohibited the use of all forms of contraception. The only family planning advocated and permitted was the natural method of the safe period, or the Billings method. Information on other forms of family planning methods was not allowed even in circumstances where another pregnancy was dangerous.

Sterilisation for contraceptive purposes was not permitted. The ethos allowed for "indirect sterilisation" where the primary purpose was for medical reasons, although the end result was that the woman could no longer become pregnant. The accepted practice in Catholic hospitals was to "isolate the diseased organ" by removing the uterus. Tubal ligation - i.e. the tying off a woman's fallopian tubes to prevent the passage of ova to the uterus for fertilization - was not acceptable.

5.2 There was an abundance of evidence that indicated the unwritten ethical code was rigidly applied. For many years, Dr. Neary and Dr. Lynch had sought clarification from the Department of Health, the Medical Defence Union and the Health Board of their legal position with regards to patient choice on offer in other hospitals. They never received what they considered adequate answers from any source, and they were obliged to operate in a grey area of "indirect sterilisation". It seemed to us that a tubal ligation for medical reasons was more likely to raise queries than the number of peripartum hysterectomies.

6   THE MISSING DOCUMENTS

6.1   We are satisfied that a person or persons unidentified, who had knowledge of where records were stored and who had easy access to those records, was responsible for a deliberate, careful and systematic removal of key historical records which are missing, together with master cards and patient charts. Three alterations to the maternity theatre register detected by the Inquiry appear to be made in the same hand and apparently were made after complaints were made against Dr. Neary. Most of the missing records refer to Dr. Neary's patients. Someone with a misplaced sense of loyalty to Dr. Neary or the unit is probably responsible.

7   THE WITNESSES

7.1   **THE MEDICAL MISSIONARIES OF MARY**

The first witnesses were sisters from the Order of **MMM.** Many of the key players were working in Africa and had to return in early September. We found these women to be of unusually strong character. They had endured much hardship in their chosen careers as providers of medical care in Africa and elsewhere. They were women of strong disposition, education and ability, who had dedicated their lives to a cause they believed in. Surprisingly, they said that it was their training as nurses never to question a consultant, but to carry out his/her orders. They worked in a hierarchical convent life and accepted carrying out orders without question. It was part of their training and discipline.

They had no worries with regards to the ability of any of their consultants. They had no concerns about the Maternity Unit. When it became apparent that they would not have the personnel within the MMMs to continue managing the hospital, it was sold to the Health Board. Their mission was Africa, and they chose to send their best missionaries there. They preferred to fulfil their founder's objectives in Africa.

7.1.1   The sisters had built up a hospital with a good reputation for providing excellent care and training but they had no choice but to sell to the Health Board. After October 1998 they were shocked at the revelations - they had been unaware of the extent of the peripartum hysterectomies. In general, they did not accept that the prohibition on sterilisation for contraceptive purposes, or the non-availability of contraceptive advice apart from natural methods, played any part in the number of peripartum hysterectomies. It was their belief that the strict Catholic position on sterilisation did not prohibit the carrying out of a tubal ligation for medical reasons. This position was not accepted as fact by the Matron of the Maternity Unit or by the two consultants working there while the hospital was still in the ownership of the MMMs.

7.1.2 Some of the MMMs, especially the non-medical sisters, had a good relationship with Dr. Neary and enjoyed his strong personality. Some of the administrators had problems with his manner and his volatile and erratic moods and gave him a wide berth. There was a feeling that one could never win an argument with Dr. Neary. They recounted some extreme examples of his erratic mood to the Inquiry. They had no such concerns about Dr. Lynch who they found the easiest to get on with. They were fully aware of Dr. O'Brien's exacting personality.

They left the management of the Maternity Unit to the Matron and ventured very infrequently into the unit. Relations between the two Matrons were professional – if perhaps prickly. A "Berlin Wall" existed between the two units, which were managed as two separate hospitals.

7.1.3 Many of the nuns in the convent are now in retirement and too elderly to have accurate or reliable memories of the unit. None of the MMMs were aware of any complaints relating to clinical care, although Dr. Neary and Dr. O'Brien were reprimanded on a number of occasions for rudeness or abrupt manner to patients and midwives. All agreed that Dr. Neary worked very hard, was always available and was very popular with patients who flocked to his ante natal clinics, as well as to his rooms in Fair Street as private patients. The nuns we interviewed had no complaints regarding any of their obstetricians and spoke well of all their consultants in the Maternity Unit.

7.1.4 I found it very difficult to understand how women of such obvious intelligence, determination and strength allowed the Maternity Unit to operate in isolation from normal standards and without any outside comparisons or audit.[8] The

---

[8] The MMMs were critical of this comment as no criticism was made of midwives, pathologists, anaesthetists and other professionals who made no comment about these peripartum hysterectomies

records were there for them to read and to collate and compare with figures at their other Maternity Unit in Waterford. I accept that obedience within a religious order and obeisance to hierarchy can produce a collective acquiescence, but I found it hard to understand that the MMMs really believed that consultants could not be challenged in their clinical judgement. Although they said they would never question a consultant in his clinical judgement there was no evidence that Dr. Neary was protected by the sisters of the MMM.

7.2   THE MIDWIVES

7.2.1   It was mid July before we heard from the first midwives, including the midwife who had so bravely voiced her concerns to the Health Board Solicitor in October 1998.

7.2.2   Very few midwives volunteered to speak to us. We had to establish their identity and role from the maternity theatre register and from lists provided to us by the North Eastern Health Board. When invited to attend, they were very cooperative, but were clearly uncomfortable at coming to terms with their lack of appreciation or concern at the number of peripartum hysterectomies in the unit until 1996 onwards. Even then, their concerns were in relation to the youth of the patients undergoing hysterectomy who they suspected could not have been "consent sterilisations". Many of the senior midwives were deeply resentful of criticisms which had been made by the Review Group regarding their lack of awareness of practices in the Maternity Unit. They felt that until we spoke to them, "*no one had sought their views*".

7.2.3   The midwives received training for routine obstetric procedures and care. They had no training in the range of surgical techniques which form part and parcel of the repertoire of a fully trained theatre nurse. For economic reasons, they were asked to act as theatre nurses for caesarean sections from 1986 onwards.

---

until the late 1990s. They say that these individuals were in a far better position, both professionally and proximately, to challenge procedures in the theatre.

The '80s were difficult economic times in Ireland. Investment in Health was low. Many wards and hospitals were closed as a result of rationalisation plans. We heard evidence that funding was always a problem in this hospital, and perhaps in the region. Many witnesses described a "make-do-and-mend" philosophy and spoke of equipment that was always promised, but slow to materialise.

The lack of full training as theatre nurses may well have played a part in the midwives' acceptance - without question - of all procedures carried out in theatre. Similarly, the separation of the two hospitals before 1991 may have isolated the theatre nurses from the reality of an unexpected caesarean hysterectomy. Also, the undiscussed suspicion that hysterectomies were covert sterilisations played a significant role in the culture of acceptance.

7.3 THE ANAESTHETISTS

7.3.1 The cooperation of the anaesthetists past and present was full. The Institute Review Group had interviewed three of the anaesthetists previously in early 1999. Their views had changed little since then. The anaesthetists who worked at the Lourdes Hospital prior to 1996 had no concerns about any of the obstetricians or their practices. Most of them had some obstetric training before taking up their position as consultant.

7.3.2 They all used the term a "safe pair of hands" to describe Dr. Neary. He never lost a patient, his patients recovered well from his surgery, and they enjoyed working with him. He was a dry worker - meaning he did not tolerate much bleeding. Similarly, Dr. Lynch was professional and competent, a quick worker and a clean worker. They were appalled at the manner of Dr. Neary's suspension, and especially at the public nature of the revelations. They had never ever seen Dr. Neary doing anything untoward in theatre, and they seemed genuinely upset at learning the extent of the hysterectomies carried out by him.

Having had a great deal of time to ponder the information now being revealed, they thought in retrospect that Dr. Neary may have been a little hasty to resort to hysterectomy. One anaesthetist suggested that the obstetricians had now gone the other way, waiting until the patient was almost moribund before they resorted to hysterectomy.

7.3.3 All of the older anaesthetists were conservative in giving blood to a woman delivering. None of them was consulted by the obstetricians before a hysterectomy was carried out, nor would they expect to be. For the most part, the anaesthetists who worked in the unit between 1974-1998 did not provide any meaningful insight into how unusual practices were accepted without comment for so long. There was no question of the anaesthetists covering up the numbers. They were simply too busy to reflect on the practice of caesarean hysterectomy.

7.4 THE PATHOLOGISTS

7.4.1 The pathologists and the scientists in the laboratory were fully cooperative with the Inquiry. They described how they saw many uteri being sent down, but how there were gaps of months between specimens. They were all aware of the ethos of the hospital, and assumed that some hysterectomies were sterilisations. Dr. Neary's reputation as a committed practitioner provided a comfort zone to those that assumed that caesarean hysterectomies were carried out for good reason.

7.4.2 None of the pathologists was aware of the cumulative number of the hysterectomies carried out in the Maternity Unit. In the absence of annual reports or clinico-pathological meetings, they had no way of knowing. The pathologists had no concerns regarding the other surgeons carrying out caesarean hysterectomy. Neither was any of them aware of any benchmark figure to use as a comparator.

7.4.3 They were all aware that negative histology findings did not equate to inappropriate reasons for removing the uterus. However, the newest pathologist was curious, concerned and alarmed at the number of uteri and ovaries he saw in the laboratory in the 9 months he was there, and he resolved to discuss the issue with Dr. Neary.

7.5 THE JUNIOR DOCTORS

7.5.1 Many of the junior doctors at the Lourdes were non-nationals and very reluctant to criticise any Irish consultant. They were highly dependent on references to advance in their training. They were all very complimentary of the three consultants working in the unit, although it was obvious that they felt special gratitude to Dr. Neary for his generosity of time in assisting them with obstetric emergencies. Many emergency caesarean sections were carried out by the registrars. If they ran into difficulty, they tended to call Dr. Neary who invariably came in to assist. They all enjoyed their time at the Lourdes Maternity Unit, and praised the midwives and the friendly and homely atmosphere there. Very few registrars admitted to carrying out a caesarean hysterectomy and had few clear memories of the procedures.

7.5.2 None of the obstetric registrars felt any tension or fear about working with Dr. Neary or Dr. Lynch. They were not intimidated or cowed, and they denied any atmosphere of fear on the part of the midwifery staff. They were extraordinarily complimentary of Dr. Neary's surgical skills and for the most part had no real concerns about the hysterectomy rate. Several junior doctors said that patients had requested hysterectomy but were now denying this.

7.5.3 Many of the doctors who had trained in Saudi Arabia and parts of North Africa had witnessed maternal death from ruptured uterus. They also witnessed the death of many babies in utero because of the cultural reluctance to carry out caesarean section. They accepted, but were a little perplexed, by the ethos of the hospital with regard to family planning.

7.5.4 The Irish junior doctors we interviewed did not have such a rosy view of the unit or its consultants. Many of these witnesses described consultants who practised in quite separate and distinct ways, and in accordance with their own unwritten protocols. Many also described unhappy experiences with all of the consultants. They were disturbed by the lack of meetings, teaching and discussion.

7.5.5 For the most part, Dr. Neary was not the worst of their experiences although several Irish junior doctors suggested to us that Dr. Neary had a personality disorder rather than a skills deficit. They, in common with some of the midwives and anaesthetists, described how Dr.Neary could not adapt to new procedures, nor did he find it easy to delegate. He always had a reason for what he did, and this was invariably based on personal experience rather than on objective evidence. Not one of these witnesses believed or suspected that Dr. Neary was deliberately harming patients. Very few Irish candidates worked as obstetric registrars in this unit.

7.6   THE PATIENTS

7.6.1   For the most part, this group presented as sound women accompanied by supportive spouses. The vast majority but not all were former patients of Dr. Neary. They were able to present their history without either high emotion or rancour. They accepted whatever their consultant told them and, until media reports at the end of 1998, they had no suspicion that they may have been subjected to unnecessary hysterectomy.

7.6.2   Many of the women used modern family planning to space their families. They accepted the Catholic ethos of the MMMs, but they did not let it interfere with their personal decision about family planning.

7.6.3   Some of the former patients had been told by independent obstetricians that there was no criticism of their treatment but others had been told that the decision to move to hysterectomy was very precipitous. A considerable number of these former patients were unable to have a review of their case notes, as they had mysteriously disappeared. These women were unable to find closure as they would never know if their hysterectomy was for valid reasons or not.

7.6.4   We found it quite extraordinary how many of the cases, when taken on their own, appeared to be acceptable obstetric practice, and we had to keep reminding ourselves that the number of these procedures was extraordinary. Only one former patient interviewed by the Inquiry admitted to a consent hysterectomy, and the patient charts in two cases contained written consents. Several patients described how Dr. Neary had refused to carry out a gynaecological hysterectomy requested before they became pregnant, only to find themselves undergoing caesarean hysterectomy later. We heard very few horror stories, and we noted a pattern of conduct. For the most part, the patients were not told of their hysterectomies until some time had elapsed. Dr. Neary tended to tell his patients himself, explaining in dramatic language that they had lost a great deal of blood and were lucky to have survived. It was clear that blood replacement was not relied upon to cope with haemorrhage. Several patients we met had a caesarean hysterectomy following their first baby.

7.6.5 Most patients were happy to keep attending Dr. Neary even after the caesarean hysterectomy. Very few of the patients questioned Dr. Neary for carrying out the hysterectomy but those who did, found that his attitude became defensive and unfriendly when he was challenged.

7.6.6 Several patients reported very positive experiences with Dr. Neary compared to their experiences with other obstetricians. Several patients were absolutely convinced that their lives had been saved by Dr. Neary. Some patients criticised him for his flippant remarks but others seemed to enjoy his sense of humour. For every adverse comment we heard about him, we heard at least one in his favour.

7.6.7 The most common complaint we heard from patients was how doctors carried out procedures on them without discussion beforehand. Very little was explained. We heard the same comment from so many patients that we have included recommendations on how to deal with poor communication skills.

7.7 MANAGEMENT

7.7.1 Again cooperation was excellent. We interviewed past and present managers, as well as former directors of nursing. One theme was common: this was a very busy hospital with perpetual funding and staffing problems. The medical and nursing staff worked very hard and with great loyalty. Change was rarely embraced with enthusiasm and the takeover by the Health Board was frequently but not invariably viewed as unwelcome.

7.7.2 It was next to impossible to establish where exactly the power in this hospital lay. The consultants and most of the administrative staff felt that it lay with the MMMs, and later in Health Board headquarters in Kells. The managers felt that the consultants, especially the older consultants ran the hospital. Older members of staff remembered that the first four foundation consultants had almost unlimited power. Few people actually knew who management was or where to voice concerns. Almost no one knew any of the members of the Medical Board and The Hospital Board was a remote and unidentified group. Managers did not feel that they had the authority to challenge consultants. No person in management knew anything about clinical practices until a Medical Director was appointed in 1992. His efforts to engage with consultants on behalf of management were viewed with suspicion and some hostility by many of his colleagues. There was and is no permanency or continuity in the top management position in the hospital. The Medical Board, made up of consultants, was unaware of what went on in the separate Maternity Unit. Any questioning was regarded as interference and there was evidence of very acrimonious correspondence between the Medical Director and the Maternity Unit consultants.

7.7.3 There was no real management of the Maternity Unit. Dr. Neary was the spokesman, and frequently viewed as the dominant rather than the senior obstetrician until Dr. O'Brien retired in 1996. The Matron and her assistant confined their attentions to midwifery and administrative matters. Each consultant attended his private patients, which at times constituted 50% of obstetric patients. They each had their own lists and their days on duty and worked in parallel lines. The role of the consultants was to provide services in the public system and to fill beds in the private system. They were not subject to any review until the health system began a bed occupancy review in the '90s. General management of the hospital received no cooperation from obstetric unit consultants and Dr. Neary robustly rejected any attempts to review their bed use practices.

7.7.4 We have been unable to comprehend the management vacuum in authority over, or accountability for, practices in the Maternity Unit on the part of the MMMs who were the owners and employers of the obstetricians.

There continues to be lack of continuity in management at CEO level and lack of training in hospital management before taking up the post of CEO.

7.8 THE OBSTETRICIANS

7.8.1 We interviewed all the obstetricians, other than Dr. Lynch, at length and over several days. It was obvious that although they were individually very helpful, they were unaware of each other's practice. We would have welcomed an interview with Dr. Finian Lynch. Originally, he was quite willing to speak to us. We suggested deferring the meeting until a later date, as we were aware that his wife was gravely ill. When he was invited to speak to us following his wife's death, he declined for legal reasons, which I accept. He responded in a limited fashion to our queries and we remain at a disadvantage without his full cooperation. He was unaware of Dr. Neary's rate of hysterectomy and had no concerns about his ability or practices until made aware by media reports. He had supported Dr. Neary fully when the complaints were first made and at that time saw no substance in the complaints. He, in common with Dr. Neary, agitated for clarification on their position as obstetricians if public patients sought tubal ligation.

7.8.2   None of the obstetricians who worked in the Lourdes Maternity Unit was aware that there was a culture of early resort to hysterectomy and were unaware of their own unit's numbers.

8 THE FUTURE

8.1   Much has changed. Much needed to change. Much remains to change. The most important change in the unit is awareness of the past, leadership in the present and strong ambition for the future. The incidence of peripartum hysterectomy has fallen precipitously and accords with national rates. The midwives have attended skills updating and management courses. They now play an important team role with consultants in providing a maternity service. Senior midwives collate figures and outcomes in the Maternity Unit and conduct audits on specific subjects and are encouraged to ask questions at daily handover meetings. There are many new and highly qualified consultants in place to bring the hospital close to specialist training status in most fields. Obstetrics and gynaecology have not yet achieved this level of recognition for training but have hopes for the future. Regular multidisciplinary meetings are held and attended where discussions on outcomes takes place. Every two months the radiologists and pathologists meet with the obstetric department to review cases. The anaesthetists do not yet attend on a regular basis as the meetings have not been structured to allow them to meet their other commitments. There are now seven consultant obstetricians and this in itself should facilitate clinical audit and clinical governance. It is expected that changed practices in relation to communication and the acceptance of the importance of leadership will, with any luck, bring this hospital forward into full university training status soon.

8.2   Management's initial response to the revelations about Dr. Neary's practice was prompt and appropriate. It is acknowledged that this was a very complex management task but the decisions made and the procedures introduced to deal with the situation at the time were courageous and correct. It is unfortunate that confidential and very sensitive information was leaked to the media causing unnecessary distress to patients and to Dr. Neary.

8.3   Management's role and actions in addressing the major structural, operational and personal deficits in the Maternity Unit and the hospital since 1998 have been slow and unsatisfactory. The overall plan and strategy has merit but the implementation has been compromised by a lack of management continuity and consistency and by failures in leadership and direction. The magnitude of the task of effecting root and branch change did not seem to have been appreciated at the very highest levels of management in the Health Board and perhaps the Department of Health. As a result, the necessary operational and structural changes in the Maternity Unit have taken much longer to realise and only now in 2006 are most of the elements in place. Audit is still not seen as an immediate imperative by management. The tools for audit are not available. No protected time is set aside for hospital wide monthly audit. It is not recognised that audit requires time and space and an audit coordinator.

8.4   Not everything in the Maternity Unit has improved. Statistics are kept but are not easily accessed. There is a lukewarm application of risk management amongst some consultants. Many do not understand what clinical governance means. Not all consultants share the burden of teaching and conducting audit. Private patient care still takes up a lot of consultant time. Two consultants have been absent over extended periods with no sign of replacement. There is still no computerised data collection system in place. No elective major gynaecology operations are carried out although theatres, staff and clinicians are in place with the requisite skills and equipment as there are no dedicated gynaecology beds available for elective operations.

8.5   The facts we uncovered revealed that any isolated institution which fails to have in place a process of outcome review by peers and benchmark comparators can produce similar scandals as those which occurred in the Lourdes Hospital. Support systems must be in place to conduct regular obligatory audit. There must be mandatory continuing professional development and skills assessment at all levels of healthcare. Senior ward sisters ought to attend updating of skills and methods programmes and should be able to recognise that procedures change in accordance with evidence based research. Outmoded and unnecessary practices ought to be recognised as such and changed as soon as information is available. Hospital management should have more authority and training and should have medical input. Clinical independence should no longer be interpreted as a licence for arrogance, disregard for patient choice, dignity and need or freedom from accountability.

EPILOGUE

I want to reiterate that this was a Maternity Unit that was to some extent caught in a time warp. There was no badness or cover up. Interviews with professionals involved in clinical governance and risk management abroad lead me to believe that similar problems have occurred and do occur in other hospitals. It took a series of high profile inquiries in the UK to realise that organised resourced systems must be in place to evaluate outcomes and competence and to act on unusual results. All those inquiries took place after Dr. Neary was suspended. They established that hard questions must be asked when the unexpected happens too often. There must be learning from mistakes. There must be functioning monitoring professional bodies. While the numbers of the procedures established in this Maternity Unit may be startling, they have to be understood in the context in which they occurred. I hope this report assists in coming to that understanding. It must be understood that good hardworking decent people can unwittingly enable bad practice when support and safety systems are not in place.

Finally, this report would not have been effective without the assistance of so many obstetricians including Dr. James Feeney who provided me with their own experience of peripartum hysterectomy or without the unstinting time given by the current and former staff of the Lourdes Hospital and the North Eastern Health Board. Sheila O'Connor of Patient Focus enabled me to see the human angle of the aftermath of the operations and the effect of ongoing and frequently irresponsible reporting of those events. The almost complete cooperation the Inquiry received from witnesses restores my faith in the effectiveness of a private non adversarial inquiry. The quality of my legal and support team made the task pleasurable. I hope that readers and those affected by the events giving rise to this Inquiry find the report informative, comprehensive and fair.

January 25th 2006

TERM 1

TO EXAMINE THE RATE OF PERIPARTUM HYSTERECTOMY AT OUR LADY OF LOURDES HOSPITAL, DROGHEDA ("THE HOSPITAL") WITH PARTICULAR REFERENCE TO THE PERIOD COVERED IN THE REPORT OF THE FITNESS TO PRACTISE COMMITTEE OF THE MEDICAL COUNCIL ("THE REPORT") AND THE PERIOD SINCE THE PUBLICATION OF THAT REPORT AND TO DETERMINE HOW THIS RATE COMPARED WITH THE RATE IN OTHER MATERNITY UNITS OF SIMILAR STATUS.

1 THE RATE IN THE LOURDES HOSPITAL

1.1 All available hospital records have been fully examined and checked against each other for consistency to determine the numbers of peripartum hysterectomies carried out between 1974–2004.

The first source examined was the Maternity Department **Clinical Reports** for the period 1960-1984. From these reports, we determined the number of reported cases of caesarean hysterectomy. We are fairly confident that these very detailed reports cover all cases of caesarean hysterectomy. For the most part, the reasons why a caesarean section ended in hysterectomy were not stated.

It was more difficult to establish numbers for hysterectomy following vaginal delivery and post partum haemorrhage, as they were not covered under a special heading in these clinical reports. These procedures were frequently reported under stillbirth or uterine rupture.

We next considered the **maternity theatre records**.

The most critical records in a maternity hospital archive are the theatre registers and the birth registers. All operations carried out under anaesthesia are detailed in the theatre registers. The register usually spans at least a decade – probably two decades in a middle sized hospital such as the Lourdes Hospital of the '70s and '80s. The theatre register is an important source document because it records patient details, the date and time of the operation, the names of the surgeon, the assisting doctors, the anaesthetist and assistant, the theatre nurses and whether any specimen was sent to pathology. The early theatre registers were missing. It was generally reported by theatre staff that there had only ever been two theatre registers in existence before 1998. The only theatre register we were able to consult was the 1991-2003 register.

The **birth registers** record details of the mother's name, age and previous parity, the time of delivery, the name of the medical attendant or midwife who delivered the baby, the details of the baby's sex, weight and condition. The birth register also recorded if any additional procedures were carried out to the mother and the condition of both baby and mother on discharge. Many of the birth registers were missing. Our efforts were seriously hampered by the absence of these critical records. Fortunately, we were able to check various secondary records, and we were assisted by many of the women who had undergone peripartum hysterectomy and who attended for interview.

An analysis of the **secondary records** enables us to be confident that we have accurately determined the numbers of peripartum hysterectomies carried out in the Lourdes Hospital between 1960-2004. In the final numbers, we included 2 patients whose term of pregnancy may possibly be pre-28 weeks, and 1 who was pre-28 weeks but on whom a hysterectomy was carried out.

We have presented our findings in the tables, which follow.

These tables indicate the figures for the period 1960-2005. This lengthy period is broken down into three sections: –

- A selected sample time prior to Dr. Neary's employment in the unit
- The time period of Dr. Neary's employment ie.1974-1998
- 1999 to the present

1.2 TABLE 1A: THE LOURDES HOSPITAL 1960-1973

The statistics for the period 1960–1973.

During this time there were two consultants, the foundation obstetrician Dr. Gerard A. Connolly, and Dr. Liam O'Brien (from 1964).

Note: for ease of analysis, adjusted figures have been used - biennial statistics from the clinical reports have been divided into separate years; hysterectomies following laparotomy have been included in figures for hysterectomy following vaginal delivery. Nature of delivery in one case is unknown.

Year	Deliveries	C/S	% c/s of del	Peripartum Hysterectomy	% Hysterectomy per Delivery	Caesarean Hysterectomy	% c/h per c/s	Hysterectomy following vaginal delivery
1960	1542	45	2.92%	0	0.00%	0	0.00%	0
1961	1347	44	3.27%	2	0.15%	1	2.27%	1
1962	1442	44	3.05%	3	0.21%	2	4.55%	1
1963	1656	43	2.60%	2	0.12%	1	2.33%	1
1964	1925	64	3.32%	1	0.05%	1	1.56%	0
1965	2072	63	3.04%	2	0.10%	0	0.00%	2
1966	2274	76	3.34%	1	0.04%	0	0.00%	1
1967	2369	76	3.21%	8	0.34%	6	7.89%	2
1968	2518	92	3.65%	2	0.08%	1	1.09%	1
1969	2528	91	3.60%	1	0.04%	0	0.00%	1
1970	2631	100	3.80%	5	0.19%	1	1.00%	4
1971	2562	99	3.86%	2	0.08%	1	1.01%	1
1972	2623	93	3.55%	1	0.04%	1	1.08%	0
1973	2490	93	3.73%	1	0.04%	0	0.00%	0
TOTAL	29979	1023		31		15		15

- total for deliveries in the period **29979**.
- total of caesarean sections **1023** (3.41%).
- total number of peripartum hysterectomies for this period **31**, **15** of which **followed caesarean section**
- the rate of peripartum hysterectomy averaged over the period was **1 per 967 deliveries (0.1%)** and **1 caesarean hysterectomy per 68 caesarean sections (1.47%)**

TABLE1B(i): THE LOURDES HOSPITAL 1974-1998

This table illustrates the Maternity Unit statistics for all operators in the Maternity Unit 1974-1998, which is the period when Dr. Neary worked in the hospital. (Note: one of the hysterectomies recorded for October 1998 was performed while Dr.Neary was on administrative leave and not working at the hospital.)

Year	Deliveries	C/S	% c/s of del	Peripartum Hysterectomy	% Hysterectomy per Delivery	Caesarean Hysterectomy	% c/h per c/s	Hysterectomy following vaginal delivery
1974	2499	102	4.08%	1	0.04%	1	0.98%	0
1975	2636	101	3.83%	2	0.08%	2	1.98%	0
1976	2648	111	4.19%	5	0.19%	4	3.60%	1
1977	2787	111	3.98%	3	0.11%	2	1.80%	1
1978	2750	140	5.09%	8	0.29%	8	5.71%	0
1979	2892	141	4.88%	9	0.31%	7	4.96%	2
1980	2839	178	6.27%	6	0.21%	4	2.25%	2
1981	2685	169	6.29%	6	0.22%	6	3.55%	0
1982	2396	170	7.10%	5	0.21%	4	2.35%	1
1983	2326	184	7.91%	7	0.30%	7	3.80%	0
1984	2099	243	11.58%	2	0.10%	1	0.41%	1
1985	1842	222	12.05%	12	0.65%	10	4.50%	2
1986	1887	194	10.28%	9	0.48%	7	3.61%	2
1987	1716	180	10.49%	8	0.47%	6	3.33%	2
1988	1761	224	12.72%	7	0.40%	6	2.68%	1
1989	1657	211	12.73%	6	0.36%	6	2.84%	0
1990	1743	201	11.53%	3	0.17%	3	1.49%	0
1991	1660	288	17.35%	12	0.72%	11	3.82%	1
1992	1685	334	19.82%	8	0.47%	8	2.40%	0
1993	1607	306	19.04%	15	0.93%	12	3.92%	3
1994	1583	317	20.03%	9	0.57%	9	2.84%	0
1995	1699	389	22.90%	11	0.65%	10	2.57%	1
1996	1725	469	27.19%	14	0.81%	11	2.35%	3
1997	1889	479	25.36%	10	0.53%	10	2.09%	0
1998	1972	528	26.77%	10	0.51%	8	1.52%	2
TOTAL	52983	5992		188		163		25

- total for deliveries in the period **52983**.
- total number of caesarean sections **5992** (11.31%).
- total number of peripartum hysterectomies **188, of which 163 followed caesarean section.**

-   the rate of peripartum hysterectomy averaged over the period was **1 per 282 deliveries (0.35%)** and **1 caesarean hysterectomy per 37 caesarean sections (2.72%)**

Later in this chapter, we deal with the rates of peripartum hysterectomy reported in other provincial Maternity Units. In making comparisons, it will be seen that figures from other hospitals as presented in this report do not distinguish between caesarean (whether elective or emergency) and non-caesarean hysterectomies, although some hospitals did supply this breakdown. As it was impossible to distinguish between the figures for caesarean hysterectomies and the more inclusive peripartum hysterectomy, we made our calculations on the basis of peripartum hysterectomy relative to deliveries. For comparative purposes, when taking all hysterectomies into account, the rate in The Lourdes Maternity Unit during the period 1974-1998 was 1 hysterectomy per 282 deliveries.

In examining the rate of peripartum hysterectomy, we noted that clusters of procedures were performed within a very short time period. A 'cluster' was defined as two or more hysterectomies in one month, or three or more over an approximate time period of two months. The following clusters were noted:

TABLE 1B(ii): CLUSTERS OF PROCEDURES 1976 – 1998

Year	Total Peripartum Hysterectomy For Year	Clusters
1998	10	5 mid-January to mid-March 3 in October
1997	10	2 in January 3 mid-May to mid-July 3 in October - 2 in one day 2 in December
1996	14	6 in January 3 mid-April to mid-May 4 from end of July to end September
1995	11	3 in January 3 in one month – February/March 3 in one month – June/July 2 in one month – October/November
1994	9	2 in February (3 over February/March) 4 end June to end August (2 in July) 2 in one week – end November/early December
1993	15	4 late February to late April (2 in April) 2 in September 2 in October 4 in December
1992	8	3 in late February to early April 3 in May/June (2 in May)
1991	12	2 in April 2 in May 2 in July 5 end September to late November (3 in November)
1990	3	2 in September
1989	6	3 in late June to early August
1988	7	3 in August
1987	8	3 mid-August to early October
1986	9	3 over April/May 3 over August/September 2 in December
1985	12	3 in April/May (2 in April) 3 in August/September (2 in August) 3 late October to early December
1983	7	4 end August to mid-October 3 in December - 2 in one day
1982	5	3 in March/April (2 in April)
1981	6	3 end July to mid-September
1980	6	3 in October – 2 in one day
1979	9	6 in July/August
1978	8	4 mid-January to mid-March (2 in February)
1976	5	3 in July/August (2 in July) 2 in November

Given these patterns, it was surprising that witnesses told the Inquiry that they were unaware of the numbers because of the time lapse between procedures.

TABLE 1C: THE LOURDES HOSPITAL SINCE 1998

Between 1999 and 2004 (the most recent year for which statistics are available to us) 6 peripartum hysterectomies were carried out in the Maternity Unit., representing a rate of about 1 each year for an average of 2,849 deliveries per annum. There has been a large increase in the delivery rate brought about by the closure of the Maternity Units in Monaghan and Dundalk in 2001, the opening of Mosney as a major reception centre for refugees and asylum seekers and the continuing trend, in common with other Maternity Units, for rising delivery rates.

NOTE: 2 hysterectomies were performed in 2005.

Year	Deliveries	C/S	% c/s of del	Peripartum Hysterectomy	% hysterectomy per Deliveries
1999	2031	490	24.13%	0	0.00%
2000	2099	513	24.44%	2	0.10%
2001	2963	681	22.98%	0	0.00%
2002	3254	813	24.98%	1	0.03%
2003	3389	817	24.11%	2	0.06%
2004	3357	902	26.87%	1	0.03%
2005*	3460	918	26.53%	2	0.06%
TOTAL	20553	5134	24.98%	8	0.04%

* 2005 figures were provided by the Lourdes in January 2006.

One peripartum hysterectomy for every 2,849 deliveries (0.0351%) compares well with the **national figures** for obstetric hysterectomy collected by the Hospital In-Patient Enquiry system (H.I.P.E.) and made available to the Inquiry by the ESRI. While these are based on total births (as opposed to total deliveries) they nevertheless give a good indication of the national incidence:

Year	Number of births nationally	Number of obstetric hysterectomies	Hysterectomy per births
1999	53,924	14	1 per 3852
2000	54,789	17	1 per 3223
2001	57854	22	1 per 2630
2002	60,503	13	1 per 4654
2003	61,517	15	1 per 4101
2004	n/a	15	n/a

The dramatic fall in peripartum hysterectomy rates indicates that lessons were learnt very quickly in The Lourdes Hospital - once the rate in the unit became apparent.

In early November 1998, Dr. Neary returned to work on condition that he was assisted by a locum consultant for caesarean sections and that no peripartum hysterectomy would be carried out without first calling in another consultant. No peripartum hysterectomies were carried out during this period. It is difficult to avoid the conclusion that practices and attitudes in the Maternity Unit changed especially when it became apparent that there was nationwide alarm at the then known rate. Obviously, far greater efforts were made to preserve a woman's uterus, even when faced with massive obstetric haemorrhage. The earlier practice of removing the uterus either because of its friable condition or for sterilisation purposes was clearly discontinued. The other changes that took place are more fully documented under Term 6 in this report.

The Medical Missionaries of Mary objected to the finding by the Inquiry that the uterus would previously have been removed because of its friable condition or for sterilisation purposes on the basis that *"no evidence was put to any member of the MMMs who were questioned by the Inquiry as to the fact that the removal of the uterus in such a context occurred. The MMMs would like it specifically stated in the report that they were not given any specific* *information in regard to the fact that this occurred, though it appears to be accepted by the Inquiry."*

In reference to this, they make the point that even if there was a basis for the suggestion that the ethos of the hospital had any connection with peripartum hysterectomies, they failed to see how there could be a connection between the ethos of the hospital and the reason why Dr. Neary was allowed to continue for so long. Secondly, they wished to make the point that whereas Dr. Neary clearly exhibited flawed clinical judgement there was never any issue in relation to his poor training as far as they were concerned. They found it odd that the Inquiry should have chosen to highlight Dr. Neary's flawed clinical judgement without making reference for example to his known fear of blood, the size of his clinical practice and his particular personality traits which have been dealt with at length by the Inquiry.

After Dr. Maresh's report and Dr. Neary's subsequent suspension became widely disseminated in various forms of the media, an effective and valuable tool in staunching otherwise intractable haemorrhage, i.e. caesarean hysterectomy, was demonised. It is probable that this had a significant impact on obstetricians and Maternity Units across the country. There is a widely held perception with obstetricians and anaesthetists who were interviewed that delay or reluctance to carry out hysterectomy because of fear of litigation or adverse publicity has contributed to several maternal deaths from haemorrhage. The Inquiry believes that it is appropriate to repeat the advice the Inquiry received from Dr. Maresh of St. Mary's Hospital Manchester.

> *"1. Caesarean hysterectomy is performed because of uncontrollable haemorrhage from the uterus at caesarean section following the delivery. It is performed when the various measures which have been taken to control the bleeding have failed and there is concern over the woman's life. Such a decision is taken by a consultant. In view of the rarity of the problem and the difficult manoeuvres required to try to stop the bleeding another consultant may sometimes be called in to assist, as the registrar helping the consultant is unlikely to have ever had experience of the procedure.*

2. Caesarean hysterectomy prevents the woman ever having any more children and therefore in young women, who have not completed their family, great efforts must be taken to avoid this. However delaying performing a hysterectomy with continued bleeding will cause its own problems. Excessive bleeding is associated with reduced clotting of the remaining blood and therefore haemorrhage may increase. Giving a blood transfusion on its own will not correct this. Accordingly the decision to abandon conservative measures to save the uterus and proceed to hysterectomy is difficult, another reason why today a second opinion should be considered."

We have been made aware, and have read reports of high morbidity, including kidney failure if the decision to carry out a peripartum hysterectomy is delayed too long. It would be wrong for the pendulum to swing too far in the other direction because of the events in Drogheda.

The Inquiry heard much anecdotal evidence suggesting that women's lives have been lost since 1998 because of reluctance to carry out appropriate obstetric hysterectomy. The Inquiry obtained figures from the Central Statistics Office for maternal deaths involving haemorrhage. These showed three deaths for the decade of the '90s, and one death in 2001. Figures supplied by the Chief Medical Officer in the Department of Health, Social Services and Public Safety for Northern Ireland show that there were two maternal deaths in the '90s, two in the year 2001, one in 2002 and three in 2003 attributable to 'pregnancy, child birth and the puerperium'. In spite of our best endeavours, we were unable to obtain a more specific cause of death or for the apparent rise in maternal deaths in the new millennium. The figures for both jurisdictions cover a short time span, and thus we were unable to confirm or deny the assertion made by several consultant witnesses that deaths have occurred because of an extreme reluctance to carry out peripartum hysterectomy in the aftermath of events in the Lourdes hospital. We were told of a particular maternal death in 2004 which we were told was associated with haemorrhage but were unable to confirm the facts.

1.3 TABLE 1D: PERIPARTUM HYSTERECTOMIES– CONSULTANT BREAKDOWN

The second table shows the operating surgeon for each peripartum hysterectomy carried out in the Lourdes between 1964 and 2005. Dr. Gerard A. Connolly was the first consultant appointed to the Lourdes Maternity Hospital. He was joined by Dr. Liam O'Brien in 1964. Both consultants worked in the hospital at a time when GPs quite frequently attended at the hospital for private patient deliveries. As far as we could determine, only the consultants performed operations. During this time, caesarean sections never exceeded 4% of total deliveries.

The table below shows the number of peripartum hysterectomies carried out, year on year, by the consultant obstetricians and unidentified registrar obstetricians ("R") from 1964 to 2005. Where the pre-1991 maternity theatre register was missing, this information was derived from secondary sources such as the annual reports, the maternity admissions register, pathology records and available birth registers.

Year	Number	Consultant Breakdown
1964	3	1 - Dr.Connolly; 2 – Unattributable
1965		
1966	9	5 - Dr.Connolly; 3 - Dr.O Brien; 1 – Unattributable
1967		
1968	3	1 - Dr.Connolly; 1 -Dr.O Brien; 1 – Unattributable
1969		
1970	5	2 - Dr.Connolly; 3 - Dr.O Brien
1971	2	1 - Dr.Connolly; 1 - Dr.O Brien
1972	2	1 - Dr.Connolly; 1 – Unattributable
1973		
1974	1	Dr.Connolly
1975	2	1 - Dr.Connolly; 1 - Dr.Neary
1976	5	1 - Dr.Connolly; 4 - Dr.Neary
1977	3	Dr.Neary
1978	8	3 - Dr.Connolly; 5 - Dr.Neary
1979	9	1 - Dr.Connolly; 7 - Dr.Neary; 1 – Unattributable
1980	6	1 - Dr.Connolly; 5 - Dr.Neary
1981	6	1 - Dr.O Brien; 5 - Dr.Neary
1982	5	Dr.Neary
1983	7	5 - Dr.Neary; 2 - Dr.Lynch
1984	2	Dr.Neary
1985	12	10 - Dr.Neary; 2 – Dr.Lynch
1986	9	6 - Dr.Neary; 3 - Dr.Lynch
1987	8	Dr.Neary
1988	7	5 - Dr.Neary; 2 - Dr.Lynch
1989	6	4 - Dr.Neary; 2 - Dr.Lynch
1990	3	1 - Dr.Neary; 2 - Dr.Lynch
1991	12	7 - Dr.Neary; 5 - Dr.Lynch
1992	8	4 - Dr.Neary; 3 - Dr.Lynch; 1 – Registrar

1993	15	1 – Dr.O Brien; 9 - Dr.Neary; 5 - Dr.Lynch
1994	9	3 - Dr.Neary; 6 - Dr.Lynch
1995	11	7 - Dr.Neary; 3 - Dr.Lynch; 1 – Registrar
1996	14	10 - Dr.Neary; 1 - Dr.Lynch; 2 – Dr.Wehab; 1 – Dr.Barde
1997	10	6 - Dr.Neary; 3 - Dr.Lynch; 1 – Dr.Wehab
1998	10	7- Dr.Neary; 1 – Dr.Lynch; 2 - Dr.O Coigligh
1999	0	
2000	2	1 - Dr.Lynch assisted by Dr.O Coigligh; 1 - Dr.O Coigligh assisted by Dr. Jones (urologist)+ registrar
2001	0	
2002	1	Dr.Rabee assisted by Dr.Milner and Dr.Doyle
2003	2	1 - Dr.Milner assisted by Dr.O'Coigligh; 1 – Dr.Milner assisted by Dr. O'Coigligh and Dr. Doyle
2004	1	Dr.Milner assisted by Dr.Barde
2005	2	1 – Dr.Rabee assisted by Dr.Higgins and Dr.Jones (urologist); 1 – Dr.Lynch assisted by Dr.O Coigligh and Dr.Akpan

From 1974 to 1982, the consultants attached to the Lourdes Hospital were Drs. Connolly, O'Brien and Neary. Dr. Connolly retired in 1982, and Dr. Finian Lynch was appointed in the same year.

Dr. O'Brien retired in 1996 and was replaced by Dr. Sami Wehab, a locum consultant until Dr. Seosamh O'Coighligh was appointed in September 1997. Dr. Haifae Rabee was appointed as locum consultant to work with Dr. Neary pending investigations into the complaints and she is still at the Hospital. Dr. Maire Milner joined the Lourdes in 1999; Dr. Etop Akpan in 2004; Dr. Rosemary Harkin in 2003; and Dr. Shane Higgins commenced in December 2004.

Dr. Miriam Doyle worked as a locum consultant from 2001-2004. Recently, more consultant obstetricians were appointed and those now working in the Lourdes Maternity Unit are:

Dr. Etop Akpan
Dr. Rosemary Harkin
Dr. Shane Higgins (lead clinician)
Dr. Finian Lynch
Dr. Maire Milner
Dr. Seosamh O'Coighligh
Dr. Haifae Rabee

A total of **129** peripartum hysterectomies can be attributed to Dr. Neary over a 25 year period.[9] **40** peripartum hysterectomies are attributed to Dr. Lynch over the 16 years from 1982-1998. Since 1998, Dr.Lynch carried out 1 such procedure. Over the period of 1974 –1996 Dr. O'Brien carried out 2 peripartum hysterectomies. 8 peripartum hysterectomies were carried out in the period of 1999-2005. On each occasion at least 2 and usually more consultant obstetricians were involved in the operation.

There was a difference in profile between Dr. Neary's patients, and those of Dr. Lynch. Analysis of patient details indicates that Dr. Lynch's patients tended to be older women and of higher parity. Dr. Neary's patients were often young women, many of whom were having their first baby (25) or had only one previous child (26). Dr. Lynch's figures are 2 women having their first baby and 4 women with one previous child (but 2 with one previous pregnancy). These differences are illustrated in **Table 1E: Age Profile & Parity Comparison**, and will be commented upon further later in this report. Parity is a well known word and concept in midwifery and obstetrics. It indicates an obstetric history; thus a patient with a parity of 2+1 at time of admission means a patient who before the delivery in question has had 3 pregnancies with 2 live babies delivered and one further pregnancy which did not end in a live birth (usually a miscarriage). Thus a mother with a parity of 2+1 would be in her fourth pregnancy and delivering her third child. For a more accurate determination of the number of live children born to a mother before her peripartum hysterectomy we treated parity as the number of children this mother had at the time. In two instances the parity was unknown, and in five instances the mother's age was unknown.

We therefore resorted to layman's language when trying to accurately depict the number of children a mother had when hysterectomy was carried out.

---

[9] DR. NEARY DISPUTES SOME OF THESE FIGURES AND PRESENTED THE INQUIRY WITH A DIFFERENT TABLE OF CASES AFTER HE HAD BEEN FURNISHED WITH A COPY OF THE DRAFT REPORT. HE SAYS THAT FOR THE PERIOD **1992-1998** HE PERFORMED **35** HYSTERECTOMIES.

TABLE 1E – AGE & PARITY PROFILE

Year	Consultant	Total per Consultant	Patient's age at time of hysterectomy	No. of Children at time of Hysterectomy
2000	Dr.Lynch	1	30	
1998	Dr.Lynch	1	29	1
1997	Dr.Lynch	3	42	2
			37	4
			40	3
1996	Dr.Lynch		39	8
1995	Dr.Lynch	3	27	6
			38	4
			32	4
1994	Dr.Lynch	5	32	7
			29	2
			45	10
			33	3
			39	4
			37	7
1993	Dr.Lynch	5	40	3
			36	4
			38	5
			40	12
			43	6
1992	Dr.Lynch	3	41	14
			32	4
			34	1
1991	Dr.Lynch	5	32	2
			30	3
			44	7
			33	3
			33	3
1990	Dr.Lynch	2	25	4
			38	11
1989	Dr.Lynch	2	37	4
			27	3
1988	Dr.Lynch	2	41	5
			42	5
1986	Dr.Lynch	3	41	5
			37	7
			32	8
1985	Dr.Lynch	2	38	3
			35	6
1983	Dr.Lynch	2	27	7
			19	2

Year	Consultant	Total per Consultant	Patient's age at time of hysterectomy	No. of Children at time of Hysterectomy
1998	Dr.Neary	7	20	1
			23	3
			37	4
			32	4
			33	2
			26	3
			19	1
1997	Dr.Neary	6	40	4
			27	1
			36	2
			32	2
			34	3
			38	4
1996	Dr.Neary	10	35	1
			25	2
			34	5
			20	1
			29	0
			37	3
			25	4
			28	1
			28	2
			32	
1995	Dr.Neary	7	29	2
			29	3
			35	2
			39	6
			33	3
			36	3
			26	2
1994	Dr.Neary	3	25	1
			28	3
			32	3
1993	Dr.Neary	9	31	1
			37	4
			35	1
			25	1
			29	5
				2
			26	4
			27	3
			32	3

Year	Consultant	Total per Consultant	Patient's age at time of hysterectomy	No. of Children at time of Hysterectomy
1992	Dr.Neary	4		3
			40	4
			41	4
			27	1
1991	Dr.Neary	7	37	3
			33	3
			33	3
			42	1
			28	4
			25	3
			35	3
1990	Dr.Neary	1	36	3
1989	Dr.Neary	4	37	2
			42	4
			44	4
			36	5
1988	Dr.Neary	5	35	5
			33	2
			40	7
			32	2
			36	2
1987	Dr.Neary	8	42	6
			33	10
			25	2
			44	2
			31	4
			30	5
			27	3
			37	4
1986	Dr.Neary	6	19	0
			32	4
			44	11
				6
			37	2
			29	4

Year	Consultant	Total per Consultant	Patient's age at time of hysterectomy	No. of Children at time of Hysterectomy
1985	Dr. Neary	10	28	1
			31	5
			34	1
			26	4
			38	5
			31	2
			31	2
				5
			35	6
				2
1984	Dr.Neary	2	34	5
			32	4
1983	Dr.Neary	5	32	6
			40	3
			27	6
			27	1
			39	9
1982	Dr.Neary	5	39	13
			35	5
			40	5
			37	6
			26	4

SYNOPSIS OF AGE COMPARISON AND PARITY COMPARISON BETWEEN PATIENTS OF DR.NEARY & DR.LYNCH

AGE COMPARISON

Age Range	17 – 20	21 – 25	26 – 30	31 - 35	36 - 40	41 - 45	Total
Dr.Neary	5 (4%)	11 (9%)	30 (24%)	43 (35%)	26 (21%)	9 (7%)	124*
Dr.Lynch	1 (3%)	1 (3%)	7 (18%)	9 (23%)	14 (35%)	8 (20%)	40*

Note: Age was not available in some instances

NUMBER OF CHILDREN

Range of Parity at Time of Hysterectomy	0 – 1	2 –3	4 - 5	6 – 7	8-9	10 - 15	Total
Dr.Neary	26 (21%)	51 (41%)	32(+1?) (26%)	10(+1?) (8%)	1 (1%)	4 (3%)	124(+2?)*
Dr.Lynch[10]	2 (5%)	12 (30%)	12 (30%)	8 (20%)	2 (5%)	4 (10%)	40

Note: Parity was not available in some instances

COMPARATIVE RATES I

1.4   PRE LOURDES HOSPITAL INQUIRY

When the North Eastern Health Board initially investigated Dr. Neary's practices, they did so in secrecy, as a matter of urgency, over a weekend.   On 24th October 1998, Ms. M.D., Director of Nursing, and Mr. Finbar Lennon, Clinical Director, checked the available maternity theatre register for the period 1st January 1996 onwards. They found 27 caesarean hysterectomies, 21 of which were attributable to Dr. Neary. (We have now established, with the benefit of months of research, that there were 34 such operations in this period, 23 of which we attribute to Dr. Neary).

---

[10] The figures for Dr. Neary range from 1974 to 1998; the figures for Dr. Lynch range from 1983 to 1998.

When Mr. Lennon and M.D. carried out their first examination of the theatre register, they found a small note fixed by Sellotape to the end of the page for 1996. This note included a tot of caesarean sections, and whether they were emergency or elective procedures. The note stated that there was 1 hysterectomy in the theatre in 1995. Mr. Lennon and M.D. looked to see if there was a similar note at the end of the 1994 period, and there was a note indicating that there was 1 hysterectomy for that year too. We could find no explanation for this careless addition but it explains why it was initially believed that caesarean hysterectomy was not a problem until 1996.

When the Health Board carried out its preliminary inquiries, there were no readily available national statistics against which these figures could be compared. The Health Board believed at this stage that the rise in hysterectomies only occurred in 1996.

On the basis of the information collected over the weekend of 24th October 1998, Dr. Ambrose McLoughlin, Deputy CEO, and Mr. Finbar Lennon contacted eminent obstetricians in Northern Ireland and in the UK and asked them about the expected rate of obstetric hysterectomy. They were told that obstetric hysterectomy was a rare event, and that the numbers of such operations in the Lourdes Hospital appeared alarming and required explanation.

Dr. McLoughlin then requested Dr. Declan Bedford, an epidemiologist employed by the North Eastern Health Board, to carry out some urgent research on the norms for such operations, and how frequently such procedures should occur in a well-regulated provincial hospital in Ireland.

Dr. Bedford furnished a report on 6th November 1998. His research indicated that there were no national statistics available, and he had to resort to the Internet. He found that no national statistics were kept for obstetric hysterectomy in the United States or the United Kingdom. He reviewed the literature, which largely consisted of individual hospital studies, and found the rate varied from a high of 1 obstetric hysterectomy per 645 deliveries, to a low of 1 per 5,953 deliveries. The highest rate in the available studies was in Brigham Women's hospital, Boston, covering the period 1983 to 1992. The lowest rate emerged from The Coombe Women's Hospital, Dublin (the only Irish study of that time) entitled 'Peripartum Hysterectomy' Report of

11 cases undertaken by Gardeil F, Daly S, Turner M.J. and published in Rev. Fr. Gynecol Obstet, 1995 Oct; 90(10):431-4' (published in French with a summary in English).

The Coombe report covered the period 1982-1991 and identified 11 emergency hysterectomies in 10 years for 65,488 deliveries. It found no hysterectomies in the 21,998 primipara, the incidence in multipara being 1 per 3,954 deliveries, and the overall rate being 1 per 5,953 deliveries. Dr. Bedford checked more recent Coombe statistics for the three year period 1996-1998 and found 10 peripartum hysterectomies, a rate of 1 per 2,737 deliveries; 1 of these was a primigravida.

Studies from Birmingham Maternity Hospital (1968–1983) showed 47 hysterectomies, or 1 per 1,429 deliveries; 12 of these procedures were planned (i.e. for cancers).

Louisville General Hospital (1953 -1977) showed 1 per 4,348 pregnancies.

Milan (1980-1990) showed 1 per 833 deliveries: 7 of the 50 cases were elective.

Southern California (1 per 769 deliveries) evidenced various in between results.

Dr. Bedford then checked the other Health Board Maternity Units in the region covering the years 1995-1997.

Cavan General Hospital reported 1 hysterectomy for 2,517 deliveries and 460 caesarean sections;

In Monaghan there were 2 for 1,034 deliveries and 160 sections;

In Louth there were none for 1,456 deliveries and 280 sections.

Dr. Bedford reported 32 hysterectomies for the same period in the Lourdes hospital for 5,313 deliveries and 1,339 sections, and concluded –

"As can be seen from the tables, the rate of obstetric hysterectomy in Our Lady of Lourdes Hospital for the period 1995 to 1997 inclusive was 1 per 166 deliveries. The rate for the three year period for other NEHB hospitals combined was 1 per 1,669 deliveries."

When the Health Board received this alarming report, it sought best available advice and engaged Healthcare Risk Resources International (HRRI), a health care risk assessment agency based in the UK with branches in the United States. This agency briefed Mr. Michael Maresh MD FRCOG, a distinguished practising Consultant Obstetrician/Gynaecologist and lecturer from St. Mary's Hospital, Manchester, to review a number of patient records and to advise on the appropriateness of Dr. Neary's clinical decision to carry out a hysterectomy in each case.

Mr. Maresh subsequently became one of two principal expert witnesses to be called by the Medical Council before the Fitness to Practise Committee in the hearing of complaints against Dr. Neary. Dr. Maresh's evidence in all of the ten cases which were heard by the Fitness to Practise Committee was accepted. In his first report to the Health Board of 8th November 1998, Dr. Maresh dealt briefly with the expected norm as follows:

"Hysterectomy at the time of caesarean section has to be performed occasionally and one might expect one case in a year at a hospital this size. In view of the random nature of problems the rate might vary between 0-3, but more often than not between 0-1."

1.5 INTERNATIONAL STUDIES

The extensive research undertaken by this Inquiry, the experience in the Lourdes hospital since October 1998, and other international studies all tend to confirm this statement of Dr. Maresh for the period during which we are concerned. Dr. James Feeney, medical adviser to the Inquiry furnished a considerable volume of publications on the subject of peripartum hysterectomy throughout the English speaking world. The Inquiry considered all of this literature. There is little doubt that until relatively recently hysterectomy associated with pregnancy had fallen to very low levels. We were made aware of rising rates of peripartum hysterectomy recently associated with repeat caesarean sections and consequent increase in placenta previa in association with placental adherence. We were made aware of a paper on unplanned peripartum hysterectomy at Melbourne Royal Women's Hospital where there had been 8 peripartum hysterectomies in a six-month period. Three of the patients were nullipara. The paper referred to the rising peripartum hysterectomy rate in the State of Victoria, which was recorded at 12 in 1992, and 48 in 2002.

At the Fitness to Practise hearings Dr. Neary referred to studies from St. Mary's in Manchester where Dr. Maresh currently works. A study of all postpartum hysterectomies between 1987 and 1995 disclosed 28 cases, a rate of 1 per 1,904 deliveries. 8 of these were "*elective*" hysterectomies (planned in advance for cancer), 6 followed rupture of the uterus, 11 followed postpartum haemorrhage and 3 were associated with placenta previa. However, an earlier study from the same hospital in the period 1972 to 1982 showed a rate of 1 per 1,552 deliveries, and the incidence was found to have fallen by about 23% in the second series (Wenham and Matijevic, "Postpartum hysterectomies: revisited", J. Perinat. Med. 29 (2001) 260-265).

A series in Paris from 1983-1998 disclosed 10 peripartum hysterectomies for 34,453 deliveries, (a rate of I per 3,445 deliveries). A series in Bergin, Norway for 1981-1996 covering 70,546 deliveries showed 11 hysterectomies, or 1 per 6,413 deliveries, or 1 per 137 caesarean sections.

In reviewing the literature on caesarean hysterectomy, we became aware that the operation had a long and controversial history. There was its very early history, when the operation may have been hailed as a success but the patient inevitably succumbed to puerperal sepsis. In the 1960s and 1970s it became apparent that in countries where a full range of family planning methods was available, hysterectomy at time of caesarean section for gynaecological complaints was acceptable practice. Hence, the mention in some early studies to **elective** hysterectomies as opposed to **indicated** hysterectomies.

It was also apparent that in the United States prior to 1970, obstetric hysterectomy was used as a form of sterilisation. This was at a time when tubal ligation had an unacceptable failure rate. When the tubal ligation procedure was improved, the operation of caesarean hysterectomy for sterilisation fell from favour. Pletsch and Sandberg ("Caesarean Hysterectomy for Sterilisation", 1963 Am. J. Obst. & Gynec.

Vol.85, p.254-259) studied 27,680 obstetric deliveries, including 1,806 caesarean sections in Stanford University Hospital/Palo Alto-Stanford Hospital between 1949 and 1961. Of 169 hysterectomies, only 9 were "*indicated*" i.e. removal of the uterus was necessary to preserve the life of the patient, and 160 were elective sterilisations. In what is now an interesting historical commentary, the authors stated:

"*Until rather recently removal of the uterus at the time of caesarean section was considered a somewhat heroic undertaking. Now that the technical aspects of this operation appear less formidable, it may be desirable to expand its use with a view to offering maximum benefits in a programme of comprehensive obstetric care. A relatively minor operation cannot now be justified if a more extensive procedure can be shown to offer greater advantages to the patient without unduly increasing the risk to the patient.*

In the past most sterilisation procedures in the female have involved merely manipulation of the fallopian tubes. Now that more extensive surgical procedures can be undertaken with relative impunity, there has been an increasing interest in, and a growing utilisation of, uterine excision for purposes of sterilisation. This practice has been condemned by some as excessive surgery – a larger procedure than necessary to accomplish the task. Increasing numbers of physicians, however, feel that in selected women removal of the uterus offers advantages that are not obtained through simpler sterilisation methods. More experience with this operation, as well as frequent evaluation of all the factors involved, will aid in determining the validity of these concepts."

The authors opined that "*morbidity occurred with about equal frequency following caesarean hysterectomy and caesarean tubal ligation*", with failure in sterilisation occurring in 3% of cases, and significant gynaecologic problems in 24% following tubal ligation. It concluded that tubal ligation should be chosen for short term goals, but that caesarean hysterectomy (for patients rigidly selected) should be the procedure of choice for effecting sterilisation.

The authors also reviewed the American literature since 1950. They found reports of 1,819 caesarean hysterectomies (including the ones in their study). They reclassified these according to their concept of *"elective"* or *"indicated"*, and stated *"it appears that 1,278 procedures were elective and only 265 were indicated"*, thus demonstrating the extent to which sterilisation by caesarean hysterectomy was commonplace in the United States and how relatively rarely the *"indicated"* operation occurred.

In the 1970s, the debate continued. In 1970 Hofmeister published an article entitled "Tubal Ligation versus Caesarean Hysterectomy", based on studies in the Lutheran Hospital of Milwaukee, Wisconsin. He noted that in the previous 30 years *"tubal ligation has gained momentum as an elective method of family planning"* but added *"one can sense a trend among some obstetricians to consider primary caesarean hysterectomy as a method of choice when sterilization is indicated."* His extensive study and comparison led him to comment: –

> *"Our approach is guided by the age of the patient and her husband, the number of children, the health of the living children, the presence or absence of disease (uterine fibroids, vaginal relaxation, uterine prolapse, symptoms of dysmenorrhoea or menorrhagia and urinary incontinence) and the attitude and understanding of the patient and her husband. Unnecessary surgery is avoided. Hysterectomy in association with section should not be done unless hysterectomy is indicated. A primary caesarean section is never performed without obstetrical indications only to permit a tubal ligation. The potential of creating one problem to avoid a future potential problem is, in most instances, poor medical practice. Even a routine prophylactic appendectomy is being challenged today."*

In that study, it is clear that while the authors disapproved of hysterectomy for elective sterilisation, or indeed the resort to caesarean section in order to carry out a tubal ligation, they fully accepted the place of hysterectomy at time of caesarean section for gynaecological disorders. This, it was argued, obviated the need to carry out a second operation for hysterectomy several months after recovery from caesarean section.

 As the '70s progressed and anaesthesia by spinal block as opposed to general anaesthesia became routinely available and tubal ligation failure rates dropped, the place of tubal ligation as the medically preferred method of sterilisation seems to have become obvious from the literature. Park and Duff, Walter Reed Army Medical Center, Washington D.C. ("Role of Caesarean Hysterectomy in Modern Obstetric Practice", Clin. Ob. And Gynae., Vol. 23, No. 2, June 1980) undertook a comprehensive review in 1980 and advised –

> "*Even with increasing experience and improved surgical techniques on the part of the clinician, caesarean hysterectomy will remain an operation with a high complication rate. Therefore we believe that its use should be restricted to situations where there is a valid indication both for abdominal delivery and for uterine removal. More liberal use of the operation, especially for the simple provision of sterilisation, is not justified and exposes the patient to an unacceptably high risk of increased morbidity and mortality.*"

Later articles tend to assume that obstetric hysterectomy should only be carried out when medically indicated, and not for sterilisation purposes e.g. Thonet "Obstetric Hysterectomy – an 11-year experience" (B.J.O.G., Aug.1986, Vol.93, pp.794-798), the study dealing with St. Mary's Hospital, Manchester.

The debate eventually concluded that obstetric hysterectomy was no longer medically acceptable in modern Western European or U.S. hospitals where it previously had been offered and undertaken for sterilisation purposes. We are not convinced that this advice was accepted or followed in Ireland, where the same range of contraceptive products and services was simply not available.

We have dealt with the history of family planning in Ireland under Term of Reference 3. We believe that time stood still for decades in the Lourdes Maternity Unit where transparency was absent. Practices acceptable in the 1970s continued up to and perhaps beyond, the time of Dr. Neary's suspension.

1.6 THE INSTITUTE REVIEW

In December 1998, by agreement with Dr. Neary and his advisors, and Dr. Harith Lamki, President of the Institute of Obstetricians and Gynaecologists, the North Eastern Health Board established a Review Group consisting of three obstetricians;

Professor Graham Harley (Belfast), Dr. Dermot MacDonald (Dublin) and Dr. Edgar Ritchie (Cork).

Their task was to review Dr. Neary's clinical practice and to assess all cases of peripartum hysterectomy carried out by him since January 1992. Their Report of April 1999 states:

> "On the data available to the Review Group, Dr. Neary performed 708 caesarean sections from 1992-1998 inclusive and 39 peripartum caesarean hysterectomies. This gives a peripartum caesarean hysterectomy rate of 5%, i.e. one for every 20 caesarean sections….. This is 20 times the rate recorded in one Dublin maternity hospital [Holles St.] where 38,816 were delivered between 1992 and 1996, and eight mothers had peripartum caesarean hysterectomies, giving an incidence of one in 441 caesarean sections …."

From its extensive review of source materials, the Inquiry has established that 46 hysterectomies should be attributed to Dr. Neary from 1992-1998 inclusive. During the same period, Dr. Lynch carried out 22 peripartum hysterectomies and 9 were carried out by other consultants. The Review Group went on to state:

> "In one Canadian study of peripartum hysterectomies over 10 years in two Manitoba tertiary centres, the overall incidence was 0.4 per 1,000 births….This would probably be more in keeping with international figures (USA and Europe) than with those for the Republic of Ireland."

The Review Group also addressed Dr. Neary's assertion that in 8 cases between 1996 and 1998, he carried out hysterectomies for the purpose of sterilisation, after discussion with the patient beforehand. This was contrary to what he told the Medical Council Fitness to Practise Committee, namely that he did not carry out sterilisations and that there had to be a medical reason for hysterectomy. He told the Inquiry that he adhered to the ethos of the MMMs and only carried out medically indicated sterilisations.

After considering the hospital's Code of Ethics (developed when it was owned and run by the Medical Missionaries), which permitted "*Indirect sterilisation.....which is the consequence of a procedure indicated on medical grounds*" (clause 5.3(iv)), they concluded –

"In previous years in Ireland, some patients may have had a peripartum hysterectomy as a method of sterilisation and, although some of Dr. Neary's patients may have fulfilled the criteria for indirect sterilisation, in the opinion of the Review Group the choice of peripartum hysterectomy for the purpose of sterilisation is not now acceptable.

Sterilisation by simple occlusion of the fallopian tubes is an easier procedure and carries a much smaller risk of mortality and morbidity than peripartum hysterectomy. The decision to have a sterilisation procedure requires careful consideration by the patient and her partner well in advance of the operation. Sterilisation is a planned operation, which means that the decision is well thought out before the procedure. Peripartum hysterectomy is usually an emergency operation, which implies that the patient does not have time to consider and decide whether to have a sterilisation procedure.

In addition peripartum hysterectomy is an irreversible procedure as regards sterilisation compared with any other method."

The Inquiry regards this as an authoritative medical statement applicable to the 1990s in Ireland, and one which applied with perhaps less vigour in the 1980s. We repeat that whatever the appropriate and acceptable practice approved by the Institute of Obstetricians and Gynaecologists, tubal ligations were prohibited in this hospital.

1.7 MEDICAL COUNCIL COMMITTEE

The Report of the Fitness to Practise Committee of July 2003 shows that that Committee received a considerable body of statistical evidence, much of it from Dr. Neary. On pages 7–8 they compare figures for the Coombe and Holles St. hospitals with figures from the Lourdes Drogheda during the period 1993-1998 inclusive.

Their Table shows;

- The Coombe averaged 1 hysterectomy per 4,373 births

- Holles St. 1 per 3,847 births

- The Lourdes Hospital 1 per 179 births.

The Report then states:

"As will be seen from the above table hysterectomies in association with pregnancy were carried out over 20 times as frequently in Drogheda in the period 1993 to 1998 as they were in the Coombe or in the National Maternity Hospital. Clearly such a substantial deviation from the norm must be a source of very serious concern. The figures indicate that caesarean hysterectomies were carried out with what was an unacceptable degree of frequency in Drogheda during the relevant period. The Committee considers that the practice in Drogheda, as demonstrated by these figures, fell very substantially outside the range of what might be accepted. From these figures the Committee can only conclude that it is highly probable that the procedures carried out in Drogheda were largely unnecessary.

"It must be immediately conceded, however, that the 1 per 179 figure is the figure for the unit in Drogheda as a whole and is not Dr. Neary's own personal rate. However, he agreed that he could not have personally attended 50 per cent of the deliveries of the hospital."

The Committee proceeded to find that Dr. Neary's personal rate was a lot higher. This was based on a document exhibited by Dr. Neary, which the Committee considered *"accurate"*, showing *"deliveries personally carried out by each consultant in the years 1993 to 1998"*. It showed deliveries *"attended by Dr. Neary"* over the period as 1,897 and his hysterectomies for those years as:

- 4 in 1993

- 2 in 1994

- 6 in 1995

- 7 in 1996

- 6 in 1997

- 6 in 1998

a total of 31, indicating *"that Dr. Neary carried out one Caesarean hysterectomy for every 59 deliveries that he attended."*

The Inquiry has established the figures in this document for Dr. Neary's hysterectomies were understated for every year but one. The correct figures are:

- 9 in 1993
- 3 in 1994
- 7 in 1995
- 10 in 1996
- 6 in 1997
- 7 in 1998

a total of 42.

Accordingly, Dr. Neary's rate per delivery might appear to be even higher than one per 59 deliveries. However the Inquiry considers that the Fitness to Practise Committee, in calculating this figure, was not comparing like with like as it did not have evidence of figures for deliveries personally attended by consultants in the Coombe or Holles St., or their personal hysterectomy rates, and indeed no such figures were available for any comparable unit.[11]

The Committee was on firmer ground when it went on to consider the hysterectomy rate as a proportion of caesarean sections – comparing the Coombe, Holles St., Drogheda, and Dr. Neary's personal rate for the same five year period (page 9/10 of their Report). The Inquiry regards this as a fairer basis for comparing units/operators as a large majority of obstetric hysterectomies follow on caesarean section. Some caution must be exercised, however, as such comparisons exclude – or should exclude – hysterectomies following vaginal delivery e.g. for secondary postpartum haemorrhage.

The Committee found the rate of hysterectomy per section at

- The Coombe: 1 per 600 caesarean sections

---

[11] As previously stated Dr. Neary disputed our figures. The Inquiry figures come from the Maternity Theatre register and the Birth registers where he is recorded as the surgeon. It may be that he was called in to assist a registrar and was therefore the surgeon in charge. Dr. Neary asserts that in some cases the clamps were already on when he came in to assist.

- Holles St: 1 per 405
- Drogheda   1 per 42
- Dr. Neary: 1 per 20.

This was based on Dr. Neary carrying out 31 such operations in that 6 year period, but this Inquiry attributes 42 peripartum hysterectomies in that time, of which 36 occurred at the time of caesarean section.   With this adjustment the Inquiry finds that for this six year period Dr. Neary did 1 hysterectomy for every 17 caesarean sections.

During the same period Dr.Lynch appears to have been the operating surgeon in 19 instances, of which 17 were caesarean hysterectomies. He carried out approximately 359 caesarean sections in the same period, and accordingly his rate was approximately 1 hysterectomy per 21 caesarean sections.

COMPARATIVE RATES II
1.8   COMPARISONS WITH NON-DUBLIN MATERNITY UNITS IN IRELAND
The Inquiry took the view that to compare the Lourdes with the large Dublin maternity hospitals would not be to compare like with like – particularly having regard to the geographical location of the hospital, the relatively small size of the unit, the number of consultant obstetricians and anaesthetists and the lack of a haematologist.

Accordingly, while personal investigation was outside the time and financial resources of the Inquiry, we wrote to most of the provincial Maternity Units to obtain details of their incidence of peripartum hysterectomy. A member of the Inquiry team visited a few hospitals to assist in collecting the data. We exclude the figure of some units where the hysterectomy rates appeared suspiciously low, or where the data was incomplete or not easily accessible.

Overall, the Inquiry had an excellent response from units requested to supply data. We collected statistics from Midland Regional Hospital, Portlaoise; Midland Regional Hospital, Mullingar; Sligo General Hospital; Letterkenny General Hospital; Mayo General Hospital; Portiuncula Hospital, Ballinasloe; Erinville and St Finbarr's Hospitals, Cork; Daisy Hill, Newry; Fatima, Airmount and Waterford Regional Hospital (Waterford Combined); St Luke's Hospital, Kilkenny; Tralee General Hospital, Kerry; University College Hospital, Galway as well as the 3 main Dublin

Teaching Hospitals – the National Maternity Hospital, Holles Street, The Coombe and the Rotunda.

The results appear in **TABLE 1F: TABLE OF COMPARATIVE PROVINCIAL HOSPITAL STATISTICS**, which also show figures from The Lourdes. It was clear from an analysis of the figures we received that the rates in the Lourdes Hospital were consistently dramatically higher than those from any of the other provincial Maternity Units.

TABLE 1F: TABLE OF COMPARATIVE PROVINCIAL HOSPITAL STATISTICS

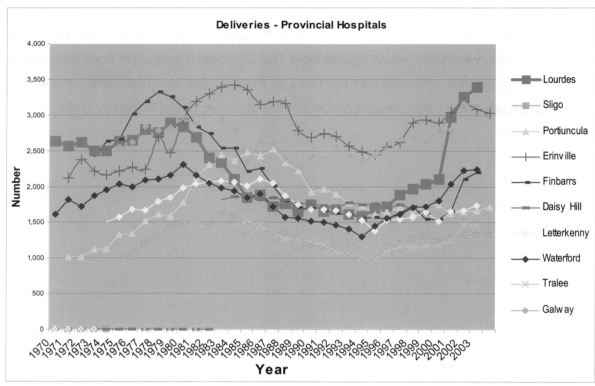

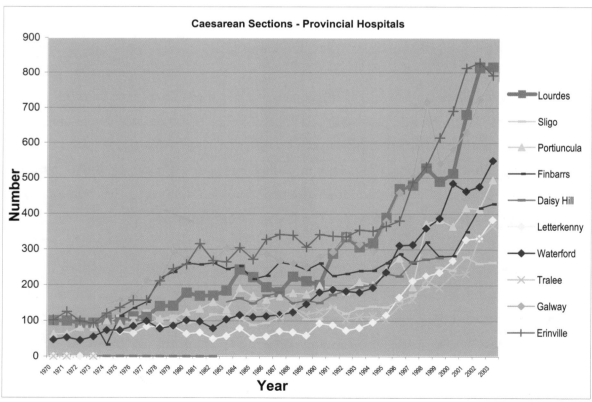

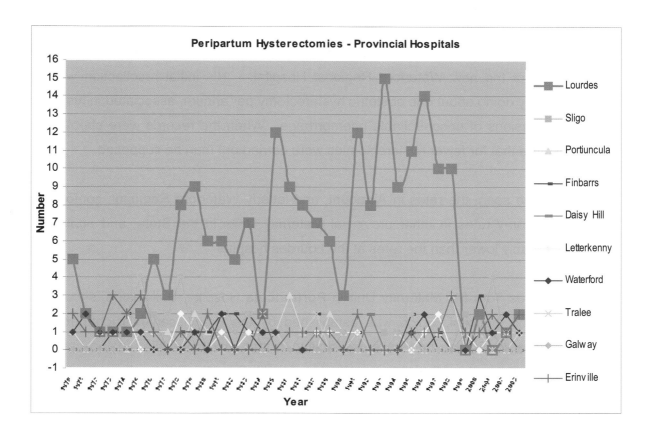

A number of these units warrant particular comment.

We sought figures from **Daisy Hill** Hospital, as it is a Maternity Unit located only 40 miles from Drogheda and is likely to be subject to the same geographic influences in wind, tide and Sellafield discharges. We found, for the limited years that figures were available, that the rates prevailing in Daisy Hill were similar to those in other Maternity Units of similar size in the Republic of Ireland during the '80s and '90s, and very much lower than the figures in The Lourdes Hospital.

We particularly checked the figures at **Airmount** in Waterford, as it was a hospital owned by the MMMs and managed according to the same religious ethos. It was established in 1952, and continued until 1995 when it, along with Fatima Hospital, was closed and subsumed into Waterford Regional Hospital. For total deliveries in the region of 61,929 from 1970 - 2003, there were 6,309 caesarean sections and 21 hysterectomies, i.e. 1 hysterectomy for every 2,949 deliveries and 1 hysterectomy for every 300 caesarean sections.

There were, for the most part, only two consultant obstetricians working in Airmount. We spoke to one of those consultants, now retired. He described under-manning and heavy workloads in a very outdated hospital while awaiting, for many years, the opening of the new Waterford Regional Hospital. His initial recollection was of personally doing about one obstetric hysterectomy per annum, associated in his mind with occasions of uncontrollable haemorrhage. When the records were checked, it transpired that far fewer hysterectomies were carried out than he supposed.

As can be seen, the rates in Airmount, and latterly Waterford Regional, conform to hysterectomy rates in other provincial Maternity Units in the State, and again are considerably lower than the rates at the Lourdes hospital.

The figures from the Maternity Unit in **Portiuncula** Hospital, Ballinasloe, should be noted. This hospital, which was established by the Franciscan Missionaries and opened in 1945, also had an ethos similar to that which prevailed in the Lourdes Hospital. It was transferred to the Western Health Board in 2001. It is attached to University College Hospital, Galway and geographically is removed from that city in much the same way as the Lourdes Hospital is from Dublin. The Maternity Unit in Portiuncula was slightly smaller, with deliveries of 1,349 in 1975, reaching a high of 2,523 in 1986 and averaging under 1,800. Caesarean section rates are also comparable. It had, for the most part, two consultant obstetricians and for a time a "*rotation*" registrar by arrangement with the Coombe. It did not have a School of Midwifery.

Portiuncula had excellently recorded statistics, largely due to the efforts of Dr C.C. From their data, it emerged that for 60,787 deliveries between 1970 and 2003 inclusive, there were 6,603 caesarean sections and 26 hysterectomies – i.e. 1 per 2,338 deliveries and 1 per 254 caesarean sections. Also notable is the even spread of the hysterectomies. Over the study period there were 8 in the 1970s, 11 in the 1980s, 6 in the 1990s, and 1 in the current decade.

We compiled comparative Tables for the Lourdes, Waterford (Airmount) and Portiuncula hospitals because of their many similarities in terms of provincial geography, religious management and ethos, number of deliveries, and purchase by a Health Board in the 1990s. A very major difference in those Maternity Hospitals emerged when speaking to 2 retired obstetricians who worked for many years in those two hospitals. Both hospitals operated the practice that no obstetric hysterectomy would be carried out by one consultant without first seeking the second opinion and if possible the assistance of another consultant.

DELIVERIES 1970 – 2000

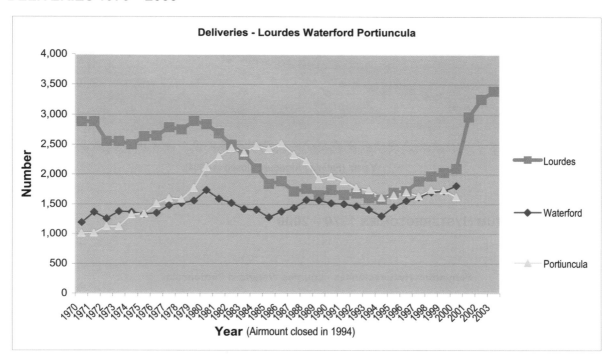

CAESAREAN SECTIONS – 1970 – 2000

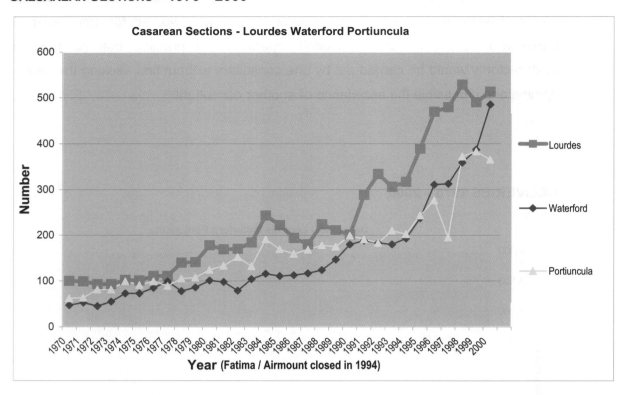

PERIPARTUM HYSTERECTOMIES 1970 – 2000

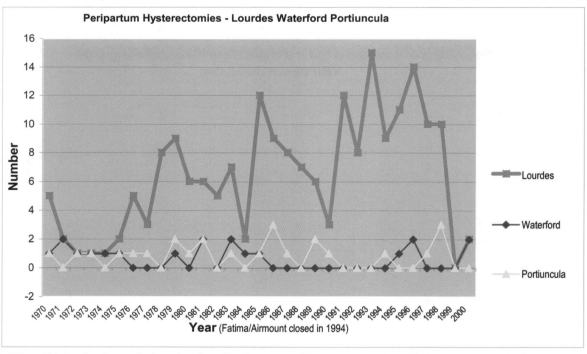

* The Waterford statistics in the Peripartum Hysterectomies Table include 2 from Fatima in '71 & '85 and 3 from Waterford Regional in '95 and '96.

The Inquiry believes that the figures shown for Cork's Erinville and St. Finbarr's are useful comparisons, even though they are situated in a city and are university hospitals.

St. Finbarr's had 67,893 deliveries for the years 1973 - 2003, of which 7,555 were by caesarean section, and 24 resulted in hysterectomy, ie.1/2,829 deliveries and 1/315 sections ended in hysterectomy. The spread between years and decades was relatively even.

From 1970-2003, Erinville had 37 hysterectomies for 94,343 deliveries (of which 11,660 were by caesarean section). This equates to 1/2,550 deliveries and 1/315 sections per hysterectomy. Again the spread over years and decades was remarkably even.

While great credit is due to the doctors and midwives working in some other hospitals e.g. Mayo General Hospital and St. Luke's, Kilkenny, we took the view that the very low numbers of hysterectomy in these hospitals might not be fair comparisons for the Lourdes Hospital for reasons such as the referral of more difficult cases to other units.

1.9 DUBLIN MATERNITY HOSPITALS

Despite the observations above on the appropriateness of the comparison, we did research the figures for the three large Dublin Maternity Hospitals (the Coombe, the Rotunda and the National Maternity Hospital, Holles St.). We felt these should be mentioned in this report as these units are generally acknowledged as "centres of excellence", and therefore suggest the standards that should be aspired to by other units. We did not consider Mount Carmel Maternity Unit because it caters exclusively for private patients and different considerations apply.

TABLE 1G: COMPARISON WITH DUBLIN HOSPITALS.

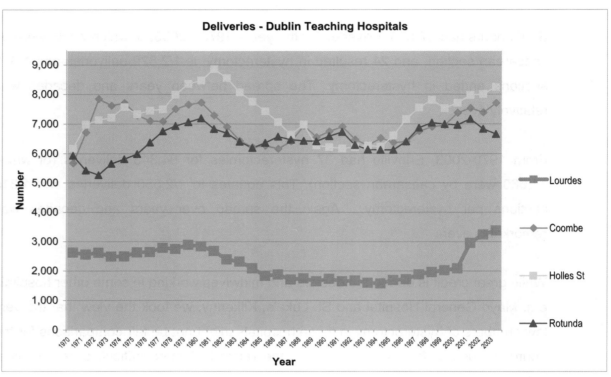

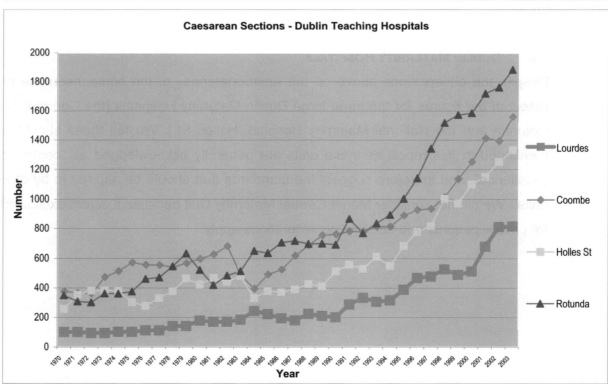

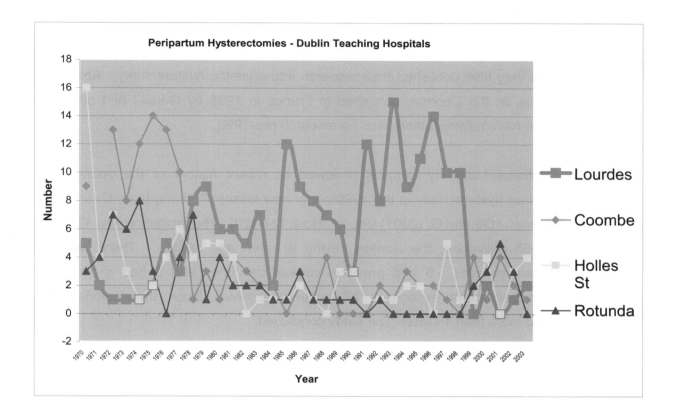

During the 1980s and 1990s the rate of peripartum hysterectomy at Lourdes Hospital far exceeded the worst figures at the three Dublin Maternity hospitals, even though rates of delivery in each of the Dublin hospitals were three times higher.

For the 1970s the rate in the Coombe was notably high. The Inquiry accepts that of the 70 hysterectomies carried out there in the period 1972-1977, some 35 of them were compassionate procedures for sterilisation purposes – a subject which will be discussed later in this Report.

It was noted that the rate of peripartum hysterectomy dropped during the '80s and '90s throughout the country, unlike at the Lourdes Hospital, where it increased.

The incidence in Drogheda is particularly high after 1990 – 12 in 1991, 8 in 1992, 15 in 1993, 9 in 1994, 11 in 1995, 14 in 1996, 10 in 1997 and 10 in 1998.

It was not until after the rate in the Lourdes Hospital came under scrutiny in late 1998 that the incidence subsided. Since that time it compares favourably with the rates experienced elsewhere in the State, including the big Dublin teaching hospitals.

1.10   IRISH RESEARCH INTO OBSTETRIC HYSTERECTOMY

There is very little published Irish research into obstetric hysterectomy. Apart from the article on the Coombe published in France in 1995 by Gardeil and others, to which we have referred, there was no research pre-1998.

The National Maternity Hospital reviewed its recent history of the operation in "Peripartum hysterectomy in the 1990s: any new lessons?" [Langdana, Geary, Haw and Keane, J.Ob.and G. (2001) Vol. 21, No.2 121-123]. The incidence was 17 cases for 64,563 deliveries, the women having a mean age of 34. There were no nulliparous patients. 6 had previous vaginal deliveries and 9 had a history of previous caesarean sections. All patients received blood transfusions, 74% receiving more than 10 units. The study concluded:

"Emergency peripartum hysterectomy is a rare operation often performed as a life-saving procedure for massive haemorrhage. Fortunately, in this series there was no maternal mortality but even in the last decade of the twentieth century, the associated maternal morbidity and perinatal mortality were high. We identified a history of at least one previous caesarean section in over half the cases. This is important, as the caesarean section rate is increasing worldwide. Many factors are associated with this but there has been recent emphasis on maternal request for elective caesarean section in the absence of any clinical indication..........This may ultimately lead to an increase in the incidence of peripartum hysterectomy.

In order to help reduce the problem of peripartum hysterectomy, we would recommend that caesarean section should be performed only for valid clinical indications. In addition when peripartum hysterectomy is required, the early involvement of an experienced obstetrician should help to minimise the operative morbidity."

Since then a study entitled "A 27-Year Review of Obstetric Hysterectomy", by Rishi Roopnarinesingh, Louise Fay and Peter McKenna, has been published in the Journal of Obstetrics and Gynaecology in 2003. The study reviews the 52 cases which occurred in the Rotunda between 1.1.1975 - 31.12.2001. This article was an exhibit considered by the Medical Council Fitness to Practice Committee hearing of complaints against Dr. Neary. The summary states:

"A retrospective case-review of 52 mothers who had a peripartum hysterectomy over the past 27 years was conducted at the Rotunda Hospital, Dublin, Ireland. The chief indications were uncontrollable haemorrhage due to rupture of the uterus, placenta previa and uterine atony. Obstetric hysterectomy is a formidable operation, usually performed for life-saving measures and requires expert surgical dexterity in order to minimise the significant morbidity that is unique to this procedure. The benefits of the subtotal operation appear to be superior to total hysterectomy. Counselling all patients having a caesarean section of the possibility of hysterectomy is advisable, particularly those who have had previous uterine surgery."

A third study on the related subject of controlling postpartum haemorrhage was published in 2004 (Rizvi, Mackey, Barrett, McKenna and Geary: "Successful reduction of massive Postpartum haemorrhage by use of guidelines and staff education" B.J.O.G., May 2004, vol.111, pp. 495-498), based on a six month study in the Rotunda in 1999. The summary states:

"We reviewed all cases of massive primary postpartum haemorrhage greater than 1000 ml over a six month period in 1999 to establish the incidence, identify aetiological factors and implement change. Fifty-four cases (1.7%) were identified. We classified four as 'near-miss' maternal mortality. Over 60% were delivered by caesarean section. Seventy-six percent were due to uterine atony, 9% due to genital tract trauma and 15% were associated with significant ante partum haemorrhage from placenta previa or abruption. No obvious labour or delivery risk factors were identified but deviation from hospital guidelines was common. Following revision of the guidelines, dissemination to staff and use of practice drills, we repeated the study on a prospective basis over the same time period in 2002. There was a significant reduction on the incidence of massive postpartum haemorrhage to 0.45%, and 100% adherence to the guidelines,

which resulted in a significant reduction on maternal morbidity. We believe
that this approach can be replicated in other units."

The Inquiry believes that this study demonstrates the benefits of proper clinical audit
and the experience and advice given in the article should be required reading for all
Maternity Unit staff, clinicians, midwives and risk managers. It is a very good
example of *"closing"* the loop.

The dearth of research on peripartum hysterectomy in this country could be
explained by the rarity of the operation, although there is a lurking suspicion that the
operation may have been underreported in some hospitals. There is little doubt that it
is a rare but known complication of pregnancy, but the suspicion remains that
because of cultural objection to tubal ligation, resort to hysterectomy may be more
common than statistics indicate.

Prior to 1998 most Maternity Units did not routinely collect or include statistics which
showed the numbers of peripartum hysterectomies carried out. In some reports
cases were referred to under sections dealing with "Postpartum Haemorrhage",
"Rupture" or "Secondary Postpartum Haemorrhage". Even close scrutiny of these
chapters did not necessarily provide a total of such procedures in a given year.

Another possibility is that, because some of the procedures were compassionate
sterilisations, there was underreporting of the cases and a reluctance to delve too
deeply into such operations. This appears to have been the case in the Coombe in
the 1970s, where the full number only emerged in the seven year review undertaken
when Dr. Clinch was Master.

Ironically, it was the Lourdes Hospital reports, particularly those prepared by Dr.
Neary, that were most consistent and open in publishing total numbers for caesarean
hysterectomies.

The search for statistics in provincial units for comparative purposes generally
involved laborious sifting through maternity theatre registers and birth registers and
while the Inquiry on occasions provided some assistance, we are very grateful to
these hospitals for their considerable contribution to our work.

The Lourdes Hospital is the only hospital whose documents were scrutinised and whose staff and patients were interviewed. The Inquiry believes that it identified all peripartum hysterectomies carried out in the unit. We came across a small number of hysterectomies carried out in association with a failed pregnancy and this caused us some concern. These were outside of our Terms of Reference.

It is difficult to believe that similar adverse outcomes and outdated practices that we uncovered were confined to this unit. The rates of caesarean and peripartum hysterectomy reported to us for provincial units were frequently very low or non existent. Our experience with HIPE figures (used to determine public funding of hospitals, and based on systematic computerised returns from all public hospitals covering all in-patient operations – figures which we found to be accurate) makes us somewhat wary of relying totally on other hospitals' records. As against that argument, many obstetricians interviewed, and many who answered our questionnaire, said they had never assisted at or carried out an obstetric hysterectomy.

We were made aware of a series of recent reports and articles on rising rates of peripartum hysterectomy associated with repeat caesarean sections. In particular we were directed to a paper on unplanned peripartum hysterectomy at Melbourne Royal Women's Hospital where there had been 8 peripartum hysterectomies in a six-month period. Three of the patients were nullipara. The paper referred to the rising peripartum hysterectomy rate in the State of Victoria, which was recorded at 12 in 1992, and 48 in 2002.

OBSTETRICIANS SURVEY RESULTS

At the start of this Inquiry, some obstetricians suggested to us that the number of hysterectomies carried out at the Lourdes Maternity Unit was not so out of line with figures from other Maternity Units where resources were limited and only 2-3 obstetricians were employed.

It was also suggested that Dr. Neary was carrying out no more hysterectomies than many of his overworked colleagues in similar situations. The Inquiry decided to test this proposition, not as a scientific survey, but as an estimation of the experience of the obstetric community in relation to peripartum hysterectomy. In November 2004, the Inquiry wrote to 124 obstetricians whose names appeared in the current Irish Medical Directory. The letter enclosing a questionnaire outlined the preliminary findings of peripartum hysterectomies attributed to the obstetricians working at the Lourdes Maternity Unit. We received 78 replies (two failed to answer the questionnaire) representing a 63% return rate. The Inquiry is grateful for the assistance of the obstetric community who took the time to respond. Many very helpful comments were received. Many of the Obstetricians offered to make themselves available to discuss their experiences. It was not possible to talk to all of them as the Inquiry had a finite budget and was subject to time constraints.

A number of respondents warned against over estimating hysterectomy numbers as several respondents could refer to the same operation. We bear that in mind.

While the survey was anonymous, 38 obstetricians signed their returns or responded with an accompanying letter. The spread of these responses makes us confident that replies came from a cross section of the obstetric community.

QUESTIONNAIRE
76 REPLIES

The following figures are approximate as some figures received were estimates

INFORMATION RETRIEVED REGARDING HYSTERECTOMIES PERFORMED BY CONSULTANTS

In our survey we asked consultants

(i)   the number of peripartum hysterectomies personally performed,

(ii)   the method of delivery,

(iii)   the reason for the hysterectomy performed, and

(iv)   whether the diagnosis was confirmed by histology.

(i) TOTAL HYSTERECTOMIES

The total number of hysterectomies performed as consultants was 176.

- 17 consultants never carried out a peripartum hysterectomy
- 44 consultants said they had performed between 1 and 3
- 12 consultants said they had performed between 4 and 7

- 3 consultants said they had performed 8 or more (maximum number was 10).

(ii) TYPE OF DELIVERY

- Caesarean section 114.
- Vaginal delivery 57.
- 5 cases were not specified.

(iii) REASONS AND CONFIRMATION BY HISTOLOGY

The most common reason for performing hysterectomy was primary post-partum haemorrhage (PPH) (151 out of 176). 102 of these were primary PPH alone, 27 involved ruptured uterus and 22 involved placenta accreta. 27 out of the 102 cases involving primary PPH alone were confirmed by histology. The main reason cited for this was that histology would not be able to confirm primary PPH. The majority of cases involving ruptured uterus were confirmed by histology (17 out of the 27). 4 were not confirmed. Clarification was not given in relation to the remaining 6 cases. Similarly, the majority of cases involving placenta accreta were confirmed by histology (18 out of 22). 1 was not confirmed. The remaining 3 were not clarified.

A much less common reason for performing hysterectomy was found to be secondary PPH (13 out of 176). Almost two thirds of these cases were confirmed by histology (8 out of 13). 3 were not confirmed. Clarification was not given in relation to the remaining 2 cases. As with cases involving primary PPH, consultants stated that again this was because histology would not be able to confirm secondary PPH.

A small number of hysterectomies were performed because of disease such as fibroids or cancer (9 out of 176). The majority of the cases involving diseases were confirmed (7 out of 9). Clarification was not received regarding 2 cases.

The remaining hysterectomies (3 out of 176) were performed because of a complication after delivery not covered by the previous categories. 1 was confirmed on histology, 1 was not confirmed and clarification was not received in relation to the remaining case.

HYSTERECTOMIES WHERE THE RESPONDENT ASSISTED AS REGISTRAR OR SHO

In our survey we asked the consultants the same questions as were posed earlier except that this time the responses related to peripartum hysterectomies at which they assisted. Information given was less detailed.

TOTAL NUMBER OF HYSTERECTOMIES

The total number of hysterectomies performed as junior doctors was 91.

29 respondents did not assist at any hysterectomies,

42 respondents assisted at between 1 and 3 hysterectomies,

3 respondents assisted at between 4 and 7,

2 respondents assisted at 8 or more.

Many of the respondents had spent time in training outside Ireland. The figures for the junior doctors include hysterectomy carried out in UK, Australian, Canadian and other hospitals.

TYPE OF DELIVERY

Very few responses clarified the mode of delivery. Of the cases clarified –

- 21 cases of hysterectomy followed caesarean section
- 16 followed vaginal delivery.

Most of these responses did not clarify the details of the hysterectomy, as the junior doctor would rarely be the surgeon making the diagnosis or decision.

REASONS AND CONFIRMATION BY HISTOLOGY

Of those that were clarified, the most common reason for hysterectomy was primary PPH (58 out of 91). Of these hysterectomies, 32 involved primary PPH alone, 13 involved ruptured uterus and 13 involved placenta accreta. Only 2 out of the 32 cases involving primary PPH alone were confirmed by histology. 4 cases were not confirmed. The histology status of the remaining 26 were not clarified by the respondents. Only one case involving ruptured uterus was confirmed by histology. The remaining 12 were not clarified. Only 2 cases involving placenta accreta were confirmed by histology. The remaining 11 were not clarified.

Secondary PPH was the reason for hysterectomy in a small number of cases (4 out of 91). Clarification was not received in relation to any of these.

Just 1 hysterectomy was performed because of disease and 2 were performed because of another complication at or after delivery. Clarification as to whether these were confirmed by histology was not received for any of these cases.

THERAPEUTIC OR OPERATIVE PROCEDURES

In the questionnaire we asked what therapeutic or operative procedures were followed before proceeding to hysterectomy.

The most common procedures referred to by the consultants in response to this question are use of -

oxytocic agents (33),

prostaglandin analogues (21),

Blood transfusion (19),

Packing of the uterus (13),

Tying the internal iliac arteries (11),

Suturing (unspecified) (8),

B Lynch suture (7),

Tying uterine arteries (4).

DETAILS OF PATIENTS WHO HAD HYSTERECTOMY PERFORMED

Consultants were asked to provide relevant obstetrical history of patients who underwent hysterectomy under the following four categories:

(i)   Parity

(ii)   Prior caesarean section – how many

(iii)   Placenta Previa

(iv)   Other – please specify

Many details were not remembered due to lapse of time.

(i) PARITY

- 10 patients were primigravida
- 44 patients had a parity of between 1 and 3
- 33 patients had a parity of 4 or more (1 patient had a parity of 10).
- Clarification was not received for the remaining 180.

(ii) PRIOR CAESAREAN SECTIONS

- 34 patients had no previous caesarean section
- 64 patients had 1 or more previous caesarean sections (maximum prior caesarean sections was 7).
- Clarification was not received for the remaining 169.

(iii) PLACENTA PREVIA

46 hysterectomies involved this diagnosis.

(iv) OTHER

There were very few comments under this category, the majority of which appeared only once. Examples include prolonged labour, fibroids, dead fetus, prior D&C, twins, introverted uterus, trauma.

From this small survey, we saw that the majority of obstetricians who responded had carried out no more than 3 peripartum hysterectomies. 3 had carried out more than 7, and 12 had carried out between 4 and 7. 67 respondents were involved in 267 hysterectomies. Many of these hysterectomies were carried out abroad and the same hysterectomy may have been referred to by more that one respondent. Some respondents had more than 30 years experience and several had been Masters in the Dublin hospitals. Many respondents were practitioners in outlying Maternity Units. A very crude analysis of figures would indicate that each consultant who responded was involved in an average of 4 peripartum hysterectomies in a lifetime of obstetrics.

It may be that those who carried out a great number of hysterectomies did not respond. There is no database for peripartum hysterectomies before the HIPE system against which we could establish the number of peripartum hysterectomies carried out in the State. The system of recording perinatal statistics on a national basis was introduced in 1999 and those figures were integrated into HIPE a year later.

This limited survey indicates that the number of hysterectomies attributed to Dr. Neary and the Unit is far in excess of those in other hospitals including in smaller outlying hospitals where the workload was heavy and access to second opinion was not always available.

TERM 2

TO ASCERTAIN WHAT SYSTEM OF RECORDING OF PERIPARTUM HYSTERECTOMY TOOK PLACE AT THE HOSPITAL; TO ASCERTAIN WHETHER ALL EXPECTED RECORDS ARE NOW EXTANT; AND IF NOT, TO INQUIRE INTO WHAT HAS BECOME OF SUCH RECORDS

1 HOSPITAL RECORDS

1.1 The Inquiry inspected and examined the systems of recording hysterectomy. We examined the various source documents outlined in Term of Reference 1. The midwifery staff, the sisters of the Medical Missionaries of Mary, the staff in patient liaison and the records departments of the hospital were of great assistance to us.

1.2 When a peripartum hysterectomy was performed, it was noted in several places. Its first notation was in the **maternity theatre register,** where all operations were recorded. The patient's chart accompanied her to theatre. The senior of the two midwives in theatre is called the scrub nurse and her assistant is described as the runner or circulating nurse. We were told that normally the scrub nurse recorded the details, which included the date, the patient's name, the patient's age and parity, the operation, the names of the operator and medical assistants, the names of the anaesthetist and registrar, the identity of the two theatre nurses, and whether any specimen was sent to pathology. Frequently, but not invariably, these nurses were accompanied by two student midwives who observed and learned.

1.3 Examination of the maternity theatre register indicated that almost every patient entry demonstrated more than one person's writing. Clearly, more than one midwife, and perhaps even the students were regularly involved in completing the record.

1.4 Maternity theatre registers, and indeed all theatre registers, are immensely important and valuable documents. They are a primary historic record of all operations carried out in the maternity theatre and a record of those present. Theatre registers remain in the recovery room adjacent to the theatre until required to record details of the next operation. Any doctor or nurse present in the operating theatre can examine the register and observe if a hysterectomy is noted there. We were told that the register was regularly consulted to determine dates of procedures, as well as to check the records of emergency out of hours surgery, to assist in validating special payments to the on call anaesthetists. We were told that it does not leave the recovery room area.

1.5   Following recording in the theatre register, the details of the patient's operation and condition were recorded in the **patient chart** and by the surgeon in his surgical history sheet which was then inserted into the patient's chart.

1.6   The midwife who witnessed the birth recorded similar details in the **birth registers.** These birth registers similarly are primary historic documents, and generally do not leave the hospital archives. The birth registers at this Maternity Unit were unusual documents. They had the appearance of school copybooks with manila covers, and were described as An Bord Altranais Register of Cases. Each of these A4 notebooks had room for 250 birth entries. All books used in any given year including the unfinished book at the end of the year were put together within an outer folder which recorded the year on its spine and was bound with a thick rubber band. These folders and books were stored in an unlocked office close to the records office and could be accessed by all hospital staff.

1.7   The birth registers were meticulously filled in, and any hysterectomy or subsequent procedure to the mother was generally recorded. In addition, the details of the baby were recorded; the birth weight, the sex and the condition at birth and on discharge.

1.8   It seemed to us that it would have been preferable to record births in a hardback annual register, rather than in the rather amateurish looking bundles of notebooks. This system, which followed the same format since 1949, was replaced in 2001.

1.9   The standard of recording of details in the birth registers was more even than the recording in the theatre register which was of poor quality.

1.10   Details from the birth registers were transferred to a large good quality ledger called the maternity register, referred to by most witnesses as the **maternity admissions register**. This ledger was used to record admissions to the unit. We learned that secretarial administrative staff filled in these details with medical details often filled in by midwives. The birth details were extracted from the birth registers which administrative staff informed us was the more definitive document.

1.11   When the patient and her chart arrived in the postnatal wards, details of any hysterectomy were entered each day in the ward daybooks. Thus, every nurse and doctor on the ward would be aware of every patient who had undergone a peripartum hysterectomy from consulting the daybooks. Every midwife tasked with filling in the daybooks was obviously also aware of each hysterectomy.

1.12   As peripartum hysterectomy was carefully recorded in 3 primary source documents – the theatre register, the birth register, and the patient's chart, one would assume that determining the number of such procedures would be a relatively easy task. Unfortunately this was not so, as many of these source documents were "*missing*".

1.13   The Inquiry thus went to secondary records and documents to determine the number of peripartum hysterectomies. These were the maternity admissions registers, ward daybooks, student personal notebooks, Sr. D's notebook of cases for the attention of the public health nurses, periodic clinical reports, pathology department specimen ledgers and pathology reports. We also checked all the gynaecology theatre registers.

2   MATERNITY THEATRE REGISTERS

2.1   Maternity theatre registers are immensely important and valuable documents, being primary historical documents.

PRE-OCTOBER 1991 REGISTER

In July 1990, the new maternity hospital was opened for business. This followed a move from the old maternity hospital which had been housed a good 5 minute walk away, in another separate building. The old hospital was originally a fine Georgian residence. It had been extended, adapted and modified, first to a maternity nursing home, then to a hospital, and finally to the Maternity Unit of the general hospital. When it was vacated for the move into the long awaited new Maternity Unit located in the general hospital and joined by a link tube corridor, the records and registers were carefully carried over to the new premises.

2.2   The evidence received was that the old register which covered all operations since at least the 1960s was still in use for the first 15 months after the move to the new Maternity Unit. Some witnesses believed that this register was the only maternity theatre register before October 1991, and thus may have covered operations back to 1957. A new maternity theatre register was opened in October 1991.

2.3   Some midwives recalled seeing the old register which was a large long book of considerable size and weight in the new labour ward, where it was kept on a shelf in a locked press in the labour ward superintendent's office. They believed that it remained there until at least late October 1998. The keys to the press were kept in an open cupboard at the labour ward nurses' station, and these keys would have been readily accessible to a considerable number of nursing and administrative staff.

2.4   Extensive searches had already been undertaken to locate the register. By 20th January 1999, it was clear that the register could not be found, and this fact was formally reported to the Health Board in a letter dated the 10th February 1999. The Inquiry has had no success in its searches for this register.

2.5   The HRRI or Healthcare Risk Resources International (now Capita) witnesses informed us that they were very surprised at the absence of such crucial hospital records which are normally never moved off the premises and they sought an explanation. They told us that no explanation was offered, other than that they were not available.

2.6   No witness has admitted any knowledge of how the register is missing. The removal of this register required knowledge of its whereabouts – i.e. that it was kept in a locked cupboard in the Labour Ward superintendent's office. It required knowledge that the keys to this cupboard were in the Labour Ward nurses' station in another press. It was not a small book and could not have been easily concealed.

2.7   The disappearance of the pre-1991 register is highly suspicious, and the Inquiry believes that it was deliberately taken from the Hospital shortly after October 1998. The Inquiry was unable to detect who was or might have been responsible for this action. Dr.Neary denied any knowledge of the taking of this register. He denied ever seeing the register after it left the theatre. He explained that consultants and non-consultant medical staff never filled it in, and that he personally had no reason to consult it. Whoever removed this register was familiar with hospital records and well aware that this register was the best record of pre-1991 hysterectomies.

2.8   The Inquiry is critical of the storing of this important historic archive in the Labour Ward. It would have been wiser to store the register in a locked office that offered limited access.

2.9   **OCTOBER 1991-2004 MATERNITY THEATRE REGISTER**

The Inquiry has been furnished with this register which runs from 7th October 1991 to 19th June 2004. The current maternity theatre register commenced in June 2004.

The 1991-2004 register disclosed that 72 peripartum hysterectomies were carried out in the maternity theatre between these two dates.

Some very alarming alterations were detected in this register. These alterations indicate deliberate attempts to prevent a full determination of the numbers of peripartum hysterectomies carried out in the unit.

2.10 **ALTERATIONS IN 1991-2004 MATERNITY THEATRE REGISTER**

Alterations to the record were made. It is possible to pinpoint the period when these alterations were made, as we know that the date on which the maternity theatre register was first examined by Mr. Finbar Lennon, Clinical Director and M.D., Director of Nursing was the 24th October 1998. The examination of this register was the first step taken by the NEHB when carrying out a preliminary investigation of the complaints made against Dr. Neary.

2.11 When cases of hysterectomy were identified, Mr. Lennon noted the names of the patients on a separate sheet and put an "X" in the margin of the register beside the hysterectomy record and close to the operating surgeon's name.

2.12 Within the next week to ten days, a senior midwife and practice development nurse, who was relatively new to the unit but trusted by hospital management, was requested by M.D. to recheck the register. This midwife listed the hysterectomies that she found and furnished her list to M.D. who compared it with the list made on the 24th October 1998 by Mr. Lennon. She compared both lists against the maternity theatre register. In so doing, she noted that two cases from 1993 that had originally appeared as hysterectomies on Mr. Lennon's list were recorded in the register as caesarean sections, followed by "RSO" (right salpingo-oophorectomy). There was no "X" in the margin. It was assumed that a mistake had been made with the first list and the names of these two patients were eliminated from the list of hysterectomy patients.

2.13 When the Inquiry team first examined the register we were unaware of the changes or of the existence of the two lists. We noted what seemed to be evidence of erasure or change in 2 places. As many recordings had been cancelled, written over or tippexed our suspicions at that time were minimal. Quite fortuitously, one of the first witnesses was a former patient who had undergone caesarean hysterectomy in 1993. When we sought to identify her operation in the maternity theatre register we found that her case was one of the entries where we thought the record had been changed. We noted that the original entry had been altered and only a caesarean section was recorded. We then scrutinised the 2 suspicious entries and noted the faint impression of the original 'Xs' in 2 places and the change in the description of the procedure.

2.14   The Inquiry then obtained the original notes of the 24th October from the Director of Nursing and confirmed two names of those patients whose entries had been altered on that list. The names were not on the later list. The alterations must have been carried out in the 10 day period between the two examinations of the maternity theatre register.

2.15   A handwriting expert was engaged to advise. He carefully examined the alterations and advised that the original entry was almost certainly hysterectomy before it was altered.   The character of the writing and alterations in both entries was very similar.

2.16   The Inquiry subsequently came across a third case of hysterectomy, this time for the year 1995, where the entry in the register had been altered in a similar manner. In this case the reference to hysterectomy had been replaced by "LSO" (left salpingo-oophorectomy). However, in this case, there had never been an "X" placed in the margin at the time of the first investigation by M.D. and Mr. Lennon.

2.17   The pathology laboratory records confirm that each of these three patients did indeed have a hysterectomy on the recorded dates, as a uterus identified to each patient had been received for histological examination.

2.18   It was disturbing to note that the records in these three cases were also missing. In the case of the two patients from 1993, their entire charts are missing. In the case of the third alteration, from 1995, the obstetric chart for the delivery in question is missing, but a chart for a previous delivery is extant. **In all three cases, the birth registers are also missing.** The selective nature of the type of missing documents is strongly supportive of a deliberate 'culling' of the records.

2.19 As previously stated, only the two maternity theatre registers covering periods from the 7th October 1991 onwards are extant. The register commenced in 1991 and was completed in June 2004, when the current register commenced.

2.20 Theatre arrangements changed on 1st January 2003. All elective/planned caesarean sections and tubal ligations are now carried out in the gynaecology theatre which operates 2 registers – one for recording elective caesarean sections and tubal ligations and the other for all other gynaecological operations. These current registers are extant. This second theatre is adjacent to the maternity theatre which is now kept available uniquely for emergency caesarean sections or other obstetric emergencies.

2.21 **COMPLETENESS OF MATERNITY THEATRE REGISTER 1991 - 2004**

The Inquiry has established that 86 peripartum hysterectomies were carried out in the Lourdes Hospital in the period covered by the maternity theatre register being 7th October 1991 to 19th June 2004. The Inquiry concludes that 78 hysterectomies were carried out in the maternity theatre, and 8 were carried out in the gynaecology theatre in the general hospital.

2.22 72 cases are recorded in the maternity theatre register as peripartum hysterectomies; 3 more are the cases where the original records referred to hysterectomy, but were subsequently falsified. In the remaining 3 cases, the caesarean section is recorded but the hysterectomy is not recorded. In 2 of these cases the hysterectomy is recorded in the gynaecology theatre register.

2.23 The other sources considered by the Inquiry, and in particular pathology records, confirm that a hysterectomy was carried out in all of these cases.

2.24 The two examinations of the maternity theatre register carried out on behalf of the NEHB on 24th October 1998, and in the following week to 10 days established that 69 peripartum hysterectomies occurred between 1st January 1992 and 27th October 1998. The two cases from 1993 where the record was altered were initially included, but were dropped from the list due to the alterations of the register. This demonstrates the value of the register as a primary source document, and that the early examination by NEHB staff was thorough. One hysterectomy carried out at the end of October 1998 after Dr. Neary was asked to take administrative leave was carried out in the general hospital and thus not recorded in the maternity theatre register.

2.25   Mr. Lennon and M.D.'s working notes at the time of the examination of the register identify the consultant/operator, and details of whether the hysterectomy followed caesarean section, whether the caesarean was emergency or elective, or followed vaginal delivery. Thus by 27th October 1998, when the representatives of the NEHB put the midwife's concerns to Dr. Neary, they had reasonably accurate information of the incidence of peripartum hysterectomy for the previous three years, and within another week or so they had, with 90% accuracy, identified the figures for all operators from the start of 1992 onwards from this register.

2.26   In October/November 1998, copies of the charts of 3 patients, identified from the theatre register as being the most recent cases of peripartum hysterectomy, were sent to Healthcare Risk Resources International (HRRI) for external consideration.

2.27   Mr. Michael Maresh, MD FRCOG, Consultant Obstetrician and Gynaecologist in St Mary's Hospital, Manchester was engaged to advise in this and subsequent HRRI reviews. HRRI observed in their first report of 8th November 1998 that appropriate review of the available data for 1996 (as could be gleaned from this maternity register) should have raised concerns in the Hospital.   Unfortunately no annual reports were being produced for the Hospital at that time, and no meaningful annual review of outcomes was taking place.

2.28   During the process of seeking comments from parties mentioned in the draft report we became aware from Dr. Neary that he had a photocopy of the 1991 Maternity theatre register. We were curious why no one in authority had mentioned the photocopying of this important document to the Inquiry. We determined that the Medical Council had not photocopied it before 2004 when the inquiry into the complaints against Dr. Neary was already completed. The senior officer in Patient Liaison was unaware that it had been photocopied and expressed surprise that such a procedure had been carried out without her knowledge. Similarly, other members of staff in this office denied any knowledge of photocopying this document. Members of administrative staff who were questioned similarly had no knowledge of any request to photocopy the register in 2001. The Director of Nursing, The Labour Ward Superintendent, the former Assistant Director of Nursing, the Hospital CEO and the Medical Director were all unaware of the photocopying of this register and expressed shock that such a procedure could be carried out without their knowledge or permission.

2.29 Dr. Neary informed the Inquiry that he had received the report from "a colleague in 2001". We determined from the Solicitors acting for Dr. Neary on behalf of the MDU that Dr. Neary had provided them with a copy of the photocopy which had been furnished by a "colleague" in September/October 2001. We wrote to Dr. Neary's two obstetric colleagues who both denied any knowledge of the photocopying of this register.

2.30 Dr. Neary attended a third time at the Inquiry premises bringing the photocopy with him. He was informed that his colleagues knew nothing of the photocopying and had not furnished him with the document. Dr. Neary then said that by the word 'colleague' he meant anyone who worked in the hospital. He was unable to give an adequate explanation for why he did not ask his solicitors to write to the hospital authorities looking for a copy of the Maternity theatre or why he obtained a copy himself. He could not recall the circumstances in which he asked for or received the photocopy other than that he had gone through patient liaison or personnel and had probably collected the copy himself from reception.

2.31 The Inquiry is very suspicious about the circumstances in which this photocopy was obtained. There is nothing wrong *per se* with such a photocopy being obtained and furnished to Dr. Neary in order to assist him in preparing statistics for the Fitness to Practise Committee of the Medical Council. However there is something seriously wrong when neither the

Director of Nursing, the Assistant Director of Nursing, the Labour Ward Superintendent nor the then Patient Liaison Officer was aware of any request to photocopy such register. It is worrying that the register was removed, copied and returned without any security relating to the preservation of the integrity of the register being in place. It was necessary to use A3 paper which required an appropriate photocopier and a supply of A3 paper. The photocopying took place at a time when it was common knowledge in the hospital and especially the Maternity Unit that the earlier Maternity theatre register had disappeared and that many other key documents were missing.

2.32   The photocopy of the 1991 maternity theatre register was made after the alterations had been carried out as the alterations were contained in the photocopy. The photocopy with which we were furnished runs to the end of 1998. Dr. Neary's solicitors received the copy in October 2001. It was clearly photocopied by at least two women, as photographs of the fingers of two different hands were clearly visible on a number of pages. One of the hands was wearing nail varnish which we are informed would make it extremely unlikely to be those of a midwife or surgical nurse. The photocopying took at least one hour, which we are told would cause the absence of a midwife from the floor to be investigated. Again, it seems that someone with sympathies to Dr. Neary was prepared to assist him without informing the parties who should have been informed.

3   LABOUR WARD STATISTICS SHEETS

3.1   We have learned that some basic statistics were always collated for returns to the Department of Health. These included records of bed occupancy, deliveries and stillbirths and caesarean sections. In addition figures were kept of all occasions when labour ward midwives were called to assist in the maternity theatre. There was a growing perception that, although birth rates were falling throughout the 1990s, the caesarean section rate was rising and that staff numbers were inadequate for the workload. Matron and senior staff sisters kept records of activity in order to make the case for increased permanent staff.

3.2   The Labour Ward Superintendent also collected statistics in 1996. Her note for January reads *"6 patients in Jan had hysterectomy = 4%"*, but her notes do not refer to any of the other hysterectomies in that year.

3.3   The labour ward staff always maintained comprehensive statistics of activity in the labour ward. All births and deviations from normal spontaneous vertex deliveries were recorded on a daily basis and totted up at the end of each month. Each month's statistics were recorded on a separate sheet contained within a plastic folder and pinned on the notice board behind the nurses' station on the labour ward. At the end of each year an administrative assistant brought the sheets of paper to the Matron of the Maternity Unit. Up to 1997, hysterectomies were not recorded on these sheets, although caesarean sections were noted.

3.4   From 1997 onwards the monthly tables of statistics, completed on a daily basis, included a line for *"hysterectomies"* where monthly totals were recorded. The statistics sheets for 1997 show all of the 10 hysterectomies carried out that year. We were unable to ascertain who decided to add the entry for hysterectomy, nor the purpose for keeping statistics of that procedure. We suspect that the recording of the hysterectomies may well have been to advance the argument that more staff was required. Certainly, no senior midwife or administrator told us that the recording of hysterectomies was associated with any concerns that too many of those procedures were being carried out.

3.5   The figures appear not to have been analysed or reviewed on an annual basis or any other basis, nor did they give rise to any realisation or discussion on the rate of obstetric hysterectomy. The statistics remained in the Maternity Unit and were not shared with the Director of Nursing or previous Matrons of the general hospital.

4   MINUTES OF MIDWIVES/OBSTETRICIANS MEETINGS

4.1   The Matron of the Maternity Unit was aware of the rising hysterectomy rate which she suspected was associated with the rising caesarean section rate.

There were occasional *"midwives/obstetricians meetings"*, and there are minutes of seven such meetings between March 1984 and April 1997.

4.2   The former Matron of the Maternity Unit gave evidence that she would not have dared to mention the word "hysterectomy" at any of these meetings. She said that she did try to raise the subject indirectly by raising discussion on the increasing rate of caesarean section in the unit.

4.3   Minutes for the meeting dated 31st January 1994, and also for the next meeting on 21st April 1997, confirm that caesarean section subject was discussed. Most caesarean sections were then being carried out by Dr. Neary, followed by Dr. Lynch, as Dr. O'Brien had been ill and on sick leave for much of the period from 1993. Dr. O'Brien was known to be very conservative about caesarean section and favoured natural childbirth. This could also explain why so many patients seeking caesarean section sought out Dr. Neary. At one of these meetings, the Matron of the Maternity Unit reported that she sought the view of Dr. O'Brien over the rising caesarean section rate. She felt sure that she could count on his support because of his known position on caesarean section. Instead, he stated that,

"The only caesarean section he ever regretted was the one he didn't do".

4.4   Thus she felt unsupported in her concerns relating to the connection between high rates of caesarean section and the risk of hysterectomy. The Matron of the Maternity Unit also stated that at another of these meetings Dr. Neary reacted angrily when the question of rising caesarean section rates was raised, and he left the meeting muttering that he knew that this meeting was to *"get him"*. The minutes of 21st April 1997 confirm that Dr. Neary left the meeting at the point when caesarean section rates were being discussed. Once again, it appears that her efforts to raise the issue were rebuffed and the minutes lend weight to her evidence. The Matron's concerns are dealt with in more detail in Term of Reference 3.

5 GYNAECOLOGY THEATRE REGISTERS

5.1 In the vast majority of cases a peripartum hysterectomy is recorded in the maternity theatre register, as most such procedures are performed following a caesarean section. As already mentioned, all caesarean sections were carried out in the maternity theatre.

5.2 On some occasions, the operation followed a return to theatre after normal vaginal delivery in the labour ward and following post partum haemorrhage. On these occasions, the hysterectomies followed examination under anaesthesia and were carried out in the gynaecology theatre in the main hospital building and were recorded in the gynaecology theatre registers.

5.3 13 peripartum hysterectomies were recorded in the gynaecology theatre registers covering the years 1974-2004. 2 more patients (whom the Inquiry has confirmed had peripartum hysterectomies) are recorded in the gynaecology theatre registers for operations such as laparotomy or oophorectomy, but not for hysterectomy

6 TEMPORARILY MISSING GYNAECOLOGY THEATRE REGISTER

6.1 The Inquiry eventually saw a complete set of gynaecology theatre registers covering the period from 1st January 1966 to 27th April 2000. The Inquiry visited the hospital on 3rd August 2004. We requested sight of the theatre registers for the period of the mid 1980s, as we had established that many patient charts and birth registers were missing for this period.

6.2 The theatre nursing staff explained that the registers were stored under secure lock and key in a room close to the nurses' station, and the likelihood of removal or loss of any records was therefore remote. However, when we sought the register for the mid 1980s it was found to be missing. It covered the period 1981-1988. Searches were undertaken but the register was not found. We were told that after the Inquiry team left the hospital, further security measures were taken and the locks were changed.

6.3 In October 2004, when revisiting the Hospital, it was reported to the Inquiry that the missing register had been found – in the same storeroom and in a reasonably prominent position. This temporarily missing register for 1981-88 was found to record two peripartum hysterectomies.

6.4 The Inquiry is concerned about this temporary disappearance, and believes that the register was probably removed and returned when suspicions were aroused. However, we are unable to come to any final conclusions, as the evidence in relation to this episode was confused and conflicting.

7 THE PATIENTS' CHARTS

7.1 Every peripartum hysterectomy was documented in the patient's file or chart. Up until 2002, the basic format for a patient's chart changed little. It contained personal details, as well as obstetric history, antenatal care, midwives notes, labour, delivery (including consultant's notes following caesarean section and hysterectomy) and postnatal care. Scan results, tests, traces, pathology/laboratory tests were also kept in the chart, together with the neonatal records of the newborn infant. Midwifery care plans were included in later charts. The charts were buff coloured and recorded a brief summary of the patient's obstetric history on the outside front cover; if a hysterectomy had been carried out, it was recorded.

8 THE REGISTER OF CASES (THE BIRTH REGISTERS)

8.1 These books, referred to by midwives and administrative staff as the birth registers, are very valuable records and an historical record of all births in the Hospital. They record a running total of all births since the Maternity Unit first opened, as well as all births in a particular year. Each booklet contains 250 births. A midwife present at the birth enters the particulars. The mother's chart number, name, address, age, parity, obstetric and delivery details are recorded, as well as the identity of doctors in attendance and details of the condition of baby at birth and discharge. Where a peripartum hysterectomy had occurred at or near time of delivery, this too was generally, but not invariably, recorded in the register of cases.

9 TABLE 2A: BIRTH REGISTERS

9.1 This table shows which birth registers are extant, and which are missing for the period 1970-1998.

Note: Where more than 1 consecutive birth register missing, dates given are estimates.

Year	From	Until	Hysterectomy	Birth Register?
1998	20-Nov-98	31-Dec-98	0	Present
1998	06-Oct-98	20-Nov-98	2	Present
1998	21-Aug-98	06-Oct-98	1	Present
1998	06-Jul-98	21-Aug-98	1	Present
1998	19-May-98	06-Jul-98	0	Present
1998	05-Apr-98	19-May-98	1	Present
1998	20-Feb-98	04-Apr-98	2	Present
1998	01-Jan-98	20-Feb-98	3	Present
1997	05-Dec-97	31-Dec-97	1	Present
1997	10-Oct-97	05-Dec-97	1	Present
1997	24-Aug-97	10-Oct-97	3	Present
1997	08-Jul-97	24-Aug-97	0	Present
1997	26-May-97	08-Jul-97	2	Present
1997	10-Apr-97	26-May-97	1	Present
1997	21-Feb-97	10-Apr-97	0	Present
1997	01-Jan-97	21-Feb-97	2	Present
1996	20-Nov-96	31-Dec-96	1	Present
1996	01-Oct-96	20-Nov-96	0	Present
1996	08-Aug-96	01-Oct-96	2	Present
1996	14-Jun-96	08-Aug-96	2	Present
1996	15-Apr-96	14-Jun-96	3	Present
1996	23-Feb-96	15-Apr-96	0	Present
1996	01-Jan-96	23-Feb-96	6	Present
1995	11-Nov-95	31-Dec-95	0	Present
1995	17-Sep-95	10-Nov-95	2	Present
1995	25-Jul-95	16-Sep-95	0	Present
1995	02-Jun-95	25-Jul-95	3	Present
1995	14-Apr-95	01-Jun-95	0	Present
1995	21-Feb-95	14-Apr-95	3	Present
1995	01-Jan-95	21-Feb-95	3	Missing
1994	13-Dec-94	31-Dec-94	0	Present
1994	11-Oct-94	13-Dec-94	2	Present
1994	12-Aug-94	11-Oct-94	1	Present
1994	24-Jun-94	12-Aug-94	3	Present
1994	27-Apr-94	23-Jun-94	0	Present

Year	From	Until	Hysterectomy	Birth Register?
1994	01-Mar-94	27-Apr-94	1	Present
1994	01-Jan-94	01-Mar-94	2	Present
1993	05-Dec-93	31-Dec-93	3	Present
1993	08-Oct-93	04-Dec-93	3	Present
1993	17-Aug-93	08-Oct-93	3	Present
1993	25-Jun-93	17-Aug-93	1	Present
1993	01-May-93	25-Jun-93	1	Present
1993	01-Mar-93	01-May-93	3	Missing
1993	01-Jan-93	01-Mar-93	1	Missing
1992	16-Nov-92	31-Dec-92	1	Present
1992	16-Sep-92	16-Nov-92	1	Present
1992	23-Jul-92	16-Sep-92	0	Present
1992	04-Jun-92	23-Jul-92	1	Present
1992	15-Apr-92	04-Jun-92	2	Present
1992	19-Feb-92	15-Apr-92	3	Missing
1992	01-Jan-92	19-Feb-92	0	Present
1991	23-Nov-91	31-Dec-91	2	Missing
1991	27-Sep-91	23-Nov-91	4	Missing
1991	05-Aug-91	27-Sep-91	0	Present
1991	10-Jun-91	05-Aug-91	2	Present
1991	02-May-91	10-Jun-91	2	Missing
1991	25-Feb-91	02-May-91	2	Missing
1991	01-Jan-91	25-Feb-91	0	Present
1990	03-Nov-90	31-Dec-90	0	Present
1990	10-Sep-90	03-Nov-90	1	Present
1990	17-Jul-90	09-Sep-90	1	Present
1990	05-Jun-90	17-Jul-90	0	Present
1990	18-Apr-90	05-Jun-90	1	Present
1990	26-Feb-90	17-Apr-90	0	Present
1990	01-Jan-90	26-Feb-90	0	Present
1989	20-Nov-89	31-Dec-89	0	Present
1989	22-Sep-89	20-Nov-89	0	Present
1989	24-Jul-89	22-Sep-89	3	Missing
1989	10-Jun-89	24-Jul-89	1	Missing
1989	15-Apr-89	10-Jun-89	1	Missing
1989	25-Feb-89	15-Apr-89	1	Present
1989	01-Jan-89	25-Feb-89	0	Present
1988	30-Dec-88	31-Dec-88	0	Present
1988	08-Nov-88	29-Dec-88	1	Present
1988	24-Sep-88	08-Nov-88	0	Present
1988	31-Jul-88	24-Sep-88	3	Missing
1988	17-Jun-88	31-Jul-88	1	Present
1988	22-Apr-88	17-Jun-88	1	Missing

Year	From	Until	Hysterectomy	Birth Register?
1988	23-Feb-88	22-Apr-88	1	Present
1988	01-Jan-88	23-Feb-88	0	Present
1987	20-Nov-87	31-Dec-87	1	**Missing**
1987	23-Sep-87	20-Nov-87	3	**Missing**
1987	21-Jul-87	23-Sep-87	1	Present
1987	02-Jun-87	21-Jul-87	1	**Missing**
1987	14-Apr-87	02-Jun-87	0	Present
1987	25-Feb-87	14-Apr-87	1	Present
1987	01-Jan-87	25-Feb-87	1	**Missing**
1986	03-Dec-86	31-Dec-86	2	**Missing**
1986	08-Oct-86	03-Dec-86	0	Present
1986	27-Aug-86	08-Oct-86	2	**Missing**
1986	10-Jul-86	27-Aug-86	2	**Missing**
1986	25-May-86	10-Jul-86	1	Present
1986	07-Apr-86	24-May-86	1	Present
1986	15-Feb-86	07-Apr-86	1	Present
1986	01-Jan-86	15-Feb-86	0	Present
1985	09-Dec-85	31-Dec-85	0	Present
1985	15-Oct-85	09-Dec-85	3	**Missing**
1985	26-Aug-85	15-Oct-85	2	Present
1985	15-Jul-85	26-Aug-85	1	**Missing**
1985	24-May-85	15-Jul-85	2	**Missing**
1985	02-Apr-85	24-May-85	2	**Missing**
1985	13-Feb-85	02-Apr-85	0	Present
1985	01-Jan-85	13-Feb-85	2	**Missing**
1984	17-Dec-84	31-Dec-84	0	Present
1984	30-Oct-84	17-Dec-84	0	Present
1984	20-Sep-84	30-Oct-84	0	Present
1984	04-Aug-84	20-Sep-84	0	Present
1984	21-Jun-84	04-Aug-84	0	Present
1984	09-May-84	21-Jun-84	1	Present
1984	26-Mar-84	09-May-84	1	Present
1984	12-Feb-84	25-Mar-84	0	Present
1984	01-Jan-84	12-Feb-84	0	Present
1983	17-Dec-83	31-Dec-83	3	**Missing**
1983	05-Nov-83	17-Dec-83	0	Present
1983	30-Sep-83	05-Nov-83	1	**Missing**
1983	23-Aug-83	30-Sep-83	3	**Missing**
1983	15-Jul-83	23-Aug-83	0	Present
1983	09-Jun-83	15-Jul-83	0	Present
1983	01-May-83	08-Jun-83	0	Present
1983	16-Mar-83	30-Apr-83	0	Present
1983	05-Feb-83	16-Mar-83	0	Present

Year	From	Until	Hysterectomy	Birth Register?
1983	01-Jan-83	05-Feb-83	0	Present
1982	08-Dec-82	31-Dec-82	0	Present
1982	28-Oct-82	08-Dec-82	1	**Missing**
1982	21-Sep-82	28-Oct-82	0	Present
1982	10-Aug-82	21-Sep-82	0	Present
1982	05-Jul-82	10-Aug-82	0	Present
1982	23-May-82	05-Jul-82	0	Present
1982	18-Apr-82	23-May-82	1	**Missing**
1982	13-Mar-82	18-Apr-82	2	**Missing**
1982	08-Feb-82	13-Mar-82	0	Present
1982	01-Jan-82	08-Feb-82	1	Present
1981	04-Dec-81	31-Dec-81	0	Present
1981	30-Oct-81	04-Dec-81	1	Present
1981	27-Sep-81	30-Oct-81	1	**Missing**
1981	20-Aug-81	27-Sep-81	2	**Missing**
1981	21-Jul-81	20-Aug-81	1	Present
1981	16-Jun-81	21-Jul-81	0	Present
1981	12-May-81	16-Jun-81	0	Present
1981	07-Apr-81	12-May-81	0	Present
1981	07-Mar-81	07-Apr-81	1	**Missing**
1981	03-Feb-81	07-Mar-81	0	Present
1981	01-Jan-81	03-Feb-81	0	Present
1980	20-Dec-80	31-Dec-80	0	Present
1980	18-Nov-80	20-Dec-80	0	Present
1980	13-Oct-80	18-Nov-80	0	Present
1980	12-Sep-80	13-Oct-80	3	**Missing**
1980	07-Aug-80	12-Sep-80	0	Present
1980	06-Jul-80	07-Aug-80	0	Present
1980	05-Jun-80	05-Jul-80	1	Present
1980	04-May-80	05-Jun-80	0	Present
1980	05-Apr-80	04-May-80	0	Present
1980	09-Mar-80	05-Apr-80	0	Present
1980	04-Feb-80	09-Mar-80	2	**Missing**
1980	01-Jan-80	04-Feb-80	0	Present
1979	15-Dec-79	31-Dec-79	0	Present
1979	14-Nov-79	15-Dec-79	1	**Missing**
1979	10-Oct-79	14-Nov-79	1	Present
1979	06-Sep-79	10-Oct-79	0	Present
1979	04-Aug-79	06-Sep-79	3	**Missing**
1979	02-Jul-79	04-Aug-79	3	Present
1979	01-Jun-79	02-Jul-79	0	Present
1979	02-May-79	31-May-79	1	Present
1979	30-Mar-79	02-May-79	0	Present

Year	From	Until	Hysterectomy	Birth Register?
1979	02-Mar-79	30-Mar-79	0	Present
1979	01-Feb-79	02-Mar-79	0	Present
1979	01-Jan-79	01-Feb-79	0	Present
1978	29-Nov-78	31-Dec-78	1	Present
1978	23-Oct-78	29-Nov-78	1	Present
1978	20-Sep-78	23-Oct-78	0	Present
1978	18-Aug-78	20-Sep-78	0	Present
1978	13-Jul-78	18-Aug-78	1	Present
1978	11-Jun-78	13-Jul-78	1	Present
1978	10-May-78	11-Jun-78	0	Present
1978	07-Apr-78	10-May-78	0	Present
1978	05-Mar-78	07-Apr-78	1	Missing
1978	03-Feb-78	05-Mar-78	2	Missing
1978	01-Jan-78	03-Feb-78	1	Present
1977	26-Dec-77	31-Dec-77	0	Present
1977	19-Nov-77	26-Dec-77	0	Present
1977	16-Oct-77	19-Nov-77	1	Present
1977	16-Sep-77	16-Oct-77	0	Present
1977	16-Aug-77	16-Sep-77	0	Present
1977	14-Jul-77	16-Aug-77	0	Present
1977	14-Jun-77	13-Jul-77	0	Present
1977	11-May-77	14-Jun-77	0	Present
1977	09-Apr-77	11-May-77	1	Present
1977	08-Mar-77	09-Apr-77	1	Present
1977	04-Feb-77	08-Mar-77	0	Present
1977	01-Jan-77	04-Feb-77	0	Present
1976	11-Dec-76	31-Dec-76	0	Present
1976	07-Nov-76	11-Dec-76	2	Present
1976	02-Oct-76	07-Nov-76	0	Present
1976	27-Aug-76	02-Oct-76	1	Present
1976	25-Jul-76	27-Aug-76	0	Present
1976	20-Jun-76	25-Jul-76	2	Present
1976	18-May-76	20-Jun-76	0	Present
1976	15-Apr-76	18-May-76	0	Present
1976	13-Mar-76	15-Apr-76	0	Present
1976	08-Feb-76	13-Mar-76	0	Present
1976	01-Jan-76	07-Feb-76	0	Present
1975	14-Dec-75	31-Dec-75	0	Present
1975	06-Nov-75	13-Dec-75	0	Present
1975	30-Sep-75	06-Nov-75	0	Present
1975	25-Aug-75	30-Sep-75	0	Present
1975	23-Jul-75	25-Aug-75	0	Present
1975	20-Jun-75	23-Jul-75	0	Present

Year	From	Until	Hysterectomy	Birth Register?
1975	18-May-75	20-Jun-75	0	Present
1975	15-Apr-75	17-May-75	1	Present
1975	10-Mar-75	14-Apr-75	0	Present
1975	03-Feb-75	10-Mar-75	0	Present
1975	01-Jan-75	03-Feb-75	1	Present
1974	21-Nov-74	31-Dec-74	1	Present
1974	15-Oct-74	21-Nov-74	0	Present
1974	07-Sep-74	15-Oct-74	0	Present
1974	30-Jul-74	07-Sep-74	0	Present
1974	25-Jun-74	30-Jul-74	0	Present
1974	25-May-74	25-Jun-74	0	Present
1974	24-Apr-74	24-May-74	0	Present
1974	20-Mar-74	24-Apr-74	0	Present
1974	07-Feb-74	20-Mar-74	0	Present
1974	01-Jan-74	07-Feb-74	0	Present
1973	29-Dec-73	31-Dec-73	0	Present
1973	18-Nov-73	29-Dec-73	0	Present
1973	13-Oct-73	18-Nov-73	0	Present
1973	07-Sep-73	13-Oct-73	0	Present
1973	28-Jul-73	07-Sep-73	0	Present
1973	22-Jun-73	28-Jul-73	0	Present
1973	23-May-73	22-Jun-73	0	Present
1973	20-Apr-73	23-May-73	0	Present
1973	17-Mar-73	20-Apr-73	0	Present
1973	08-Feb-73	17-Mar-73	0	Present
1973	01-Jan-73	08-Feb-73	0	Present
1972	15-Dec-72	31-Dec-72	0	Present
1972	09-Nov-72	15-Dec-72	1	Present
1972	30-Sep-72	09-Nov-72	0	Present
1972	26-Aug-72	30-Sep-72	0	Present
1972	23-Jul-72	26-Aug-72	0	Present
1972	23-Jun-72	23-Jul-72	0	Present
1972	23-May-72	23-Jun-72	0	Present
1972	22-Apr-72	23-May-72	0	Present
1972	17-Mar-72	22-Apr-72	0	Present
1972	10-Feb-72	17-Mar-72	0	Present
1972	01-Jan-72	09-Feb-72	0	Present
1971	22-Dec-71	31-Dec-71	0	Present
1971	15-Nov-71	22-Dec-71	1	Present
1971	11-Oct-71	15-Nov-71	0	Present
1971	06-Sep-71	11-Oct-71	0	Present
1971	31-Jul-71	06-Sep-71	0	Present
1971	26-Jun-71	31-Jul-71	0	Present

Year	From	Until	Hysterectomy	Birth Register?
1971	25-May-71	26-Jun-71	0	Present
1971	21-Apr-71	25-May-71	0	Present
1971	17-Mar-71	21-Apr-71	0	Present
1971	07-Feb-71	17-Mar-71	1	Present
1971	01-Jan-71	07-Feb-71	0	Present
1970	12-Dec-70	31-Dec-70	0	Present
1970	03-Nov-70	12-Dec-70	0	Present
1970	25-Sep-70	03-Nov-70	0	Present
1970	24-Aug-70	25-Sep-70	0	Present
1970	20-Jul-70	24-Aug-70	1	Present
1970	17-Jun-70	20-Jul-70	0	Present
1970	17-May-70	17-Jun-70	0	Present
1970	16-Apr-70	17-May-70	0	Present
1970	12-Mar-70	16-Apr-70	1	Present
1970	07-Feb-70	12-Mar-70	2	Present
1970	01-Jan-70	07-Feb-70	1	Present

9.2   The Inquiry established that 266 birth registers were created during the period under examination. 40 of those were missing. These missing birth registers would have recorded 78 peripartum hysterectomies. No birth registers should be missing.

All of the missing registers would have contained details of at least one patient on whom a hysterectomy was carried out. There are no missing registers for any period during which there were no peripartum hysterectomies.

9.3   Since 1998 no birth registers are missing.

9.4   There are no missing registers for the period from 1970 to February 1978. **39 of the 40 missing registers are from the period 1978 to 1993.**

9.5   The birth registers for the periods in 1993 which correspond with two cases of altered entries in the maternity theatre register, are missing.

9.6   The final missing register (and the only one missing after 1993) is that for January/February 1995. This register would have recorded 3 hysterectomies including 1 case where the maternity theatre register was falsified to disguise the carrying out of a hysterectomy. In other words, **in the 3 cases where the Maternity Theatre register was falsified, the birth register is also missing.** They are the only missing registers for the 1990s.

9.7   **Of the 44 obstetric hysterectomy patients whose charts are missing, the corresponding birth register is also missing for 41 of those patients.** Of the 3 remaining cases of missing charts where the birth registers are extant, two patients are Dr. Lynch patients from 1988, and one patient from 1997 is a Dr. Neary patient.

9.8   The Inquiry has been unable to discover precisely when the full set of birth registers was last seen, or what has become of the missing registers. Nursing and administrative staff in the Hospital related how the birth registers were often consulted by interested parties (including nurses born in the old Maternity Unit and now working in the hospital) looking for the historical record of their birth, or that of their children or husband, particularly as the registers would also record the hour and minute of birth. One of the clerical staff came from a large family. She recalls that while working in the Maternity Unit she checked details of her siblings' births in several birth registers scanning many years. Her recollection is that this was during the short days of the winter of 1998. Approximately 2 to 3 months later she returned to verify some details to discover that many of the birth registers that she had previously consulted were missing. She noted that 40 registers had been removed. She was aware that a maternity theatre register had been reported as missing and was concerned. She removed the rest of the registers and placed them in her office, which she locked. She then notified the Hospital Manager. There is a note on the Manager's records that indicates the report in early February 1999. Thus we can deduce that the birth registers were removed between October 1998 and February 1999.

9.9   Midwives were aware that some very early birth registers were missing but they believed that all other registers were available. When the Inquiry interviewed the former Matron of the Maternity Unit, she was adamant that at the time she retired in December 1997 there was a full complement of birth registers stored chronologically in file covers (one file for the 7 to 11 booklets covering each year) on open shelves in the Medical Records Officer's room on the ground floor.

9.10 Other midwives felt that some of the birth registers from the 1940s or 1950s were missing, but that otherwise there was a full set. No one was able to tell us when it was first noted that birth registers were missing. The fact that they were missing was noted in the first HRRI report prepared in 1999.

9.11 In 1995, the Stillbirths Registration Act 1994 came into operation, and the Hospital received hundreds of requests from parents of stillborn children seeking particulars of the stillbirth so that they could in turn furnish those particulars to the Registrar of the district for registration. Ms. G, Administrative Officer, handled these requests. Ms. G. gave evidence that in order to obtain these particulars she had to search the birth registers. She had no difficulty locating any birth register. The Inquiry accepts her evidence that there was a full complement of birth registers in the hospital prior to October 1998.

9.12 When it was discovered that significant numbers of these books were missing, the room in which the remaining books were stored was secured with a lock. The Inquiry took possession of the remaining birth registers in October 2004. To date, none of the missing birth registers has been recovered.

9.13 The Inquiry is driven to conclude that some person or persons deliberately, systematically and carefully removed birth registers where obstetric hysterectomy was recorded and where the corresponding patient charts are also missing. This is particularly for the period covered by the pre-October 1991 missing maternity theatre register.

9.14 The Inquiry considers that there is a high degree of probability that the person/s who removed the old maternity *theatre register* used the information contained in that register to identify obstetric hysterectomies, the patients' names and the dates of operation. Once that person had the date of the operation and the patient's name, the *birth register* would provide the patient chart number. This would lead to the location of the chart. The older charts were stored in the old Nurses' Residence.

9.15   The Inquiry was unable to identify those responsible for the removal of the birth registers but believes it had to be one or more persons working in the Hospital who had an intimate knowledge of the recording and filing system, and whose presence with files would not cause query or surprise.

9.16   No one had any information that would assist in identifying who removed these records. Midwives told us that it was very unlikely that any consultant would know of the recording system or where the documents were stored. Dr. Neary denies having knowledge of the disappearance of these records or the alteration of the entries in the theatre register. He explained that he was greatly prejudiced by not being able to consult records to defend his position in numerous civil suits that have been filed against him. He appeared surprised at the alterations in the theatre register and spent time examining them. He also indicated a number of entries which were out of sequence and explained there had been discussion about these entries in early 1998. He indicated that several caesarean sections carried out on the same night by a registrar in January 1998 were not recorded in the register until March of the same year. Dr. Neary told the Inquiry that someone may have been trying to blacken his character by removing so many records relating to his patients.

9.17   While the vast majority of the records that are missing relate to procedures attributed to Dr. Neary, we note that the removal of all record of the patient details also obliterates all trace of those who were present or assisting at the operations. This includes details of theatre nurses, MMMs who assisted either as doctors or as theatre nurses, midwives who assisted in theatre after 1986, junior doctors and anaesthetists.

9.18   As mentioned previously the birth register generally, but not invariably, recorded a hysterectomy where this had taken place. In 6 cases where the registers were extant the hysterectomy was not recorded. In 3 and possibly

4 of these the explanation is that the hysterectomy took place some days after the birth, probably in the gynaecology theatre, and probably after the birth register was filled in by the midwife. In 2 other cases the hysterectomy is well documented elsewhere. It is clear that at the time of each operation there was no attempt to hide it, and it was the practice to record it in the birth register if it had occurred at that time.

10 THE MATERNITY REGISTERS, OTHERWISE KNOWN AS "MATERNITY ADMISSION REGISTERS"

10.1 These big ledgers were used to record admissions to the Maternity Unit and are commonly known as the maternity admissions registers. Reference to entries from maternity admissions registers were mentioned in reports prepared by HRRI and the Inquiry was anxious to review the contents. We were unable to locate the maternity admissions registers in the Hospital. No one working there seemed to know about them, and felt that they were being confused with birth registers.

10.2 The former Matron of the Maternity Unit was first interviewed at her home in October 2004. She was upset to hear of the selective and comprehensive removal of many of the records. She heard that it was difficult to establish how many peripartum hysterectomies were carried out before October 1991 without these records. She indicated that all peripartum hysterectomies ought to be recorded in the maternity admissions registers, and she was sure that we would locate them in the basement of the new unit near the nurses' changing rooms.

10.3 The maternity admissions registers were located by hospital staff who reported that they found them heaped in a corner of a storeroom off a passage in the basement of the general hospital. This room was visited by the Inquiry and was found to be full of medical supplies, but some old records, including cardex antenatal records were also seen. It was reported that the maternity admissions registers had been located in October 2004. We were aware that they had been made available to HRRI in late 1999 when they conducted their *"retrospective review of cases"* for the NEHB. We were unable to unravel this inconsistency.

10.4   On examination of the maternity admissions registers, which are very large heavy books, it was established that they comprised a complete set from 1970 up to 10th December 1998. We were informed that after December 1998, the registers were deemed to be an unnecessary duplication of information contained in the HIS (hospital information system) computerised admission record and were discontinued.

10.5   The Inquiry took possession of the registers for the period 1970 to 1998 and scrutinised them.   They typically recorded the name, address and other personal details of the patient and her partner, whether or not she was in labour (many who were not in labour were sent home until genuinely in labour and were again recorded as admissions some time later) the time of admission, the nature of the delivery, the *"complications"* (if any), the attending doctor, and details of the baby.

10.6   The Inquiry has identified the names of all 188 patients who underwent peripartum hysterectomy between 1974-1998. The registers recorded the admission of 185 of those 188 patients. The shortfall of 3 may be accounted for by women who, following delivery and discharge from the unit, were readmitted as emergency cases through the accident and emergency system with secondary postpartum haemorrhage.

10.7   Of the 185 patients whose admissions are detailed, the registers record 126 as having had the *"complication"* of hysterectomy. The hysterectomy was not recorded in 40 cases and no birth details were recorded in the remaining 19 entries, 14 of which are recorded post the date at which the maternity theatre register became the primary theatre register. There was no pattern to the omissions and the Inquiry considers that such omissions could be attributed to carelessness. The entries in these registers were made by administrative staff from other records – birth registers and the maternity theatre register - and were very much secondary to those documents. On occasions, the entries were made by midwives.

10.8   The Inquiry found it surprising that these registers were not located until it was half way through its work. If they had surfaced sooner, an enormous amount of time would have been saved.

10.9   These registers were still in use at the time the NEHB was investigating Dr. Neary's practice in October and November 1998. The Inquiry is satisfied that neither M.D., the Director of Nursing, nor Mr. Finbar Lennon, Medical Director, nor any of the other people carrying out that initial investigation, were aware of the existence of these registers. We were informed that a decision was taken in or about 10th December 1998 to discontinue using these registers to record details, but we were unable to determine who took this administrative decision.

10.10 A4 size admission books were kept on the Labour Ward until about 1996. These were discontinued, again probably because the HIS system was introduced, and the old books were destroyed at the time. The Inquiry did not regard this as suspicious.   It is probable that these books would have recorded peripartum hysterectomies.

11   POSTNATAL DAY BOOKS

11.1   Midwives in the postnatal wards kept "Daybooks". These facilitated handovers and recorded bed occupancy. Although these daybooks are not official records, the series going back to 1983 is largely intact. They record the name of the patients admitted to particular rooms in the postnatal wards from the labour ward or maternity theatre. The daybooks recorded each hysterectomy and repeated information on every day of the patient's stay in successive pages until discharge.

11.2   Up until the time that the Inquiry obtained the maternity admissions registers these daybooks were a very helpful source for identifying peripartum hysterectomy numbers for the period from 1983.   The most significant feature of these postnatal daybooks is that they contain useful summary information on every postnatal patient at any given time. Between November 1983 and the end of 1998 the Inquiry established 139 hysterectomies had been carried out. The details of 4 patients could not be checked as the daybook is missing for the relevant period. Out of the remaining 135 only 8 patients were not recorded in the daybooks at all and a further 3 patients were detailed but the hysterectomy was not recorded. This represents an 89% accuracy rate in recording hysterectomy. In the main, there appears to be no ulterior motive for failing to record hysterectomy in these books, and the operation is recorded in other hospital records.

11.3   The daybooks were read by consultants and registrars doing ward rounds and by Matron or her deputy Sr. D. when they were doing their separate rounds. Whoever removed the other documents was clearly unaware of their significance.

11.4   Several midwives said that the consultant on duty would always read these daybooks in the postnatal ward nurses' station before doing a ward round. Any consultant looking at daily entries in these books should have noted any hysterectomy carried out by other surgeons. We were told that it was not the convention for a consultant on ward round duty to visit another consultant's private patients unless specifically requested. All the consultants who gave evidence said that they visited public patients on the postnatal ward. Some registrars doubted that consultants visited public patients in the postnatal wards unless the patient required special attention. It was their view that the consultants only visited private patients.

11.5   The Inquiry is satisfied that these records, if consulted, were capable of alerting each consultant and obstetric registrar of every hysterectomy carried out in the Maternity Unit. The Inquiry is satisfied that, from this and other records and reports, the Matron of the Maternity Unit and Sister D, who was an Administrative Assistant in Maternity from 1982 -1998, would have been aware of every peripartum hysterectomy soon after it occurred.

11.6   The Matron and Sr. D. accepted that if they did rounds, they knew of each patient who had an unusual outcome. They may not have appreciated the cumulative numbers or rate or peripartum hysterectomy, or that the numbers were unusual, or that any particular operation was questionable. Before 1982, the Matron's assistant was Sr. D. She accepted that she would have learnt of hysterectomies from staff sisters but she was unaware of the rate, and believed every such operation to have been "*necessary*".

12 "PUBLIC HEALTH NURSE" BOOKS

12.1 Sr. D., Administrative Sister 1982-1998, recorded details of all mothers who she felt required early visits from the public health nurse, whether because of a stillbirth or neonatal death, the condition of the child, or the condition or personal circumstances of the mother. She used A4 size books; three covering the period 1983-1991 are extant. She covered the first two with pink gingham cloth to distinguish them from the similar hardback postnatal daybooks. The information recorded was then passed on to the relevant public health nurse. These books were not official documents.

12.2 These books record 37 women who had peripartum hysterectomies between March 1983 and May 1991. The Inquiry found that a total of 56 women in fact had this operation over that period, including all those named by Sister D. It is very probable that these 37 women received a public health nurse visit, or at least a telephone call. The entries reflect the relative seriousness attached to the operation by Sister D. We tried to determine why almost two-fifths of the hysterectomies were not noted in her books, and were told that sometimes the patient lived in another county or was returning to stay at her parent's home which was outside of the local Public Nurse's area. The Inquiry believes that some of the patients whose names were not included were patients who had planned hysterectomy because of the condition of their uterus.

13 STUDENT MIDWIFE BOOKS

13.1 Each student midwife was obliged as part her training to record births attended. Very occasionally under "*unusual cases*" students have recorded that a hysterectomy took place. The records were too incomplete to be reliable although there were some reports of peripartum hysterectomy as a complication of birth.

14 MATERNITY UNIT BIENNIAL/ANNUAL REPORTS

14.1 The maternity hospital published annual or biennial clinical reports for every year from 1952–1984. These remarkably detailed documents recorded the statistics for the unit. In the reports covering the years to 1984, the number of hysterectomies following caesarean section is set out. The reports were formally published. Reports specifically relating to the Maternity Unit were not prepared for the years after 1984, but a small section on Obstetric and Gynaecology activity was included in the general hospital's annual report from 1989 to 1992. These reports did not record peripartum hysterectomies and generally contained very little information apart from numbers of births, percentage caesarean section rate and gynaecological procedures. There were no annual reports until 2002.

14.2   This subject is more fully covered in Term of Reference 5 which is specifically concerned with 'periodical clinical reports'.

15   PATHOLOGY LEDGERS

15.1   These ledgers recorded specimens sent to the pathology laboratory from all sections of the hospital including uteri sent for examination from the maternity theatre. The ledgers record the date of receipt (usually, but not always, the date of operation), patient name, patient chart number and operator, and the word "Mat" denoted the source was the maternity theatre.   There were 12 ledgers in all, a complete set.   The Inquiry limited its search to the ledgers covering the period 1974–1998.

15.2   These pathology ledgers were of vital importance as secondary sources for establishing the numbers of peripartum hysterectomies, particularly for the pre-1991 period for which the maternity theatre register is missing.   The Inquiry used the patient chart number on the ledgers to find charts or look to other records - e.g. birth register, maternity (admissions) register - to confirm peripartum hysterectomy in cases where a uterus specimen was received from the maternity theatre.   This method traced or confirmed 184 of the 188 patients who had peripartum hysterectomy from 1974–1998.   Of the four missing cases, one of them was traced to 1974 when not all specimens were sent to the laboratory. Another case which is from 1997; there is an entry in the ledger recording receipt of a placenta, but not the uterus. The remaining 2 were unaccounted for. This ledger was extremely useful and led to the discovery of many more cases of peripartum hysterectomy.

15.3   In no case did the Inquiry rely solely on an entry in the pathology ledger as satisfactory evidence that a peripartum hysterectomy had taken place.   In all cases, the Inquiry sought some other information or record to support its findings and corroborate the validity of the pathology ledger entry.   The Inquiry is of the view that omissions in the pathology ledger had an administrative origin and were not in any way suspicious.

16   HISTOLOGY SPECIMENS

16.1   Uteri specimens received in pathology laboratories come down in a special bucket designed for receiving large specimens. The specimens are preserved in formalin and then examined in gross within the next 24-48 hours. The uterus is then dissected, and 'blocks' (small tissue samples cut from the specimen and preserved in wax blocks) are then cut into slides. These are wafer thin one cell thickness samples cut from the block by laboratory technicians in consultation with a pathologist. The specimen itself is bulky and is not retained, although in some unusual cases it is kept for a little longer to enable further inspection or further blocks to be taken. The Inquiry found that record keeping and storage of histological blocks and microscopic slides by the pathology department was of a good standard. The blocks, with a full set of slides for each block, were carefully stored in date order in the old nurses' residence. The blocks and slides in storage go back to 1952 when the general hospital was first established and was located in the old maternity hospital.

16.2   Placenta accreta is a condition where there is abnormal adherence of the placenta to the uterus. It is described medically as where *chorionic villi are adherent to the myometrium, associated with partial or complete absence of the decidua basalis and, in particular, the stratum spongiosum.* Until very recently, it invariably led to hysterectomy as it is associated with severe haemorrhage that does not respond to treatment. Placenta accreta is a rare condition except in association with placenta previa or previous caesarean section, myomectomy (removal of fibroids) and D&C. The incidence of placenta accreta is rising worldwide in association with repeat caesarean section. The Royal College of Obstetricians and Gynaecologists have recently issued guidelines on the diagnosis and management of placenta previa and placenta previa accreta. They describe that maternal and fetal morbidity and mortality from placenta previa are considerable. Women with anterior placenta previa who have had previous caesarean section are at high risk of having a morbidly adherent placenta especially if the interval between caesarean section and conception is small.

16.3   Placenta accreta with or without placenta previa or a variation of that condition was recorded some 43 times as the reason for hysterectomy in the period relevant to this inquiry, of which 9 were associated with repeat caesarean section. The Inquiry searched for and obtained the slides for all of the cases where placenta accreta was diagnosed by the obstetrician. All blocks in the sample search were present. Histological review of the accreta slides is set out in detail in Term of Reference 3.

16.4   The practical effect of the practice of retaining all histology blocks is that patients can have their histology slides reviewed, and new cuts can be taken from the block for micro examination. The secure storage of these blocks has enabled the women who had an obstetric hysterectomy but whose records are missing to at least obtain a histology report.

17   PATHOLOGY REPORTS

17.1   These were completed by the Pathologist on a Request Form, with carbon copy attached that accompanied the specimen from the theatre to the laboratory.   Dr. Neary invariably recorded his clinical diagnosis on the histology report form. The report was typed onto the lower half of the form. The original was returned to the Maternity Unit and added to the patient file. Usually, the consultant signed the report after reviewing it – which would be regarded as good practice.   Dr. Neary followed this practice. The pathology report was not always available in the patient file. Whether this was due to misfiling, carelessness or removal was unclear. Copy reports were retained in or near the laboratory. Through pressure on space, older reports were culled in or about 1990. While the pathologists entertained reservations about the shredding of older reports, it was their belief was that the original reports would still be on the patient chart. Copy reports were kept by the pathology laboratory from 1990 to April 1996.

17.2 A computerised system was introduced to the Pathology department in April 1996. A separate report is now typed and is no longer part of the request form. A separate report is prepared. This system was extended in 2001, and since then all reports can be retrieved with ease from the computer system.

17.3 Pathology reports are of limited value in determining the reason for hysterectomy. Histopathology is frequently unable to confirm a genuine clinical reason for hysterectomy.

18 PATIENT DISCHARGE LETTERS

18.1 When a patient was discharged from the hospital, a letter was written by the consultant or a registrar to her GP detailing the fact that a hysterectomy had been carried out and on occasions giving a reason for the operation and other information. The Inquiry was not able to use this source as a means to establish the rate as very few copies of these letters appear on patient charts. Despite individual requests and general advertising by the Inquiry, General Practitioners in the hospital catchment area did not contact the Inquiry. This may in part be explained by the fact that while one practice cared for two or three women who underwent this operation over 25 years, the vast majority of GPs would only have had one such patient so that they may not have recalled the event, or perhaps they thought they could add nothing to the investigation.

19 PATIENT CHARTS

19.1 The vast majority of patient charts are available and, where these were examined by the Inquiry, they always contained details and documentation recording the obstetric hysterectomy performed. Unfortunately, many patient charts were missing.

19.2 **Table 2B: Missing Patient Charts** shows the number of missing charts for obstetric hysterectomy cases in the Lourdes Hospital from 1974 to 1998 inclusive. Other patient charts (e.g. gynaecology) are also missing.

Year	Total Records	Number of Existing Records	Number of Missing Records	Consultant Breakdown of Missing Records
1998	10	10	0	
1997	10	9	1	Dr.N: 1
1996	14	14	0	
1995	11	10	1	Dr.N: 1
1994	9	9	0	
1993	15	13	2	Dr.N: 2
1992	8	8	0	
1991	12	7	5	Dr.N: 3, Dr.L: 2
1990	3	3	0	
1989	6	4	2	Dr.N: 2
1988	7	3	4	Dr.N: 2, Dr.L: 2
1987	8	3	5	Dr.N: 5
1986	9	7	2	Dr.N: 2
1985	12	6	6	Dr.N: 6
1984	2	2	0	
1983	7	4	3	Dr.N: 3
1982	5	3	2	Dr.N: 2
1981	6	3	3	Dr.N: 3
1980	6	2	4	Dr.N: 3, Dr.C: 1
1979	9	6	3	Dr.N: 2, Unknown: 1
1978	8	7	1	Dr.N: 1
1977	3	3	0	
1976	5	5	0	
1975	2	2	0	
1974	1	1	0	
TOTAL	188	144	44	Dr.N: 38, Dr.L: 4, Dr.C: 1, Unknown: 1

19.3   These numbers have been confirmed by hospital staff who assisted the Inquiry. Of the 188 patients who underwent a peripartum hysterectomy between 1974 and 1998, 44 charts, or 23.4%, cannot be found. 38 of those 44 missing charts relate to patients of Dr. Neary.

19.4   A search for a patient chart is triggered by an actual request. The fact that charts were unobtainable only came to light during specific searches following receipt of a request for a particular chart. A general search of all patient charts has not been conducted. There is no way of knowing whether any particular chart exists unless a request is made. To date, the vast majority of requests for charts have been by patients of Dr. Neary. The Inquiry sought to establish the existence of all charts concerning hysterectomy patients within its Terms of Reference, regardless of the consultant concerned. The Inquiry therefore initiated a search of all identified hysterectomies from the pathology specimen book to confirm if those patient records were available.

20 CHART RECORDING AND STORAGE SYSTEMS

20.1 We established that there was an entirely separate chart recording system in the Maternity Unit which was not managed from the patient records office in the general hospital. As far as we could ascertain the responsibility for storing charts lay with secretaries and the Matron. A separate chart and chart number was assigned to each woman on her first obstetric admission to the Maternity Unit. Prior to 1990, all obstetric patient charts were stored in the old maternity hospital. When the new unit opened in that year, the charts were transferred there. At some point in the 1990s storage space reached full capacity and the pre-1990 charts of women beyond child-bearing age were put into storage in the basement of the old nurses' residence, a building located in the hospital campus and beside offices occupied by the NEHB. In 1999, charts of women over 40 were archived and then stored in the ground floor of the nurses' residence where they could be easily accessed. The key to this building was kept behind a cold drinks vending machine in the nurses' residence.

20.2 Charts of patients who are currently pregnant and attending the antenatal clinic, are stored in the Obstetric filing room in the general hospital until the patients are discharged after delivery. Private patient notes are kept in the consultant's private rooms until admitted for delivery. All laboratory results are kept in the hospital and a chart is opened when a private patient first attends for tests or scans.

20.3 If a patient is of child-bearing age, her chart will be filed in the general filing room in the main hospital following discharge. Where a mother has passed child-bearing age, charts are stored in the old nurses' residence.

20.4 In July 1999 Morpheus Data Solutions was engaged by the hospital to organise the older obstetric files. All the files were recorded on a database and put into labelled cardboard boxes and stored once again in the basement of the old nurses' residence. The process was spread out over several months as it was reported that the charts were badly filed. Excel spreadsheets printed from the database, but not the computer database itself, are still extant. In 2002 the new CEO, Mr. D G was made aware of the anguish caused to so many former patients who were unable to obtain their charts. He decided to establish a new reliable and current database of all files in storage. A further search for known missing files was conducted but none were found. The opportunity was not taken to reconcile both databases or to determine whether any further records had been removed after the Morpheus databases was prepared. All the records were moved over from their storage place to the general hospital where each box was checked for contents. [12]

21 FINDING A PATIENT'S CHART

21.1 As technology developed, the hospital used different systems of recording admissions and filing charts. As a result, there is no one system that guarantees location of a patient's chart. The initial task is to find the patient chart number. This should appear from the master card.

21.2 This small card was opened when the patient was first admitted to the Maternity Unit and contained the basic administrative details of the patient's name, address, date of birth, date of admission for each delivery and the patient's chart number. In 1998, this system was replaced by the computerised Hospital Information System (HIS).

21.3 We followed the search for patients' charts. The master cards were stored in filing cabinets but, surprisingly, only two out of the six drawers were organised to facilitate searching. The cards were chaotically stored in the four drawers and members of the Inquiry team had to organise the cards into alphabetical order before conducting a random test survey (see below).

---

[12] It has recently been brought to the attention of the Inquiry that there is a shortfall of 165 files between the Morpheus database and the 2003 new database. As we go to press a complete reconciliation between the two databases is taking place. See further Addendum to Report.

21.4   Once a patient's chart number was identified from the master card it was necessary to search the HIS or other computer database such as NOPAS, and, for older cases, the Morpheus Excel spreadsheets, to obtain the area and box number where a particular patient's chart was stored.

21.5   If a patient number cannot be identified, the search for a file cannot proceed. For some of the 188 cases identified, no master card could be found. As the patient's name and address were available to us, the NOPAS and Morpheus databases were used to obtain the patient chart number. In several cases, the chart was located from these databases.

21.6   A further source of the file number is the birth register. We are aware that in 6 of the 44 'missing charts' cases, no patient number was ever located, and we were told that in a further 2 the number was inaccurate. We were told that in the rest of the cases (36) where a patient number was found and led to a specific box, the chart was not there and was never found in any other location in the hospital.

21.7   A second reason for a search to falter is when the chart has been removed from the correct filing box but no tracer card has been filled in and physically left in its place. Such a tracer card is meant to replace a file that is temporarily legitimately required. The person who retrieves the chart should record the name of the person removing the chart and where it has gone.

22   RANDOM SURVEY

22.1   Some witnesses suggested that patient records could be missing because of carelessness or misfiling, particularly because of the hospital move in 1990 and the culling or archiving of charts. The Inquiry carried out a random survey as a control to test the reliability of the records system in normal circumstances. Three pages of admissions recorded in the maternity admissions register were randomly selected by opening a page from pre selected years in each decade – one page from 1975, one from 1985, and one from 1995. Initial inspection of the names confirmed that none of them was on the missing records list. The 3 random pages of admissions yielded 104 patient names, and the Inquiry then tried to locate those 104 charts.

22.2   The search commenced with the master cards for the relevant chart number and this search revealed:

1975 - Of 35 patients = 12 had no master card

1985 - Of 34 patients = 4 had no master card

1995 - Of 35 patients = 1 had no master card

22.3   This result was somewhat surprising as we had been led to believe that the master cards were totally reliable for the older charts and less so for the newer charts. Our search revealed the opposite to be the case.

22.4   A chart number was recorded on all the retrieved master cards. The Inquiry then searched the Morpheus spreadsheets for those 17 patient names with the following results:

1975   –   All 12 chart numbers were located on Morpheus (0 missing)

1985   –   3 were located on Morpheus (1 missing)

1995   –   The patient was not recorded on Morpheus (1 missing)

22.5   The remaining 2 chart numbers were not found in NOPAS, a bigger and older computer database that is not restricted to obstetric patients. The remaining two chart numbers were obtained from the birth registers. Fortunately, these registers were available. Thus all 104 patient obstetric chart numbers were obtained albeit with some difficulty in 17 cases.

22.6   The next step was to establish the location of each stored chart. The computer Excel spreadsheets and Hospital In-Patient System (HIS) detail the location of patient charts. HIS (recent patients) charts were stored either in the hospital or in the old nurses' residence. Details of the location of 2 charts were not contained on these databases. Thus, 1 chart from 1975 and 1 from

1985 could not be located. Records for a further 1 patient from 1995 were located but details of the birth were not included.

22.7 Accordingly 104 charts were sought from the three random pages in the Maternity Admission Register, and 3 could not be found. This represents a 97% success rate.

22.8 As previously stated, the Inquiry had chart numbers for 36 of the 44 women who had obstetric hysterectomies and whose charts were missing. On the basis of the random survey the hospital/the Inquiry ought to have been able to find charts for all but one or two of these 36 women.

23 HAEMOVIGILANCE SURVEY

23.1 For the purposes of comparing the random survey result, the Inquiry looked at another obstetric patient records search conducted by the Haemovigilance Officer in the hospital in the year 2000/2001. This involved a search for records to determine whether any patients of the hospital not already identified by the Irish Blood Transfusion Service may have received infected Anti-D blood products from January 1990 to March 1994.

23.2 This search revealed 341 new names for whom it was necessary to check individual patient charts. The survey related that in 335 cases the search results were successful.

23.3 No information could be found on one patient. In the five remaining cases *"their charts could either not be found or the relevant information could not be located within their charts"*.

23.4 The focus of this haemovigilance search was not missing records per se but the result provides a useful comparison in relation to the search conducted for the missing hysterectomy patient records. It is worth noting that for exactly the same period as the Haemovigilance search, January 1991 to March 1994, a total of 7 obstetric hysterectomy charts cannot be located.

23.5   The Inquiry was also directed to another search for files conducted earlier in the general hospital and not involving obstetrics. Almost 200 requests for files were made and only one file was not located. In that case there was an innocent explanation for the unlocated file.

24   WHAT HAS BECOME OF SUCH RECORDS?

24.1   The current whereabouts of the missing maternity theatre register and birth registers, master cards or patient records is unknown. The pre-1991 maternity theatre register has not been seen since October 1998.

24.2   The fact that significant numbers of birth registers were missing was not appreciated until end December 1998/beginning January 1999. Unsuccessful searches conducted in the hospital confirmed that they were missing as of 20th January 1999.

24.3   When some patient records were first sought, they were missing from their storage boxes, but a tracer card was in place. In every such case, the tracer card led to recovery of the charts.   There were no tracer cards for any of the 44 'missing charts'.

24.4   Obstetric, gynaecological and general hospital patient charts were and continue to be archived separately. A different coloured file cover has always been used to readily distinguish obstetric charts. For reasons of lack of space, older charts are culled, microfiched and destroyed on a regular basis. This applies only to gynaecological and general hospital charts. It is believed unlikely that obstetric charts would have been mixed up in such files, although it remains a possibility that this may explain the loss of one or two files.

24.5   The Inquiry became aware that in 2004 An Garda Siochana commenced an investigation into missing patient records following a formal complaint by the hospital management. The Inquiry is not aware that any original charts relating to peripartum hysterectomy were recovered by that investigation.   In the process of the various searches conducted by the Patient Liaison Department in the hospital, including a search prompted by the Garda

Siochana investigation, a small number of patient records originally believed missing were found.

24.6 Dr. Neary voluntarily furnished the Inquiry with his statement to the Gardai. We thus became aware that one original file had been found in his house. This case did not refer to a hysterectomy and was removed after mid 1999. Again, it was furnished by someone who had contact with Dr. Neary and who had access to hospital files. This file was included on a database of files prepared in mid 1999 and was absent from a newer database prepared in early 2003. A new database was created in early 2003 as there were reports that the 1999 database had become "corrupted". The Inquiry learned in the last few days that there was a discrepancy between the numbers of files on the original database and the current database. The only way the numbers could be checked was for some of the Patient Liaison staff to physically count the number of entries in a hand written ledger and compare this number against the computerised new database. We were unhappy at the lack of failsafe mechanisms in the creation of each of these databases. As there has been little continuity of staff either in hospital records, management or Patient Liaison since the new millennium we were unable to draw any inferences from the facts as presented. Human error played too large a part in the assessment of the numbers of files. We were informed that there was a discrepancy of 165 between the two numbers. This would, if accurate, indicate that 165 more files are missing since 1999. If this is correct, we can assume that they do not refer to peripartum hysterectomies. We know from patients who contacted the Inquiry, from Patient Focus and Patient Liaison that 44 peripartum hysterectomy files are missing and that 8 gynaecology files are also missing. The difference between these charts is that ancillary documents such as theatre registers are available even if one theatre register was temporarily unavailable. Are these 165 files really missing or have some files been missed in the transfer of chart information from the boxes that formed the subject matter of the 1999 database to the 2003 database? All we can safely say is that patient requests for files indicate that of the 44 missing files which relate to peripartum hysterectomy, 40 were not on the 1999 database so the assumption can be made that they were missing before the database was prepared. They have never been located. Of the remaining 4 cases, two were on the 1999 database and were removed since mid 1999. The other two cases appeared on the database but their box number was omitted so that locating them was impossible. See Addendum.

24.7   In our efforts to uncover missing records or determine what became of them, the Inquiry team physically searched various parts of the hospital. We identified and interviewed persons who we believe had access to records and understood the system. A handwriting expert was engaged to assist in identifying the author of the alterations in the post-1991 maternity theatre register and much time and energy was expended in this investigation. The Inquiry was not a criminal investigation but believes that even if it were invested with the most extensive investigative statutory powers, it is unlikely that it could have done any more. Regrettably, the outcome is that the Inquiry failed to recover any significant records, and failed to obtain any clear evidence of who was responsible.

25   CONCLUSION

25.1   The Inquiry has concluded that 23.4% of obstetric hysterectomy records (44 cases) are missing. The conclusion that they were intentionally identified, traced and removed from the hospital is inescapable. The Inquiry finds confirmation from the random survey carried out that the storage of documents was adequate to protect their integrity from all but mischievous intent. We believe that the charts were unlawfully removed from the hospital with the object of protecting those involved in the hysterectomies or in protecting the reputation of the hospital.

25.2   Further corroboration of deliberate systematic removal of all records of certain hysterectomies is substantiated by the fact that in 40 of the 44 cases, the birth registers are also missing. Although some master cards are missing, it is less than certain that they were removed improperly as they were not stored or filed as carefully as other records.

25.3   Disturbingly for a significant proportion of the women who had peripartum hysterectomies, their charts and other secondary records are missing. For the women who have sought their charts in vain, this is a huge disappointment and, in some instances the absence of these records has been traumatic.

They will never know precisely what happened to them and what caused the operating surgeon to proceed to hysterectomy. They will never be able to have an expert review of their file to advise whether the operation was justified or not.

25.4   Included in this group are patients who really want to have confirmation that Dr. Neary was honest with them and that he really did his best for them. Without a review of their records, they will never know. The only sources available to them are the theatre register entries (in cases pre-1992 even this is not available), the pathology laboratory blood books or expert review of their pathology slides which often provide tantalisingly little information. Some private patients whose hospital records are missing have sought and received copies of their private records from Dr. Neary.

25.5   There can be no doubt but that the bulk of these missing charts and the missing birth registers were deliberately and unlawfully removed from the hospital with a view to concealing the details of the operation performed and the treatment given. It is probable that the pre-1992 maternity theatre register was also removed with this motive in mind.

25.6   These documents were probably removed by one or more persons – and the Inquiry doubts that one person acting alone could have done this – working within the hospital and with a good knowledge of the recording systems. It takes a person of particular determination and coolness to spend hours retrieving multiple birth registers from one room, and then to use the information contained within to seek out the patient charts from the Maternity Unit records department or from a dark unheated musty basement of an unused building. Those persons must have spent hours retrieving the files without the benefit of the Morpheus database which only came into being in autumn 1999.

25.7   It has to be remembered that the miscreant/s had to be familiar with the hospital and be persons whose presence in the Maternity Unit would not raise suspicion. Keys had to be located and used. Finally, the documents had to be removed – perhaps carried openly - without causing suspicion and ultimately they had to be disposed of, destroyed or secreted.

25.8   The Inquiry doubts that any further records will be recovered at this stage or that anyone will be made accountable and deeply regrets its inability to comfort any of the patients who remain in the suspense of not knowing.

26   STANDARDS OF RECORDING

26.1   Healthcare Risk Resources International (HRRI) presented its first report to the NEHB on 8th November 1998. This report focused on 3 patients who had caesarean hysterectomies performed by Dr. Neary in that year.   Their charts were considered by obstetric and nursing/midwifery and legal experts.   The report noted the recording of operations in the patient charts as being *"adequate".* But with *"clearly room for improvement"* and commented on deficits in midwifery documentation standards.

26.2   A subsequent HRRI report to the NEHB, in December 1998, where 9 patient files were reviewed (including the original 3 above) repeated these criticisms, reporting as follows:

"Standards of records and record keeping are very variable with essential information and explanations not being recorded. There is little or no recording of dialogue with the patient and or her significant others. There are regular entries by medical staff, but unfortunately the notation is so brief and there is not a comprehensive or consistent record of all care delivered. The midwifery/nursing records are also poor, some gaps can be extracted from these but again they are not contemporary and fully comprehensive of all events. Note taking and sequence of events by PF give a very good and clear history of events. Many lessons could be learned and training given to other midwives on the importance of records and standards of record keeping. There is too much crossing out and trying to obliterate what has been written with 'error' written beside the notation but no date/time/signature.

Consent forms exists for the elective and emergency Caesarean Sections and IVP, but there is no record or notation of any dialogue regarding the emergency procedures such as hysterectomies and even the laparotomy. Consent forms are too open ended and do not have room for risks, benefits or alternatives for treatment and questions could be raised about who the witness is as most signatures cannot be identified and there is no grade or designation of the witness. All forms should be supported by full discussion and issues discussed with the patient and significant others.

The recording and prescribing of drugs leaves much to be desired with incomplete recording and uncertainties about administration of certain drugs such as Vitamin K and syntometerine. Are BCGs give as a matter of routine within this hospital or are they just where there any known contacts or exposure.

The recording and administration of blood transfusion including the taking of vital signs and responding to adverse reactions including notification and responses from medical staff are poor. Many of the charts, anaesthetic and observation sheets do not even have patient identifiers on them let alone comprehensive dates, times, sequence, signatures and legible notation with many crossings out, incomplete recording, subjective information and the use of Christian names without surnames or signatures.

Considering the nature of the conditions reviewed the fluid balance charts could certainly be improved and the recording of intravenous fluids including additives and batch numbers. In none of these cases is there record of a swab count or weighing of swabs and observation of suction jars for estimated blood loss. Poor photocopies and incomplete CTGs including illegible or non-existent notation have not helped the review of these cases......

There is a lack of a team approach to patient/family care with poor continuity, on consistency in approaches to care, lack of communication with the patient and between the professionals and poor co-ordination made worse by the record keeping".

26.3   The HRRI reports only considered obstetric hysterectomy cases of recent origin, from 1996 to1998, and their findings were therefore relevant to practices in the hospital Maternity Unit as it stood in 1998. They were prepared by appropriate experts who the Inquiry has interviewed, and the Inquiry broadly accepts the comments which they make.

26.4   Dr. Feeney has looked at many case notes going back as far as the 1960s, and noted that some changes have taken place over the years. He indicated to us that the practice where the anaesthetist wrote up most of the surgery notes seems to have ceased in the later 1970s, as thereafter the anaesthetist's notes began to appear on separate sheets. The records were often difficult to decipher and the operating surgeon's identity frequently unclear. For instance, a registrar may have carried out the caesarean section and a consultant may have performed the hysterectomy, but as the registrar may have completed the notes, the identity of the operator was uncertain.

26.5   Dr. Feeney confirmed very inadequate detail and clarity in note taking at all levels. Caesarean hysterectomy was frequently entered so casually that an innocent reader might be forgiven for thinking that hysterectomy was the purpose of the operation and not the delivery of a baby.

26.6   While caesarean hysterectomy was documented clearly, it was obvious that it was not always treated as an event of great import giving the appearance of being no more unusual than a breech delivery.

26.7   An example of this casual approach emerges from the annual totalling of operations recorded in the maternity theatre register which is noted in that register.

26.8   As previously mentioned, a note in the register of totals for the year ended 1995 gave figures for emergency and elective caesarean sections, and a total of such operations, but recorded only one hysterectomy for the year where 8, and probably 9, were clearly entered in the register in that year.

26.9 Again, for the previous year 1994, the total sections, emergency and elective, were added up but again only 1 hysterectomy was recorded at the end of the year. A total of 8 were recorded in the register.

26.10 These errors misled the initial investigation of practices in the unit in October 1998, creating an impression that prior to 1996, Dr. Neary's rate of peripartum hysterectomy was unremarkable, and giving support to the view that the illness of his wife which led to her untimely death in August 1996 adversely affected his judgement from that time on. Our findings indicate that this is simply untrue. Dr. Neary was clearly very much affected by the death of his wife from ovarian cancer but his grief did not affect his judgement in relation to the treatment of haemorrhage which remained as it was from shortly after he took up his position as consultant in 1974.

26.11 Before the complaints against Dr. Neary took centre stage in the Maternity Unit, and before any of the HRRI reviews of practices within the unit took place, M.D., the new Director of Nursing appointed by the NEHB in 1996, continued with previous efforts to integrate the Maternity Unit into the general hospital.

26.12 Several of her predecessors had expressed concern that the hospital management was unaware of what was going on in the Maternity Unit. There had been a long tradition of treating the Maternity Unit as a separate hospital during the time when the MMMs actively managed the hospital. It was clear that all attempts to review, change or modify nursing practices or standards were looked upon as interference and were not welcome.

26.13 The shortcomings in record keeping do not appear to have been recognised within the unit. At the request of M.D., the new Director of Nursing, a report on midwifery activity was prepared by senior midwives at the end of 1996. The Quality Assurance Committee – a committee of midwives formed in 1994 –

carried out interviews with midwives and collected responses to questionnaires concerning patients and reported -

"The results were very positive and very helpful.

95% felt that staff recognised their need for privacy.

91% felt that their comfort, dignity was maintained in the delivery suite.

93% were entirely happy with the care they received.

64% of primigravida mothers attended Antenatal Classes.

We have learned much from auditing our service and we anticipate an improvement when we audit in 1997. In particular we ascertained that Mothers in our Maternity Unit expect to be treated as individuals at all times. They expect their dignity and privacy to be respected. The quality of our communication and information is very important to them. Good record keeping is also a very vital element.

Quality Assurance has increased our awareness of the needs and expectations of Mothers in our care. Much remains to be done in this area and in 1997 we will broaden our approach involving a Multidisciplinary Team. This we hope will help to insure that the quality care we all aspire to can be delivered in the future."

This report contains no comment on records or record keeping, and voices no concerns over any obstetric practices.

26.14 A "Report on the Review of Midwifery Practices" in the hospital, prepared by Ms Liz Duffin, OBE, in November 1998, does not address the content and quality of midwifery record keeping concerning theatre procedures as the theatre was not one of the clinical areas visited by her.

The review recommended the avoidance of duplication of record keeping in relation to the antenatal ward but makes no reference to the quality of record keeping.

In the 'Review of Midwifery Practices' of November 1999, which looked at the implementation of earlier recommendations in the original report, there is no reference to record keeping.

26.15 It is clear that no one reviewed the contents of the patient charts or the quality of record keeping or the security of the storage systems before 1999.

26.16 The Inquiry believes, as the literature suggests, that record keeping mirrors the overall standard of practice and reflects the skill of the practitioners, be they obstetricians, midwives, anaesthetists or others, and that best practice in documentation encourages quality improvement as it provides evidence for the continual evaluation of current practice, audit, research and good clinical risk management.

26.17 Documentation or computer recording systems need to be clearly understood by professionals and should permit the collection of patient information in a concise, accurate and comprehensive manner, within frameworks that systematically identify and evaluate information and monitor the effects of healthcare interventions and policies on patient outcomes.

26.18 Conversely, inadequate recording systems compromise communication of clinical activity, stifle the opportunity for quality improvement and disempower practitioners – all of which occurred in the Lourdes Hospital. Audit is meaningless when the data is inaccurate.

TERM 3

TO INQUIRE INTO WHETHER DR. NEARY'S PRACTICE IN RELATION TO PERIPARTUM HYSTERECTOMY WAS COMMENTED ON OR ACTED UPON BY CONSULTANT OR OTHER MEDICAL STAFF, BY MIDWIVES AND OTHER NURSING STAFF WITHIN THE HOSPITAL, OR BY THE MANAGEMENT OF THE HOSPITAL.

1 CULTURE

1.1 The findings here were quite extraordinary and difficult to understand. We found an incredibly pervasive culture of acceptance and acquiescence of consultant activity. To ask why, or to comment was not a part of everyday practice. To consider that things could change seemed unimaginable.

1.2 In the first few months of interviews it seemed that, apart from the few midwives who had been concerned in 1998, no one had any knowledge of concerns about Dr. Neary or about peripartum hysterectomies in the unit. No one saw anything out of the ordinary, no one heard even a whisper of disquiet, and no one had been given any reason to say or think that any of the hysterectomies were questionable. No one added up the number of procedures and if they did, they were unaware of the rate, or what was an acceptable incidence of peripartum hysterectomy in other hospitals.

1.3 There were many reasons advanced to try and explain why the management of the hospital and the consultants and staff of Maternity Unit were unaware of the numbers and therefore unconcerned; they were not informed; they were not on duty on the days when the operations took place; they thought the operations they assisted at were the only ones; they were very busy; Dr. Neary was a very competent surgeon; Dr. Neary did more caesarean sections than any other consultant; Dr. Neary was the easiest surgeon to work with; Dr. Neary was always available; all the hysterectomies were carried out for a very good reason; the hysterectomies were sterilisations; there was no audit; there were no published figures; no one knew what an acceptable rate was and so on.

1.4 Even now, despite the glare of publicity on the unit, many of the professionals working there seemed to have no real appreciation that the hysterectomies were not confined to Dr. Neary. Even at this stage, many anaesthetists and all the pathologists were surprised to hear that, of the 188 identified hysterectomies over 25 years (1974-1998 inclusive), 59 were not performed by Dr. Neary. Their lack of awareness was surprising.

1.5   As the Inquiry progressed and it seemed to us that fears of bias or repercussions diminished, we began to hear that from about 1996 there was a definite unease on the part of some of the midwives in relation to the youth of a number of Dr. Neary's patients who had undergone obstetric hysterectomy. There is no evidence that anything tangible was discussed, any action taken or any complaints made. The main concern seemed to be the youth of the patients rather than the fact of so many hysterectomies.

1.6   We tried to understand why the midwives, who formed the largest group of health professionals involved and who were principled women of training and intelligence, did not take their concerns further. Why did they not speak to management? Why did they not bring their concerns to the Matron and her assistant? In trying to untangle this puzzle we became aware of a history of tensions between the obstetric unit and the general hospital. The maternity hospital was the first MMM hospital, starting out as a maternity nursing home. It predated the general hospital and at one stage both the maternity hospital and the general hospital occupied the same building. The Matron of the maternity Hospital then was the only Matron. The subsequent building of a much bigger general acute hospital, with its own Matron and management infrastructure, may have created resentment within the older maternity hospital of any interference from the newer separate hospital.

1.7   Whatever the origins of the tensions and separateness, the attitudes extended into later decades until it became well established that the maternity hospital had its own management structures, with its own Matron and assistant to the Matron, and was more or less left to manage its own affairs. The sad reality was that the Matron of the Maternity Unit was not given the power to properly administer the Maternity Unit. She lacked the authority necessary to question the consultants or to change procedures and she lacked the support of the MMMs if a dispute arose. Many of the midwives felt that the Matron could only do so much and so there was no point in complaining to her.

1.8 The maternity hospital was then physically at a distance from the general hospital but even when the new Maternity Unit was resituated beside the general hospital in 1990, the sense of separateness continued. It is apparent that frosty relationships existed between the Matron in the general hospital and the Matron in the Maternity Unit whose official title was Assistant Matron but who was always referred to as "the Matron". The effect of this separateness was that problems relating to the maternity hospital remained within the unit and were not discussed with the management of the general hospital. The Tripartite committee of the MMMs were the day to day management of the Lourdes Hospital but, on their own admission, they left the maternity hospital to the Matron of the Maternity Unit and her administrative assistant who was an MMM. Neither the Matron of the Maternity Unit nor Sr. D had any management training. All the evidence was that they had little authority over the consultants or registrars.

1.9 In 1991/1992, it was clear that the MMMs were seeking a purchaser for the hospital. The Tripartite management consisting of 3 MMM sisters – the Matron, the Secretary Manager and the Accountant - was disbanded over a very short period and replaced by a new Management Board consisting of a male accountant, Mr B. C, the Medical Director, Mr. Finbarr Lennon who was a consultant and Sr. A. MMM. The Matron of the general hospital Sr. C., and Sr. E., the accountant left. Sr. B. who had been the Secretary Manager remained on as CEO for a short while. No explanations were given to the nursing staff in the general hospital, and they were left to speculate why their familiar management team which had been in place for many years had left so suddenly. The sudden disbanding of the Tripartite left a management vacuum which took years to fill, and created an atmosphere of suspicion and resentment towards the new lay Matrons who replaced the MMMs. Midwives would not have taken their concerns to the new Directors of Nursing in the general hospital. This would have been seen as disloyal to the Matron and the unit.

1.10   All attempts by the new Directors of Nursing to create an all inclusive management of the entire hospital were rebuffed. The hospitals remained separate with tensions increasing. Relations between the consultants were riven by disputes involving the use of hospital beds. Dr. Neary, who was spokesman for the obstetricians, had engaged with the Chairman of the Medical Board in ill humoured correspondence on the issue. With this backdrop of tensions, it was unlikely that any concerns within the Maternity Unit would be exchanged with the management of the general hospital, who were now seen as being driven by the North Eastern Health Board. Many midwives told us that they had no idea who precisely management was.

1.11   It seemed to us sometimes as if the two parts of the same hospital were utterly separate institutions. Two odd events stand out as examples of the detachment from interest or awareness in outcomes between the two hospitals. Both of the events occurred after the glare of publicity fixed on the hospital in 1995/1996 following allegations of misconduct against a consultant surgeon. A Help Line was set up by the hospital, yet no one used it to raise any concerns regarding Dr. Neary's practices although the peripartum hysterectomy rate was rising.

1.12   The first incident involved a maternal death in 1997. We became aware of the event from a patient who recounted the details of her stay in the Maternity Unit. She had an unplanned caesarean hysterectomy and sought sympathy from the midwifery staff in the postnatal ward. She was told to consider herself lucky that Dr. Neary had been on duty that night, as a young mother had died the same night. She understood that to mean that she had nothing to complain about, as she was alive unlike the other patient.

1.13   By coincidence, another patient had undergone the same caesarean hysterectomy procedure and was in the ward at the same time. She too recounted a similar story to the Inquiry. We then consulted the birth register for 1997 and found confirmation for the death.

1.14   We put this death to a number of senior midwives and to the assistant Matron Sr. D. No one to whom we spoke could recall that a maternal death had occurred in 1997. Eventually, the matter was looked into and details were furnished. The patient had been transferred from the Maternity Unit to the intensive care unit in the general hospital where she died. Strictly speaking therefore she was not considered as a death in the Maternity Unit. It seemed to the Inquiry that if a sentinel event such as a maternal death in 1997 did not stick in the memory of the midwives, how then would procedures occurring every couple of months and which had been happening for as long as anyone could remember make an impact?

1.15   The other surprising event concerned a former patient who came alone to tell her story. Hers was not a peripartum hysterectomy and although her experience was outside of the Terms of Reference, the Inquiry listened to her. She had her hospital notes with her. She was at the time in her late 30's and her family was complete. She had what seemed to be a gynaecological problem. Dr. Neary asked her to attend as a day patient for a D&C. She was aware of the routine involved in a diagnostic D&C procedure. Her husband took the day off from his work to care for their children. The possibility of any other procedure was not discussed. When she woke in pain she knew something had happened. She learned that she had undergone a total abdominal hysterectomy with removal of her ovaries and fallopian tubes. Dr. Neary informed her that he had to carry out a hysterectomy, as he "*could not stop the bleeding*". Later she was told that she did "*not have any cancer*". This was not a possibility that had ever been discussed with her. The histology reported no disease but rather "*degenerate products of conception and a collection of endometrial polyps*". The operation notes and the request for histology indicate that Dr. Neary believed when he carried out the hysterectomy that she had advanced uterine cancer.

1.16   We found this case quite remarkable as no consequences flowed from it. A day patient had unexpectedly to be accommodated; a minor procedure requiring a short anaesthetic became major surgery with further anaesthetic involvement. A uterus, ovaries and tubes were removed for cancer, yet only degenerate products of conception or an incomplete miscarriage were found. The patient was given a booklet on hysterectomy while still an inpatient so people had to be aware that this had happened. No discussion followed, no curiosity appears to have been elicited by this event and no one mentioned it to us, nor did anyone questioned have any knowledge of the incident. We found evidence of another similar case. The normal curiosity for reasons why unusual outcomes happened simply did not occur.

1.17 After 12 months of dialogue, including two lengthy interviews with Dr. Neary, conducted over two days, two matters became apparent. No one, including Dr. Neary himself, was aware of the full numbers of peripartum hysterectomies. In addition, there was no mechanism after the maternity clinical reports had ceased, for anyone in the hospital to be aware of the cumulative annual figures unless they looked through the maternity theatre register and counted the procedures themselves.

1.18 Clinical audit as we now know it was not a feature in many provincial hospitals, and certainly no formal weekly or monthly review of throughput and outcomes occurred at this Maternity Unit. Daily figures for births and complications were always entered on a monthly statistical sheet and kept behind the labour ward nurses' station but only from 1997 did these statistic sheets include a count of hysterectomies. Adverse outcomes were not the subject of team or departmental discussions.

1.19 Meetings, known as 'Grand Rounds,' had taken place up to about 1988 where departments in the hospital took it in turn each month to present an interesting case to the entire hospital staff. This was not an analytical meeting or an audit of outcome, nor was peripartum hysterectomy ever presented as a topic. From time to time, midwives and obstetricians met to discuss common interests. There were 7 of these meetings recorded for the period 1984 to 1997, but hysterectomy was never one of the subjects of these meetings.

1.20 We heard many references to audit but it was apparent that few witnesses actually understood the process. Frequently we felt that the concept of audit and statistics gathering were confused. Audit requires an agreed topic, protected time, commitment, ability to collect data and input it into computers. It requires the insight to identify known external benchmarks and to compare those against data collected. It requires time for discussion of results and the identification of reasons for less favourable outcomes set against the comparators. Most important, meaningful audit requires a return to the same audit subject after changes are introduced so that comparison of outcomes is made to measure improvement. Audit requires that all the consultants work together with the whole maternity team to achieve best practice.

1.21   There was no evidence of anything approaching audit in this unit before Dr. Neary was suspended, and it has taken many years for audit to be accepted and implemented. The consultants still do not have protected time and tools for audit notwithstanding that the common contract for consultants offered in January 1998 introduced the requirement for audit as a condition of employment, imposing obligations on consultants and employers.

2   OBSTETRICIANS OUTSIDE THE UNIT

2.1   The periodic reports could have been a valuable and effective system of audit as the results could have been compared with those of previous years and with the results of the Dublin teaching hospitals. The contents and purpose of periodic clinical reports is discussed elsewhere in this report. It is patent from any perusal of those reports that obstetric hysterectomy was always recorded and was clear to see. We found no evidence that any of the parties to whom annual reports were sent ever raised any queries.

2.2   Dr. Neary recalled that few of the recipients acknowledged receipt of the report. He recalled that some obstetricians commented on the induction rate, but never raised any queries relating to the caesarean hysterectomy rate, where the numbers were always clearly indicated. He also told us that no one ever commented on the symphysiotomy rate either. We felt that publishing reports without having meetings to discuss and compare internally and externally was not a particularly useful exercise.

3   DR. NEARY'S OBSTETRIC COLLEAGUES IN THE MATERNITY UNIT IN THE EARLY YEARS

3.1   The late Dr. Gerard Connolly was the first obstetrician in the hospital. He took up work in his position in July 1945 at 30 years of age, and retired in April 1982, aged 67.   When he took up his post, he had already spent time in Sierra Leone and in Nigeria. He graduated in 1940. He spent a year as house officer then 6 months as a surgical SHO in Cavan Hospital, and a further 6 months studying for his Diploma in Public Health. From 1942 -1945, he worked at the MMM hospital at Anua. It has to be a natural inference therefore, that Dr. Connolly's formal and structured hospital training in obstetrics and gynaecology was truncated. He did not have the usually held Membership of the Royal College of Obstetrics and Gynaecologists (MRCOG) but held an MAO degree (Master in the Art of Obstetrics), obtained with distinction by written exam in 1948.

3.2 All questions asked of the individual members of the MMMs relating to Dr. Connolly elicited comments about his courtesy, integrity, honour, and popularity. He was a deeply religious man and was held in very high esteem by the sisters. We had the impression that the very notion of questioning Dr. Connolly's qualifications was offensive. One of the MMM Order's main objectives was to train doctors for work on the missions. It is very likely that Dr. Connolly's skills were appropriate to the training of medical personnel on African mission stations, where there were no colleagues to consult, little in the line of blood supplies and decisive action was important. The Inquiry was told that preserving fertility was of paramount importance in African culture and thus caesarean sections were a last resort. There was no evidence that Dr. Connolly worked anywhere other than Africa and the Lourdes Hospital in the period relevant to this Inquiry.

3.3 It seemed that no one would ever consider the possibility that Dr. Connolly's decisions could be reviewed. What he did was right and set the tone for the unit permanently. We heard from several nurses who worked with him that it was felt that his practices were influenced by his years on the missions. This was just accepted without any further question as to whether such influences were appropriate for the patients at the Maternity Unit in Drogheda. All reports confirm that Dr.Connolly was highly respected by the MMMs and perhaps even revered. He was described as a gentleman. His religious beliefs carried into the practice of obstetrics and were shared by his employers. Contraception was not permitted and female sterilisation by tubal ligation was not an option. Women seemed happy to have large families and symphysiotomy was carried out to facilitate this end.

3.4 Dr. Liam O'Brien came to the hospital following conventional training in Ireland and the UK, including being an Assistant Master in the National Maternity Hospital at Holles Street. He was a man of few words and fairly rigid practices. His memory is that Dr. Connolly came to Drogheda to be in charge of the MMM obstetric nursing home. He was under the guidance of the then Master of Holles Street, Dr. A.P. Barry, who visited the nursing home if there were problems. This arrangement ceased when Dr. O'Brien was appointed as the second consultant. Dr. O'Brien was not aware that Dr. Connolly had done any postgraduate training in obstetrics unless it was in Africa.

3.5 We heard evidence that Dr. O'Brien had *"no great respect"* for his senior colleague. They did not have a warm relationship. Dr. O'Brien felt that he was not treated as a consultant of equal status when he took up his position and he found himself obliged to work as Dr. Connolly's assistant for 3 years in order to be paid at all. There was also a huge difference in their formal training.

3.6 Dr. O'Brien was not a man to engage in unnecessary conversation. He held his own counsel and answered only to his own duties. He did not enjoy robust health and thus perhaps appreciated the youthful enthusiasm and willingness to work which he saw in Dr. Neary when he joined the group 10 years later. He and Dr. Connolly welcomed Dr. Neary as a positive addition to a hardworking hospital. It is apparent that soon after Dr. Neary arrived, gynaecological services in the general hospital greatly increased, although there were few opportunities to practise his skills in complicated pelvic surgery as major cancer cases were sent to Dublin where the ancillary services were located.

3.7 All the evidence we heard relating to the early days of the Maternity Unit indicate spartan working conditions. Hot water was not available and had to be brought over from the general hospital. Patients had to be carried up and down stairs to and from the theatre. There was a missionary zeal set by the founding members of the MMMs, which seemed to exhort the staff of the hospital to work incredible hours with little equipment or luxury. In spite of its many shortcomings in comfort, the maternity hospital seems to have been embraced by the women of the area and its popularity as a place to have a baby grew from year to year. There was always a sizeable private patient practice in the maternity hospital.

3.8   In 1974, the young Dr. Neary took up his position as consultant to this hard working International Missionary Training Hospital. His training barely encompassed 7 years in obstetrics and gynaecology, but he had his MRCOG exams and appeared to be a good candidate. Although he had trained in some of the best hospitals, there is a suspicion that his obstetric training was considerably less developed than his gynaecological surgery skills.

3.9   At that time in the UK, where Dr.Neary's entire specialist training took place, gynaecology was the higher status skill as midwives and junior doctors safely delivered most babies in the labour suite. NHS hospitals did not have private patients or private beds. Dr. Neary himself said that much of his training involved major cancer gynaecological surgery in modern, highly equipped and serviced hospitals. His specialist training took place under the tutelage of gynaecologists rather than obstetricians, and it is very probable that he was recruited to the Lourdes for his surgical skills in gynaecology.

3.10   Although it was probably acceptable in the past, Dr. Neary's training would nowadays be considered deficient. Having only 7 years postgraduate specialist training would not be acceptable for a consultant post. 31 years of age is now considered young to be appointed a consultant obstetrician. The system now is to spend a further 3-4 years in structured, supervised training as a specialist registrar in an approved post after obtaining the MRCOG. Although Dr. Neary was universally highly praised for his surgical skills by his supervising consultants and other doctors who trained with him, 7 years may perhaps, in retrospect, not have been enough time to develop mature judgement.

3.11   The IMTH was a voluntary hospital and as such was not subject to the same selection process for consultants as hospitals in the public sector. At the time that he was selected the MMMs and Dr. Neary's fellow consultants were delighted with their coup in attracting him into their ranks. He could after all, so they convinced themselves, have stayed in England or gone to one of the Dublin hospitals. The Inquiry believes that it is a great pity that Dr. Neary did not remain in a large centre of training working with many more colleagues where his deficiencies might have been recognized and put right and where his great self-belief might have been moulded into a little more introspection.

3.12 Dr. Neary's period of training as an obstetrician/gynaecologist in England was not always happy. He trained first in Manchester where he believed his stand as a Catholic doctor on tubal ligation and termination prejudiced the advance of his career. His undergraduate training was in Galway University, where he was mentored by Prof. Eamon O'Dwyer. Dr. Neary determined that when he went to Manchester to receive training in Obstetrics and Gynaecology, he would insist on the insertion in his contract of employment of a conscience clause permitting him the right not to carry out contraceptive sterilisations or to assist at terminations of pregnancy.

3.13 He informed the Inquiry that this stand brought him into direct confrontation with one of his consultants, who would not permit him to scrub in theatre at all. He did not receive a good reference at the end of the year and had great difficulty in obtaining another training post. Eventually, on advice, he changed the name of his referee and was fortunate, he believes, to have been offered a post at a very prestigious training hospital, St. Mary's at Portsmouth. From there, following the recommendation of Prof. Eamon O' Dwyer, he went to the Hammersmith Hospital, another prestigious establishment renowned for the teaching of gynaecology. He trained under an eminent gynaecologist who had taken a strong moral position against abortion. Many Catholic and especially Irish obstetricians trained at this hospital because of the senior consultant's views. Investigations reveal nothing untoward about Dr. Neary's practices in those years.

3.14 There is a certain irony in Dr. Neary's position. He took a stand as a Catholic doctor against routine sterilisations and terminations in the UK, therefore limiting his job prospects within the National Health system. He subsequently came to a hospital in Ireland owned and managed by the Medical

Missionaries of Mary where he knew that there would be no possibility of change from traditional ethical values but he was eventually struck off for carrying out procedures which he believes were forced upon him by the strict Catholic ethos of nuns.[13]

3.15   After Dr. Neary arrived at the Maternity Unit in Drogheda his formal training ended. He never attended for any further training or competence assessment or assurance. On arrival, he found that the conditions under which consultants worked were less than ideal. The workload was heavy and equipment was basic. As junior consultant, he was expected to carry a heavier share of the load, as Dr. Connolly eased up on his share of public practice. Although initially dismayed and shocked by the primitive conditions in the maternity hospital, he decided to rise to the challenge and took solace from the excellent facilities in gynaecology in the modern purpose built general hospital.

3.16   When asked whether any of his colleagues ever queried his obstetric hysterectomies, Dr. Neary recalled a meeting of the three obstetricians called by the Matron of the Maternity Unit regarding the high caesarean hysterectomy figures in the 1978/1979 period.   He believes that the discussion followed preparation or publication of the biennial report, which indicated 16 hysterectomies following caesarean section. There were 281 caesarean sections carried out in the unit in that two year period. This gives a rate of 1 hysterectomy in every 18 caesarean sections. Dr. Neary attributed this high rate to indirect sterilisations. We noted 4 women having their first baby in that group.

3.17   Dr. Neary's recollection is that at the meeting when the Matron talked of the high hysterectomy rate for the years 1978/1979 his colleague, Dr. O'Brien remarked that although the hysterectomy rate was high, there were no maternal deaths from haemorrhage during this two-year period. Obviously, the figure warranted further discussion and explanation – and indeed there may have been legitimate explanations available – but after Dr. O'Brien's

---

[13] **The MMMs wish to reiterate their position which is that** *"the Catholic ethos of the Hospital could not have had any bearing on the necessity to carry out peripartum hysterectomy."*

comment, none were given or further sought. Dr. Neary believes that the discussion went no further. He has no recollection of any other mention of peripartum hysterectomy to him.

3.18   Dr. O'Brien's comment seems to have put an end to the Matron's meeting. Dr. Neary believed that he enjoyed the support of his colleagues and that there was not a problem.   Of those 16 caesarean hysterectomies, Dr. Connolly carried out 4; Dr. Neary carried out 11 and 1 was unattributed. Dr. O'Brien was specifically asked about the figures for caesarean hysterectomies in the late 1970s. He told the Inquiry that he had no recollection of any concerns about the rate in those two years. He told us that as Dr. Neary was the youngest and most recent appointment, he had the biggest workload and carried out more caesarean sections than the other two obstetricians put together. The annual reports confirm that prior to Dr. Neary's arrival caesarean section was considered a high risk procedure and was avoided where possible. There were very few elective caesarean sections carried out before Dr. Neary joined the unit.

3.19   As we are now aware that the publication date of the 1978/1979 reports was in early 1982, the meeting between the Matron and the consultants may not have had the same urgency and impact as a meeting in what risk management experts describe as *"real time analysis"*. The moment seems to have passed. The Matron described to us that she felt that the consultants *"stuck together"* whenever there was any criticism and this may well have been one of those occasions. Although the Matron of the Maternity Unit has no recollection of such a meeting and doubted she would have succeeded in collecting the three obstetricians together to discuss anything, there are several items in the Matron's diary for 1981 and 1982 that note meetings with all three consultants. On balance, the Inquiry believes that some such meeting did take place but that the matter went no further.

3.20   Dr. O'Brien was not asked about the meeting with the Matron as he was interviewed well before this information became available. In a letter he recalled a meeting which he thought was in 1980, at which he attended with Dr. Connolly and Dr. Neary. He recalls that Dr. Neary left but his memory does not run to the subject of the meeting. However, he did tell us that he had a recollection of Dr. Neary speaking to him with some concern saying that he had performed 3 obstetric hysterectomies recently. Dr. O'Brien felt that this was a run of bad luck and told him not to worry as these things 'sometimes happen in threes'. He felt that this conversation took place perhaps in the mid '80s. Analysis of the earlier reports shows that Dr. O'Brien himself had such a bad run in 1970 when he performed peripartum hysterectomy 3 times in the space of 1 month. It is understandable therefore that he would give such comfort to Dr. Neary who he felt, was concerned.

3.21   Dr. O'Brien does not deny that the Matron may have spoken to him about her unease regarding Dr. Neary's high hysterectomy rate. He always assumed that if a hysterectomy was carried out after delivery, then it had to be for a legitimate reason. He was not prepared to discuss a colleague's practice with the Matron. He believed that he was not accountable for his colleague's practices. He confirmed the strict ethos relating to all family planning matters and that Dr. Connolly was very close to the MMMs.

3.22   Dr. Connolly who died in 1990 was the senior obstetrician in the unit. He appears not to have criticised Dr. Neary's caesarean hysterectomy rate. He must have been fully aware of the rate and had no concerns. The Matron of the Maternity Unit said that she spoke several times to Dr. Connolly about Dr. Neary's high rate of caesarean hysterectomy and he told her that Dr. Neary was *"afraid of haemorrhage"*.

3.23   It was suggested to Dr. Neary during interview that an analysis of each of the caesarean sections which ended in hysterectomy in that 2 year period (1978/79) may well have identified some deficiencies in the manner in which post partum haemorrhage was treated in the unit, and especially by him. He agreed that this was so. Unfortunately there was no such analysis and Dr. Neary, the junior consultant, acted on the basis that he had the support of his colleagues. He continued his practice of resort to hysterectomy at an early stage to prevent what he perceived to be imminent maternal death or severe problems with a subsequent pregnancy. It is also probable that included in those numbers, there were hysterectomies carried out which were justifiable and may have saved lives.

3.24   It is the view of the Inquiry that if there had been an analysis of Dr. Neary's hysterectomy rate in those two years, legitimate queries should have been raised as to why he was carrying out hysterectomy so frequently for *"uncontrollable haemorrhage"*. Although the incidence of caesarean hysterectomy at that time may not have been particularly remarkable, an analysis ought to have revealed a trend towards a much increased number of caesarean sections and **early** hysterectomy in **women of low parity**. It was not good enough to say that Dr. Neary was *"afraid of haemorrhage"* without more. He clearly needed retraining in the management of uterine bleeding. The Inquiry was unable to understand why Dr. Connolly did not raise queries. All reports indicate that he had the authority to question practices and that he was not intimidated by Dr. Neary. We leave aside for the moment the belief in Dr. Neary's mind that 75% of the hysterectomies, which he carried out in the first 10 years of his tenure, were justified by uterine frailty due to high parity or organ defect.

3.25   In trying to rationalise how resort to hysterectomy became systemically accepted or systemically ignored we considered the question of leadership. We are aware that designated leadership of hospital departments was probably confined to the Dublin maternity hospitals, which operate the 7 year Mastership system. During the entire period with which the Inquiry is concerned, there was no designated lead obstetrician at the Lourdes Maternity Unit. It seemed that no one had the authority to question outcomes or practices. Seniority, which was based on years of service, brought privileges, but no extra duties or responsibilities. Thus it did not occur to any of the *"senior"* consultants to review a colleague's work. Each consultant worked in his own way, at his own pace and there was no review of each other's outcomes or of outcomes generally. There was no maternity hospital manager and no one was entrusted with ensuring best clinical practice. There were no agreed protocols or practices for the maternity service. The consultants never worked in the presence of one another and rarely had the opportunity to observe their colleagues at work. We also noted that private patients seemed to occupy a different position to public patients. They were treated by the individual consultants and not seen by registrars or the other consultants except by prior arrangement. Many of the members of Patient Focus were private patients. Almost all of those members of Patient Focus who have undergone peripartum hysterectomy were operated on by Dr. Neary.

3.26 We are led to believe that it was normal in most hospitals with a small quota of consultants for the department not to review each other's outcomes. There was no recognisable peer review in this Maternity Unit during Dr. Neary's period there. With no designated lead consultant there was no system approaching the Mastership system, with its non-renewable tenure and the benefit of the introduction of new ideas to advance the practice of obstetrics and to improve the service offered to the public with each new Master. In the Dublin maternity hospitals it is the principal way in which a hospital can refurbish its ideas and keep itself up to date. This concept of changing leadership and renewal of ideas was sorely lacking in The Lourdes Maternity Hospital. None of the obstetricians employed there felt it was their duty to comment on or inquire into Dr. Neary's practice. Indeed, the evidence is that none of them was even aware of his practice of resort to hysterectomy at a relatively early stage.

3.27 If his colleagues were not aware of his practices we posed the question 'Why not?' They read the reports and they must have seen the postnatal ward daybooks. The personality of the consultants played a role. Dr. Connolly, the ageing senior obstetrician clearly saw Dr. Neary as skilled, energetic and hard working. He did not carry out tubal ligations or dispense the contraceptive pill or insert intrauterine devices. He admired his gynaecological skills and sometimes came in to observe him in his gynaecology list in theatre on Saturdays in the first year that he worked there. They appeared to get on well.

3.28 If Dr. Connolly the senior obstetrician said nothing, then Dr. O'Brien with his quiet, punctilious private manner would certainly not comment. The Inquiry concludes that during the early years of Dr. Neary's tenure, his colleagues were aware of the number of peripartum hysterectomies being carried out but they did not consider the possibility that something was wrong. They seem to have assumed that an obstetrician from Portsmouth and Hammersmith must be carrying out peripartum hysterectomy for good reason.

4   COMPARISONS WITH THE DUBLIN MATERNITY HOSPITALS

4.1   Dr. Neary told the Inquiry that he himself would from time to time wonder if the unit's caesarean hysterectomy rate was in accordance with accepted practice. He and Dr. Connolly discussed the rate and looked at the three Dublin maternity hospital annual reports for comparisons. In particular he says that they considered Dr. James Clinch's report of the 7 years of his Mastership of the Coombe Hospital in the period 1971-1977.

4.2   In that report, there is a chapter entitled *Hysterectomy with Pregnancy 1972-1977* (the records for 1971 were not complete). During this time, 70 such cases were detailed. The National Maternity Hospital at Holles Street recorded 23 hysterectomies in pregnancy for the same period. However, in 1970 there were 16 hysterectomies with pregnancy recorded in a year when only 262 caesarean sections were carried out. This rate is very similar to the rate at the Drogheda unit for the 1978/79 period. The Holles Street figures were not confined to caesarean hysterectomy and included all obstetric hysterectomy.

4.3   Dr. Neary believes that there is a possibility that the hysterectomy rate was under-reported at Holles Street as many ill mothers were transferred to St. Vincent's Hospital and may have had peripartum hysterectomies carried out there. He appeared to completely discount figures from the Rotunda Hospital although his reasoning was not clear. He told the Inquiry that he and Dr. Connolly were satisfied that their rate was not out of line with the Dublin hospitals where there were many extra pairs of experienced hands to cope with emergencies which occurred.

4.4   The total deliveries in Drogheda for the period 1971-1977 were 18,245. The total deliveries were 51,213 at Holles Street and 51,445 at the Coombe hospital for the same 7-year period. There were 15 peripartum hysterectomies carried out in the Lourdes Maternity Unit in that period. The level of peripartum hysterectomy was therefore not very remarkable when put alongside the Coombe hospital figures. The Coombe never reported such high rates again. Dr. Neary suggested that the rate was only honestly reported in Dr. Clinch's period as Master. Comparing hysterectomies to delivery rates can sometimes be misleading. Thus the rate in the Lourdes at that time was 1 hysterectomy for every 1216 deliveries while the Holles Street rate was 1 for every 2227 deliveries and the Coombe rate was 1 for every 735 deliveries.

4.5 When the reported hysterectomy rate in the Dublin hospitals fell to levels of between 1 and 3 per annum in the mid '80s, Dr. Neary attributed the fall to the availability of tubal ligation and a full range of contraceptive advice, both of which were forbidden in the Lourdes Hospital Maternity Unit. When the rates at the Lourdes Unit continued throughout the '80s to average about 7 a year, he maintained his view that their figures accorded with best practice within the unchanged ethos of the hospital. He believed then, and now, that if he had the right to advise effective contraception and tubal ligation to women whose uterus or health would make further pregnancy dangerous, his hysterectomy rate would have been reduced by 75%. The other 25% he attributed to peripartum haemorrhage.

4.6 The Inquiry heard ample evidence from Dr. Neary's consultant hospital colleagues that they considered him a skilled surgeon. They did not recognise that his judgement was flawed. They seem not to have considered what the Inquiry has been told frequently, that a skilled surgeon with flawed judgement has the potential to do more harm than a moderately skilled surgeon with excellent judgement. The Inquiry believes that somewhere along his career, Dr. Neary perceived hysterectomy as a haemorrhage preventative and lost sight of the norms operated in every other hospital in Ireland.

4.7 It is clear that Dr. Neary was unable to deal conservatively with serious bleeding and saw every haemorrhage as inevitably life threatening. He told the Inquiry that when he took up his post at the hospital he became aware of an extraordinary number of cases of Sheehan's syndrome, which he associated with haemorrhage. These women were chronically ill and unable to function as mothers and were very unlikely to have further children. He therefore had little faith in blood replacement as a method of buying time while trying to identify the source of bleeding. He did not apply procedures followed by other consultants of equal skill and training. Although very attentive to his work he was severely deficient in the capacity to critically review his own outcomes. He was visibly taken aback and shocked when confronted with the number of the hysterectomies that the Inquiry has attributed to him. He was unable to take comfort in either sterilisation or likely obstetric emergency in the table of young low parity women on whom hysterectomy was carried out. He was prepared to admit that during the 1990s his treatment of post partum haemorrhage was deficient.

5   WHY?

5.1   Although it was not a term of reference to establish why Dr. Neary performed the number of hysterectomies that he did (129), this question was frequently posed. It is relevant to why there was no comment or action taken on his rate of hysterectomy. The isolation of the unit recognised by the Medical Council played a large part in the lack of awareness that contributed to the lack of comment. The belief that the IMTH was somewhat superior to other hospitals in the area may also have played a part.

5.2   We considered whether there might have been a deficiency in his surgical technique.   Anaesthetists, junior doctors and nurses present in theatre with Dr. Neary described how he fussed about with swabbing, pressing, clipping and suturing while waiting for bleeding to stop and that he was slow to close the abdomen after caesarean section. He seemed unusually intolerant of bleeding. At the time, all those who worked with him saw this as a sign of a good surgeon.   With the benefit of hindsight, one consultant said that it was almost as if *"he anticipated the worst "*.

5.3   We considered whether he was as Dr. Connolly said, afraid of haemorrhage. One experienced father of five who had been present for all his children's births and who knew Dr. Neary well recounted a rather revealing story. Dr. Neary was delivering their fifth child. Both mother and father were quite relaxed even though the delivery was taking some time. There was some bleeding and the witness noticed to his surprise that Dr. Neary was visibly stressed with sweat flowing from his brow. He appeared agitated and suggested that the mother be taken to theatre for caesarean section. Both the witness and his wife had to reassure Dr. Neary that everything was all right but were unable to make him relax until the baby was born.

5.4   A junior doctor, now a consultant, who assisted Dr. Neary at caesarean sections, described how Dr. Neary became quite animated when he saw heavy bleeding and began to sweat profusely. He appeared outwardly calm and well in control, but the profuse sweating was for him a giveaway of inner fear. Others, with the benefit of hindsight, have recalled how Dr. Neary was quiet and tense until the placenta was out and the uterus sutured at which stage he became cheery and talkative. Dr. Neary told the Inquiry that this is quite normal as patients are awake and it is inappropriate to talk until the placenta is delivered.

5.5   Several obstetricians have advised that swabbing, dabbing and poking at the uterus and small bleeding points may have actually provoked bleeding in susceptible patients. Some patients have a propensity to bleed very briskly and heavily, and these seem to be the patients who triggered Dr. Neary's irrational anxieties. We were unable to discover the source of these irrational anxieties apart from his fear of triggering Sheehan's syndrome. The syndrome is defined as "*hypopituitarism developing postpartum as a result of pituitary necrosis; caused by ischemia resulting from a hypotensive episode during delivery*". Dr. Feeney advised that this condition is rarely seen nowadays because of treatments (including blood replacement) to maintain blood pressure and blood circulation.

5.6   The Inquiry postulates that Dr. Neary had an acutely heightened sense of danger and a morbid sensitivity to haemorrhage when carrying out surgery, especially at caesarean section. It is highly probable that fear of losing a patient approached phobic dimensions and led him to practise defensive medicine in one of its most extreme forms and probably explains why, from an early stage in his career, he expressed rather frequently to patients that the hysterectomy had "*saved your life.*"

5.7 Other examples of his heightened sense of danger are found in his reported fear that blood would not arrive in time, there would not be enough blood, or that the blood might not be fresh enough. We do not believe that Dr. Neary had any real insight into his propensity to exaggerate danger. Even at interview, he continued to say that particular patients would have died in theatre unless he prevented haemorrhage developing. He continues to believe that most of the hysterectomies, which he performed, would not have been necessary if tubal ligation had been permitted.

5.8 Although we have heard numerous accounts of Dr. Neary's attention to his patients and his capacity for hard work, we felt that there had to be some personality defect at play which prevented a competent and experienced surgeon from having insight into the effects of hysterectomy or oophorectomy on the psychological health of a woman. The dichotomy between his conservative stand on planned gynaecological hysterectomy and emergency obstetric hysterectomy was puzzling. A caring doctor should have been able to recognize that hysterectomy in a young woman was a heartbreak, even when carried out for cogent reason. He should have been able to compare his outcomes. He should have had the capacity to reflect and ask why so many of his patients ended up with hysterectomy when most patients of other consultants did not die or have hysterectomy.

5.9 We put the many media suggestions that he did not like or respect women to Dr. Neary. He responded that women were intuitive and knew if men did not like them. He said that he had a large practice and that women knew that these allegations were untrue. He furnished us with a list of midwives, nurses, doctors and doctors' wives who attended him. We asked Dr. Neary how his practices differed so much from the norm and queried why he did not keep up with changing standards. He stated that he would have welcomed the opportunity to be retrained and to observe other obstetricians at work. He worked very hard without respite for many years. He said that he was aware of the many criticisms that have been made against him in relation to his assessment of blood loss, the rate of blood loss, placental attachment, fundal defects or the effect of DIS. He said that at the time he reported his findings on the surgical notes, he genuinely believed that what he was describing was correct. When speaking to us, he appeared to have some insight into his practice of resort to hysterectomy at a low threshold generally, but he was prepared to defend individual cases. He expressed annoyance at the loss of key documents, as he was unable to defend his position without them. He suggested that someone with an agenda to harm him had removed the documents.

5.10 It was difficult not to have some sympathy for Dr. Neary when he was giving his evidence. His health is no longer strong. He is pilloried in the media and frequently referred to as a 'monster' or a 'mutilator of women' and the 'disgraced obstetrician'. The affect on his life is profound. He will never practise medicine again, and he will never be given the opportunity to see how and where he got it wrong.

5.11 **The consequences for his patients and for Dr. Neary himself make it poignantly obvious to the Inquiry that it is vital to have an objective review system in place in every hospital where outcomes are measured against accepted norms, and serious deviations are examined dispassionately for explanations.** It is not enough to be a caring surgeon or a hard working surgeon. Nice doctors are in a position to do great damage if they are inadequately trained, have poor judgement or have developed poor practices. They must go through regular retraining and skills assessment and their results must be subject to objective audit.

5.12 We spoke to other consultants who had worked in undermanned maternity hospitals. We were very impressed by the evidence of a former consultant in a typical 2 obstetrician provincial hospital in the 1970s and 80s. He described to us how from time to time he faced unexpected major haemorrhage in the small hours of the night and struggled going through his checklist of common causes for post partum haemorrhage. He (and many others) described just how terrifying uterine haemorrhage can be when blood wells up in massive volumes, or spurts in huge gushes and you wonder if you will lose the mother before your eyes. This retired consultant said that although he would know that the lab had been alerted, that the anaesthetist would soon be able to supply some blood, and that his colleague had been called, he nevertheless had to resist the very real temptation to carry out a hysterectomy while waiting to guarantee that the mother would not die. Very many obstetricians told us that their worst nightmare was that a mother would be lost in childbirth. The retired consultant told us that, contrary to what is generally believed, a caesarean hysterectomy carried out before the patient has collapsed is not a difficult operation; judgement and courage are therefore of supreme importance in deciding when it is appropriate and when one should hold on.

5.13 We learned that in a provincial hospital one did not have the luxury of a haematologist on hand; there was often only one other colleague and he or she may have been unavailable. The reassuring comfort of a second opinion, especially in the case of a young mother of low parity, was frequently not available. Obstetricians have sometimes to make hard choices between losing a patient and sacrificing fertility but there are generally guidelines worked out in advance for the management of these emergencies. In Dr. Neary's hospital, there was no protocol or guideline that required the opinion or assistance of another colleague before hysterectomy was carried out. There seemed to be no general agreement that blood and blood products would or should be used, if only to buy time until a second opinion was available. We heard no evidence to equate with that of the efforts made, or the heart stopping moments endured, before resorting to hysterectomy described by obstetricians in other provincial units. The ordinariness of the operation in this unit was disturbing.

6 **DID ANYONE IN THE LOURDES HOSPITAL COMMENT ON THE ANNUAL REPORTS BETWEEN 1974 AND 1984?**

6.1 We have found no evidence to suggest that any MMM, midwife, obstetrician or other consultant commented on the reports. Many MMMs and midwives stated that the reports were for doctors and were not made available to them. They were therefore unaware of the contents of the reports.

6.2 At the time, student nurses and midwives used a separate library to the doctors and it is possible that the annual reports were not furnished to the nurses' library. The reports were filed with the MMM archives. Many of the

MMMs were midwives or doctors. The Medical Director was an MMM. When Dr. Connolly and Dr.O'Brien were preparing the reports, they were assisted by members of staff who were MMMs. None of the MMMs to whom we spoke said that they were aware of the contents of the reports and thus made no comment and had no recollection of ever being made aware of any concerns arising from the reports.

6.3   There was concern however regarding Dr. Neary's resort to hysterectomy from two parties in the late '70s and in 1980. Thereafter, we found no evidence that any person expressed any concern until some midwives who assisted in theatre began whispering between themselves in the late '90s that there seemed to be a lot of young mothers having hysterectomies.

7   THE MATRON OF THE MATERNITY UNIT

7.1   Dr. Neary's recollections of concerns expressed regarding his rate of peripartum hysterectomy were mentioned previously. The Matron of the maternity hospital did express such concerns to Dr. Connolly, the senior consultant obstetrician but he told her not to worry, that Dr. Neary was *"afraid of haemorrhage"*. She spoke several times to him but he told her again that there was nothing to worry about and anyway that these were *"clinical matters"*. She felt that he was indicating to her that she should back off.

7.2   The Matron of the Maternity Unit tried speaking to Dr. O'Brien, the other obstetrician there, and his response was to indicate by gestures that she should not persist. He explained to the Inquiry that he was not responsible for other clinicians, he had no authority to question Dr. Neary, and any concerns that the Matron had should be raised with Dr. Neary's employers. He had to work with him.

7.3   Dr. O'Brien himself told us that he had no concerns that anything was amiss at the Maternity Unit, and he was unaware until he read about it in the newspapers that there was a high incidence of peripartum hysterectomy at the Maternity Unit at which he worked for 30 years. He was unaware of any climate of early resort to hysterectomy. He had no concerns regarding the figures in 1978/1979 or any concerns relating to any colleagues. He believes now that if he had been aware of the extent of Dr. Neary's figures, he would have been duty bound to act.

7.4   At the same time as the Matron was trying to express her misgivings to the consultants, Sr. F. a temporary midwifery tutor, also a Medical Missionary, had serious reservations relating to two caesarean hysterectomies carried out in late 1979 by Dr. Neary. It was not entirely clear whether her concerns were ethical concerns (about possible sterilisations), concerns for the patients, or a combination of both. She had been looking for interesting case histories to present to her midwifery students and had become aware that two young mothers who were patients in the postnatal ward had hysterectomies following caesarean section in and around the same time.

7.5   We believe that we have identified these cases but the charts are missing. We have confirmed that two hysterectomies were carried out in late August 1979, but the particulars in the pathology reports do not accord with the description given by the tutor. Both these patients would have been in the postnatal wards when the tutor took up her position.

7.6   Sr. F. followed up the cases and formed the view that neither the surgeon's notes nor the pathology reports revealed any findings to warrant hysterectomy. What followed afterwards is quite extraordinary. She did not contact any clinician outside the hospital to discuss her concerns; she did not discuss her concerns with the Medical Director who was a doctor and an MMM; she did not contact the pathologist; neither did she speak to the senior obstetrician Dr. Connolly. She spoke to a theatre sister, whose name she has forgotten, who indicated that Dr. Neary was resorting to hysterectomy any time he thought a patient would bleed. The tutor then tried to establish whether there were other hysterectomies being carried out, but was refused access to patient charts by secretarial staff on the basis of patient confidentiality.

7.7   When asked why she did not bring her concerns to her colleagues in the convent, this tutor told the Inquiry that in the MMM Order, there were strict rules about talking about patients, that no information about a patient could be brought over into the convent, and they were not allowed to discuss any patient at table.

7.8   She did not discuss her concerns with either of the two obstetricians who were available to her, nor did she discuss the cases with Dr. Neary. Instead, she sought advice from a theologian friend whom we subsequently learned was the Cardinal and whom Sr. F. said was *"not in Maynooth"*. He advised her that it was a matter for the doctors and that there was no legal imperative for any doctor to write any or all records on a patient's notes.

7.9   Apparently, her inquiries outside the hospital became known within the Maternity Unit and the identity of her adviser, a very senior Church figure, was recognised. The Matron called her in and admonished her for discussing problems outside the unit and was quite annoyed with her. A robust discussion ensued and the conversation eventually ended with an understanding that the Matron shared the same concerns and was taking care of the issue herself. The tutor believed that the Matron subsequently brought the issue before the Tripartite management committee of the MMMs, and that no more hysterectomies were carried out in the period for which she worked there. She left in October 1980.

7.10   The hospital was a small one, and the tutor was of the view that the obstetricians became aware that she had been looking at caesarean hysterectomy cases. She felt that Dr. Connolly went out of his way to tell her the details of a hysterectomy he had carried out subsequently, telling her that the reason for the hysterectomy was placenta accreta. He also subsequently provided her with laboratory information to assist her in teaching her students. She had no concerns about this hysterectomy. Pathology reports confirmed the clinical diagnosis of placenta accreta in the presence of placenta previa.

7.11   We met the tutor who was well educated, articulate and confident. The story is illustrative of hospital hierarchy in the past. Such a self possessed woman could not bring her concerns to the appropriate persons but felt she should seek advice from a church dignitary. She felt that she was not supported by the senior consultant and the Matron when she had the temerity to question a consultant. She expressed very deep regret that she did not follow her instincts and do more to stop Dr. Neary's practices in 1980.

7.12   The Matron of the Maternity Unit's strong and unshakeable memory of these events was that the Tripartite spoke to her about Dr. Neary's hysterectomies and asked her to check the records to ascertain the numbers. She believed that the tutor had herself raised her concerns before the Tripartite and they had thus called her in. The Matron believed that the Tripartite had called Dr. Neary before them to explain his numbers, and that he had reversed the argument by alleging that a registrar who had left the hospital recently had been carrying out covert sterilisations by tubal ligation at caesarean section. The Matron felt that the implication was that she had permitted such a state of affairs to occur, and that Dr. Neary had cleverly deflected attention away from him, forcing her to defend her position.

7.13   We spoke to the two surviving members of the Tripartite Committee for their recollections of any meeting relating to concerns about Dr. Neary's hysterectomy rate. Neither had any recollection of any meeting of the Tripartite with the tutor, the Matron or Dr. Neary about hysterectomies. They were adamant that if anyone had raised any issue over high hysterectomy rates, they would recall such a complaint. They disagreed with the Matron that any discussion had ever taken place with her regarding concerns about Dr. Neary's peripartum hysterectomy rate. They had no recollection of ever asking Dr. Neary to appear before the Tripartite. They did however have a recollection of allegations of tubal ligations carried out by the named registrar. They vaguely recalled that the allegations were investigated and disproved.

7.14   We asked Dr. Neary for his recollection of such a meeting. He was firmly of the view that he had never been asked to appear before the Tripartite for any reason, and that prior to October 1998, he was unaware that anyone had concerns about any of his practices. He did recall being called up before a meeting of what he believed to be a group of senior figures of the Order of Medical Missionaries in early 1981. The meeting he said was to warn him that he would lose his job if he were to consider carrying out a tubal ligation. He too had a recollection about the registrar and tubal ligations.

7.15   The background to this meeting with the MMMs is somewhat complex, but perhaps explains Dr. Neary's subsequent suspicious attitude towards the MMMs. The meeting was the culmination of a process, which commenced with a request from a patient with health problems for a tubal ligation to be carried out at time of caesarean section. Dr. Neary sought permission to carry out the tubal ligation at time of caesarean section, relying on affirmative advice obtained by the patient from Dr. O'C, a moral theologian in Maynooth, on the facts of the case. It is probable that this was the meeting where Dr. Neary was asked to explain his position, and that he may have raised the spectre of the registrar who was reputed to be carrying out tubal ligations.

7.16   Dr. Neary told the Inquiry that he had to give an undertaking to the group of MMMs that he would never carry out tubal ligations for any reason, and he had to apologise to the Order and to his colleagues. Dr. Neary's account of this meeting before the senior MMMs appeared a little far-fetched at first glance, but analysis proved less certain. This is dealt with later in this chapter (paragraph 15.28). Dr. Neary is adamant that such a meeting took place and provided many details. The MMM sisters to whom we spoke did not accept the veracity of this evidence.

7.17   Transparency was not a characteristic of the management of this hospital. The Matron, who occupied a very senior post, was told only what her employers the MMMs chose to tell her. She did not feel that it was her place to seek information and she did not participate in the tripartite management. In such an atmosphere, gossip and speculation thrive. Thus the Matron of the Maternity Unit believed that the tutor had informed the Tripartite and they then came to her as a result of that information. The tutor believed that the Matron of the Maternity Unit had gone to the Tripartite on her own concerns. The Tripartite members say they knew nothing about either party's concerns and were not approached by either party.

7.18   The Matron's recollection is that she was informed by the Tripartite that Dr. Neary blamed her for failing to notice that a junior doctor had been carrying out sterilisations at caesarean section. She examined all 40 caesarean sections carried out by that named doctor and found no evidence to confirm this allegation. In fact, out of 40 caesarean sections, 37 women had had subsequent babies and the remaining 3 were no longer of childbearing age. A perusal of the hospital's ethics file reveals a document that could well be the analysis of these caesarean sections, which disproved the allegations of tubal ligations.

7.19   It is probable that the request to carry out a tubal ligation had taken centre stage in 1981. The Matron of the Maternity Unit may have heard rumours that Dr. Neary had been brought up before the Tripartite and assumed that this meeting was connected to the caesarean hysterectomies, whereas he was called up before an infinitely more august body of the MMMs. The convenors of this meeting perhaps did not feel it their duty to inform the Tripartite, or indeed the Matron, who was involved in dealing with Dr. Neary's request for clarification on the tubal ligation issue. Thus it is possible that the Tripartite simply did not know.

7.20   The Matron of the Maternity Unit was interviewed a second time but was unwell at the time. She was shown portions of the transcripts from the MMMs denying any conversations or meetings with the Tripartite regarding Dr. Neary. She remained positive that she was called by the Tripartite to investigate the numbers of caesarean hysterectomies carried out by Dr. Neary in the late 1970s.

7.21   It is clear that some meetings took place before either the Tripartite or the 3 consultants but the subject is unclear although there is the strong probability that the stories have become confabulated with the passage of time. The Matron believes that Dr. Neary was aware that she was the complainant, as thereafter her life was made very difficult with him. There is confirmation that he treated with her little respect. She felt that the support that she received from the MMMs in relation to her subsequent treatment by Dr. Neary could have been stronger. She remains convinced that in spite of her efforts, she was unable to gather any support for her concerns about Dr. Neary, either from her employers or from the other consultants who always, she believed, supported each other. She also believes that many hysterectomies carried out in the unit over the period during which she was Matron were sterilisations.

7.22   In spite of the ineffectual efforts of the Matron and the tutor to raise their concerns, the peripartum hysterectomy rate continued generally to be excessive, averaging 6 or 7 per annum over the next 10 years. Dr. Neary carried out the vast majority of those hysterectomies. The Matron of the Maternity Unit felt that her efforts to bring her concerns before the Tripartite succeeded only in victimising her. If she ever mentioned anything about Dr. Neary again to the now senior obstetrician, Dr. O'Brien, he indicated by gestures that he would not enter into any discussion on the subject. She believed, as did the tutor, that the rate of hysterectomy fell after 1980. The tutor believed that no hysterectomies were carried out in the remaining twelve months of her tenure. They were both incorrect. Whatever the truth of the conversations which occurred, the hysterectomy rate remained unchanged from the late 1970s.

7.23   From time to time, the Matron of the Maternity Unit tried to raise her concerns, but she was fearful of legal consequences if she were wrong. She was not altogether confident that she was correct and sought explanations or reassurance from others. Many witnesses described to us an occasion where a patient whose husband was a doctor had a hysterectomy following her first baby. They felt that surely if anything was wrong with Dr. Neary's practice, this couple would have complained or sued. The Matron firmly believes that the Tripartite must have investigated the reason for so many hysterectomies during the late 1970s and approved as otherwise Dr. Neary would not have been able to continue. She believes that if anything needed to be done then either the MMMs or Dr. O'Brien would have taken steps to prevent any abuses.

7.24   Both the Matron of the Maternity Unit and the temporary tutor told the Inquiry that they believed that the Maternity Unit had been inspected by the Medical Council and the RCOG, and was fully accredited. The Matron believed that the Medical Council had actually investigated Dr. Neary's practices and reviewed his files.[14] Believing that her fears were not supported, she decided thereafter to concentrate on midwifery matters and the welfare of her staff. She was a valiant warrior for her nurses and took on the consultants if they were rude to the midwives or if they were too demanding. She firmly believed that the consultants' common contract allowed them total clinical independence to the extent that they were untouchable where clinical practices were concerned.

7.25   The Matron tried several more times in the mid '90s to draw attention to the caesarean hysterectomy issue within the unit by calling meetings on the caesarean section rate in the hopes of lowering the caesarean hysterectomy rate. Her attempts were apprehensive and hesitant, as she feared Dr. Neary's wrath and feared that he could sue her for defamation. Her attempts came to nothing as Dr. Neary either failed to attend the meetings, or left them in anger.

7.26   She told the Inquiry that she was aware that the hysterectomy rate was high so when finally a new consultant came to the unit, she decided to speak to him. She expressed her concern at the high rate of hysterectomy. She recounted how he listened without comment. Dr. O'Coigligh, the new Consultant who replaced Dr. O'Brien in late 1997, had no recollection of the Matron of the Maternity Unit speaking to him. He explained that if she said she spoke to him that he would not dispute it and he suggested that his reason for not remembering such a conversation with the Matron was that he could have thought that she was talking about hysterectomies in general and not caesarean hysterectomies. For some time before this, with the introduction of the Mirena coil, the modern practice of gynaecology was moving away from hysterectomy for dysfunctional bleeding in pre menopausal patients. He believed that she may have been speaking of the continuing practice of carrying out hysterectomy for dysfunctional bleeding in this group of patients. He had absolutely no idea that there was any practice of early resort to hysterectomy in the Maternity Unit and was very shocked

---

[14] The Inquiry found no evidence to support this belief. While the Unit was approved for training of SHOs and registrars, there was no evidence of any peer review of Dr. Neary's hysterectomies

and surprised when he was informed by the Medical Director of the number of hysterectomies identified from the theatre register.

7.27 The Matron of the Maternity Unit is very glad that Dr. Neary was asked to resign, but she nevertheless reminded us that he did a great deal of good as well as harm. Although Dr. Neary did not treat her well or with respect, her loyalty to the Unit was such that she found it difficult not to defend their consultants. In her period of more that 25 years as a Matron, she never attended a course in management skills, assertiveness, risk management or audit. Her long years working with the MMMs moulded her into a caring and deeply committed, but submissive nurse with no confidence to take her concerns to a higher level, or to follow through on them. Many of the nurses we interviewed fitted the same mould.

8   THE MIDWIVES

8.1 All midwifery students are subject to the same syllabus prepared and approved by An Bord Altranais. The standard textbook for midwifery students is 'Myles', published by Churchill Livingstone. Every midwife learns about post partum haemorrhage and the conditions which give rise to such haemorrhage. The textbook goes through each condition and describes the treatment. In all the editions that have been furnished to us by An Bord Altranais, post partum haemorrhage is described as one of the most serious complications in obstetrics, and the woman's life depends on the midwife's prompt, intelligent action. The textbooks state that the commonest causes of post partum haemorrhage is atonic uterus (the uterus fails to contract in the third stage of labour). They are taught massage and bimanual compression of the uterus and to call a doctor if that fails. They are made aware of placental attachment difficulties and they are taught that, except when a dire emergency arises and no medical help is available, a manual removal takes place in theatre with a registrar or consultant. The various editions of Myles Textbook for Midwives state:

"Morbid adherence of placenta – very rarely, the placenta remains morbidly adherent: this is known as placenta accreta.   If it is totally adherent then bleeding is unlikely to occur and it may be left in situ to absorb during the

puerperium if, however, only part of the placenta remains embedded, the risks of fatal haemorrhage are high and an emergency hysterectomy may be unavoidable."

8.2   The midwives are trained to look after mothers in the delivery suite. It is not part of their normal training to assist in theatre. Midwives are not therefore involved in surgical decisions on methods of treatment. Most of the hysterectomies that concern the Inquiry are associated with caesarean section in theatre where the midwives acted as theatre assistants rather than as clinical practitioners.

8.3   Obedience was part and parcel of the training of nurses and the rule in a convent. One midwife reminded us that when she was a student nurse that if you broke a thermometer, you paid for its replacement. Student nurses had to live in the nurses' home. Until the late 1990s, almost all of the tutors and the instructors were MMMs. The nurses were taught that anticipating the consultant's needs was the sign of a well-trained nurse. Nurses did not question nuns or ward sisters and they certainly did not question consultants. The nurses operated in a very hierarchical atmosphere. There were more qualified nurses than there were jobs for nurses to fill. Financial constraints in the health system meant that staff shortages were common and services stretched to the limit. Hospitals depended on student nurses to fill staff quotas on wards.

8.4   There is much to recommend hierarchy when escalation of rank is based on degrees of competence and experience. With rising rank comes rising authority and responsibility. Respect for authority, obedience to directions and accountability at every level of the chain of command are part and parcel of the orderly running of a modern hospital. Unfortunately, in this unit the training seems to have produced a large body of nurses and junior doctors who were not expected to have authority or to be accountable and who looked only at their particular task in hand and looked no further. This began to change in the Lourdes Maternity Unit only when it was clear that the Health Board was taking over and outside influences began to penetrate the hospital

8.5   If it were in the power of the Inquiry to make an award of bravery to any person, it would be to the midwife who we shall call Ann who made the first complaint to the North Eastern Health Board solicitor. She came from the North of Ireland and was trained as a nurse and midwife in the Royal Victoria Hospital in Belfast. She came to work in the Maternity Unit in Drogheda in late September 1997. Even though she had more than five years previous experience as a Staff Midwife in a very busy maternity hospital, she was engaged on a temporary basis. This is a reminder, if one were necessary, that even in 1997, the good times had not arrived and permanent nursing jobs were still a scarce commodity.

8.6   Ann painted a picture of a very inward looking Maternity Unit where intense loyalty was shown to the obstetricians working there; where midwives looked after mothers for routine deliveries and obstetricians looked after problem pregnancies or private patients. The percentage of private patient deliveries was in the region of 50%. The nurses' duties were task oriented with little continuity of patient care and the concept of patient advocacy was unknown. Some of the practices like carrying out rectal instead of vaginal examinations were new to her. She found a unit where tensions existed between Senior Sisters and Junior Nurses, and where traditional loyalties to the former owners of the hospital conflicted with Health Board administrators. In particular, she observed major tension between nursing management in the Maternity Unit and in the general hospital.

8.7   Ann made her concerns regarding a caesarean hysterectomy carried out by Dr. Neary known to her colleagues immediately after an incident in theatre, where she questioned why she should *"fetch the hysterectomy clamps"*. Her colleagues either did not wish to countenance such criticisms, or found reasons to disprove her perceptions. She did not share her colleagues' admiration of Dr. Neary and found him opinionated and difficult. She found that his practices were outdated and too interventionist. She was appalled to see that he only did midline incisions for caesarean section. He carried out episiotomies routinely on women who had already had children, he put women in the lithotomy position when she had not seen this practice for years and she was generally unimpressed by what she observed.

8.8   There was no forum for expressing her concerns. She became particularly upset when she saw that hysterectomy was carried out with some regularity, and that some of the patients were young women. Her colleagues told her that she had no evidence so she had taken to carefully documenting what she saw in theatre. She nagged her colleagues constantly and was beginning to see some shift in opinion. She was told however that there was nothing anyone could do unless a patient actually complained. It was explained to her by her colleagues that consultants were clinically independent. They could not be questioned about their procedures. In particular, one could not interfere with the treatment of private patients.

8.9   On October 22nd 1998, Ann was asked to make a statement to the Health Board Solicitor regarding an allegation that an anaesthetist on call had refused to attend and the incident was being investigated. She determined to use the opportunity to ask if clinical independence went so far that questions could not be asked about serious concerns.

8.10   We heard from the staff midwife Bridget who accompanied Ann to the interview with Mr. Gary Byrne, the solicitor for the Health Board, and who had supported Ann. We heard how the Health Board moved with speed to establish whether the perceptions held by the two midwives deserved serious consideration. When the complaints were deemed to have validity, Dr. Neary was invited to attend to discuss the concerns.

8.11   In trying to determine whether any of the midwives – apart from the Matron of the Maternity Unit - had previously raised comments or concerns on Dr. Neary's practices, we spoke to the current and former senior midwifery sisters and most of the theatre nurses who were present for many of the hysterectomies carried out in the unit. We can say generally that the midwives divided down into a number of groups:

A.   Those who had **absolutely no concerns** at any stage about any of the obstetricians in the unit or any of the operations, which were carried out. They accepted **then** and **now** that all procedures were carried out for appropriate reasons, which were given to them by the obstetricians or the registrars involved. This group forms a **small minority** of the midwives and it caused us some concern that even at this remove, they were not prepared to accept that there could be legitimate concerns surrounding many of the hysterectomies which had been carried out, and at which they had attended as theatre nurses. They never made any comments relating to Dr. Neary's frequent resort to hysterectomy and they appeared unconvinced that the Inquiry is either useful or necessary. These midwives used very similar language, which sometimes made us suspect that they had had discussions in a group in relation to what they were going to say. They described how they were *"disempowered"* by the consultants, how they were *"handmaidens to the consultants"*, how their job was to anticipate the consultants' needs and how they were trained to look after routine deliveries only. They had no concerns ever and wanted to "move on".

B. The next group of midwives, and these were by far the largest group, struck us as decent, hard-working caring women who are **now deeply shocked** at the extent of the hysterectomies. Most of these midwives were tearful when giving their testimony and blamed themselves for never even suspecting that anything was amiss. They had known, liked and admired Dr. Neary and never dreamed that there could be any questioning of the reason given for the removal of a mother's uterus. They had appreciated his kindness to them over the years and while they accepted that he had his humours and he was difficult to challenge, they believe that *"he never deliberately meant to harm anyone"*.

Some of this group of midwives who enjoyed working with Dr. Neary had much good to say of him. They described how he was always available, and how he was very kind and helpful to junior doctors even when not on call. He regularly covered for the other consultants, always gave reasons to assistants in surgery for the hysterectomy, patients loved him and he was very popular with staff and families. They described him as a very dedicated doctor who really cared about his patients. He was always willing to come in to assist. He was very good in a crisis and superb at resuscitating newborns. He was very strict about asepsis and very few of his patients had returns to theatre or suffered from infection. They also liked the fact that he was supportive of modern family planning methods and critical of church hypocrisy. He was the first consultant who knew and used their first names. He was the only consultant who helped to lift patients from the operating table to the trolley. He was a very good gynaecologist.

They described another consultant to us and told us how his strict attitude filled them with fear and dread. He did not tolerate conversation. The same applied to patients who were to be in their beds with tables tidied and blankets and sheets turned down in a certain manner when he was doing rounds. His methods in theatre were difficult. He operated in silence, insisting that each instrument he required was placed without comment on the patient's body. The job of the theatre nurse was to anticipate his needs. Mistakes were not tolerated. To these midwives, it was a relief when Dr. Neary was on duty. He treated them as humans and spoke to them. He was *"great at telling stories"*.

This group never commented, as they had no concerns until perhaps 1998. Then because of Ann and some other theatre midwives, they began to wonder if there was another way to deal with post partum haemorrhage. Some of this group wondered if perhaps some of the hysterectomies were sterilisations although very few actually assisted at such a sterilising hysterectomy. One of the midwives who had worked there for many years said of peripartum hysterectomy *"It was there when I arrived – it continued to be there – for the want of a word and I hate using it, it was accepted practice or the norm – it was part of what happened – it wasn't questioned…"*

A number of this group who never questioned, wondered or compared the number of peripartum hysterectomies with those in other hospitals, did say that they found Dr. Neary *"heavy handed"* and went to Dr. O'Brien for their own deliveries.

They described to us how it was inconceivable that a nurse or midwife at the Lourdes Hospital would dream of questioning the clinical judgement of a consultant. This was not part of their training and they were unhappy at the concept that they should be expected to question a consultant and especially one of Dr. Neary's stature.

Within this group there was another small group of midwives who were unhappy but had grown used to not being listened to. They mentioned their concerns to each other but believed that, as the Matron and her assistant were aware from the day sheets of the hysterectomies, they were the appropriate persons to do something. They believed that Matron had discussed the matter with the Medical Director and that everyone knew. They were aware that peripartum hysterectomy was necessary in certain cases and were not confident that their concerns were well founded. They described a number of reasons for why they were not confident that there was anything wrong with Dr. Neary's practices. There were two new consultants in the unit who surely were aware of current practice. The new anaesthetist had been present for hysterectomies and had made no adverse comments. The new obstetrician had carried out two hysterectomies himself. A colleague had undergone a hysterectomy and had made no complaint. In at least one hysterectomy case, Mr. Lennon a general surgeon had been called in to assist when a ureter had been nicked. He had not said anything to Dr. Neary regarding the hysterectomy. They knew that Dr. Neary did not like bleeding but not every haemorrhage ended in hysterectomy. While unhappy they had no confidence in the validity of their concerns.

C. The third small group consisted of junior midwives, some were staffed and others were on temporary contracts – not students as frequently reported - who were beginning to have some deep misgivings about the fact that many young rather than older mothers of high parity had undergone caesarean hysterectomy. The newer midwives had come from hospitals with full family planning procedures and did not countenance that hysterectomies carried out on older women with three or more children might be sterilisations. Instead they were beginning to be seriously alarmed at the number of cases of hysterectomy on women of low parity in their twenties. One of this group who had had worked in the Unit for many years accepted that women of high parity did have sterilising hysterectomies. She believed that Dr. Neary was more likely to carry out hysterectomy than the other consultants and thus chose to have her babies outside the Lourdes Maternity Unit. Several other midwives did likewise when one of their own peer group, a private patient of Dr. Neary, had undergone a caesarean hysterectomy following the birth of her first baby. This midwife was seen as *"one of Dr. Neary's favourites"*. This operation under spinal block rather than general anaesthetic, took place in the latter half of 1996.

The hysterectomy on this midwife who was seen as *"one of Dr. Neary's favourites"* caused different reactions in the midwives. Those who did not share the concerns of the younger midwives relating to the youth of the mothers having hysterectomies saw this operation as proof that Dr. Neary could not legitimately be criticised. The one or two midwives who believed that something was not right were furious. One midwife Fiona, who was a close friend of the patient, was very distressed and asked the Matron for something to be done. This operation coincided with the period during which Dr. Neary's wife died from uterine cancer, and it is very probable that natural sympathy to him combined with the lack of any complaint from the midwife who had undergone caesarean hysterectomy caused the matter to go no further.

Following the hysterectomy on the midwife, the Matron who had harboured concerns for years went with the labour ward superintendent to make enquiries of the theatre staff and anaesthetist who had been present. Although upset to see such an operation on one of their colleagues and to have witnessed her pleading with Dr. Neary not to carry out the operation, they had no concerns regarding the necessity for the hysterectomy. The anaesthetist noted heavy bleeding, and the midwives present remembered that Dr. Neary explained that there was a defect in the uterus due to the patient's mother taking diethylstilbestrol to suppress lactation. They also noted that while the patient had begged Dr. Neary not to do the hysterectomy, she and her husband had given their consent after the explanations. The senior midwives could do no more, as it seemed that all those present felt that the hysterectomy was necessary. Fiona remained doubtful.

D. In a group on her own was another midwife who shall be called Dara. She came to the Lourdes Hospital in late 1997. Her training was outside the unit and she was working as a part time practice development nurse and a temporary midwifery tutor. She had been invited by Sister D. and Director of Nursing M.D. to review some midwifery practices in the unit. She was taken aback by some of the practices that she observed there.

"There were no guidelines, no systems in place, everything was dictated by unwritten policies and most of the time you just didn't know where you stood– they said that's the way we do it around here and you just had to accept practice. Basically, it was all led by the Obstetricians. The hospital managers or the midwifery managers had very little say in how they managed the midwifery services not just the obstetric services and the practice was very, very – what I probably would have expected 20 years ago – it was like coming back – it was like coming back to work in Jervis Street, I remember that's exactly what I thought actually, that's what it was like."

"You weren't allowed to think, you weren't allowed to articulate an opinion or you weren't allowed to participate in trying to develop anything and that was the way it was – that wasn't just my initial thinking on it."

Dara noted that to her amazement, although the unit was short staffed, much valuable midwifery time was spent in sterilising and packing theatre instruments. In every other hospital in which she worked, the packs were purchased ready packed and autoclaved or nursing assistants carried out the work. She noticed that mercury thermometers were still in use. She noted the use of the lithotomy position and the practice of rectal examinations. She noted the lack of meetings. Her attempts to modernise some midwifery practices were not always well received. While most of the midwives expressed enthusiasm for change, their participation was poor. She felt that the role of practice development midwife was perceived as *"more interference from the new Director of Nursing"* in the general hospital. She tried to set up journal clubs and additional lectures on chosen midwifery subjects to encourage awareness and engender open discussion within the unit. The attendance at these talks was poor.

9   HOW DID THE STORY BREAK?

9.1   In early October 1998, Professor C.B. from the Midwifery School of Nursing at TCD attended at the hospital in Drogheda to arrange a programme of lectures to a group of 20 midwives over a period of several weeks. Towards the end of the programme, Prof. C.B. was talking to the group about assertiveness and asked if the group had any issues or dilemmas they wished to discuss. Ciara who was one of the small group of staff midwives who had concerns asked Prof. C.B. about caesarean hysterectomies and said, *"We seem to have a lot of them"*. Prof. C.B. expressed shock at what she was hearing, but the brave young midwife Ciara found herself unsupported by her senior colleagues. Some went so far as to say that they saw no problem, while most kept silent.

9.2   A desultory discussion followed but petered out as the midwife Ciara began to lose confidence in her stand. Her evidence of that meeting has been totally corroborated by Prof. C.B. who noted the divisions and discomfort in her audience. She asked if they would like her to do anything about the query but was told that they would deal with it themselves. Prof. C.B. furnished the Inquiry with a list of attendees at the course. The list included some senior midwives who the Inquiry would put in Group **A** above.

9.3   Ciara who spoke up to Prof. C.B., had been trained as a nurse and then a midwife in large Dublin university hospitals and therefore had comparators against which to measure her experience in the Lourdes. She described how she was subsequently criticised by the new Assistant Matron of the Maternity Unit, Sr. D. for being unprofessional for disclosing confidential patient information to Prof. C.B. and felt deeply upset. Sr. D. who was in office as Assistant Matron for less than 1 year denied that such criticism or conversation ever occurred. We prefer the evidence of the junior midwife, as there was corroboration from others that she had been *"picked on"* and was suspected of being the whistleblower. While it would be unfair to hold Sr. D. responsible for the unquestioning attitudes over the years, we nevertheless found that her personal attitude puts her in the group of midwives described in the **A** group above. Sr. D. recalled vivid memories of patients who had died because hysterectomy was not carried out.

9.4   Within a very short time of the lectures provided by Prof. C.B. and around mid-October 1998, the practice midwife Dara was lecturing final year midwifery students on the treatment of post partum haemorrhage. One of the students told her about a caesarean hysterectomy on a 20 year old primigravida which had taken place a week or so previously. The student's understanding was this was one of the acceptable treatments for post partum haemorrhage.

9.5 Dara had been a midwife for close to 20 years and had never experienced a caesarean hysterectomy and doubted that what the student was saying could be true. When next on the wards, she followed up on the case and discovered that everything the student had reported was accurate. Later in the week, Dara discussed her anxiety with Ann, the midwife from Belfast, Ciara, another of the seriously concerned group and Elaine, a midwife who had been working in theatre, and they exchanged views about whom they could go to with their now deep concerns about Dr. Neary. Elaine referred Dara to where she would find records of peripartum hysterectomies in the maternity theatre register. It is worthy of note that Ann, Ciara, Dara and Elaine all trained outside the Lourdes.

9.6 Dara received this information and made it her business to review the maternity theatre register and count the number of caesarean hysterectomy entries for 1998. She did not make a written record of her findings but believed that the figure was 12 or 13. She was very alarmed and decided to take the matter out of the Maternity Unit and went to M.D., the Director of Nursing. Dara was aware that Ann, with whom she had shared her apprehensions, was due to consult with the Health Board solicitor on a completely unrelated matter that day and that she planned to use the opportunity to raise the hysterectomy issue with him.

9.7 On the same day that Ann and Bridget, (the two midwives involved with the allegation against the anaesthetist) were talking to the solicitor, another hysterectomy was carried out in the maternity theatre. Ciara, the young midwife who had spoken to Prof. C.B., had some involvement in the care of this patient and determined to speak to the Assistant Matron. She brought with her to the Matron's office the patient's chart and also that of the 20 year old primigravida on whom Dr. Neary had carried out the hysterectomy earlier that month. She believed that her concerns were not treated seriously. She was not even invited to sit down. The Matron explained to Ciara that the patient was a high risk case as she had placenta previa and placenta accreta, and generally tried to allay Ciara's now serious concerns. The Matron did not appear to accept Ciara's assertion that other maternity hospitals did not have the same incidence of caesarean hysterectomy and that she had trained in a very busy Dublin maternity hospital where caesarean hysterectomy was a very rare event. The Matron tried to persuade Ciara that there could not be a problem with Dr. Neary's practices as the new consultant who had come to the unit had never seen a caesarean hysterectomy before, and yet he had done two since he came.

9.8   In fairness to that Matron, although she belongs to the group who find it hard to accept that Dr. Neary carried out unnecessary hysterectomies we know that in spite of her benevolent explanations, she had sufficient concern to bring the file and pathology report of the 20 year old patient to show to Dr. O'Coigligh and to seek his view.

9.9   Dr. O'Coigligh, who had just been made a permanent consultant, felt embarrassed at being asked to comment on a senior colleague's management of a private patient. He had already had a serious run-in with Dr. Neary, when his use of the theatre had delayed the commencement of Dr. Neary's list. Dr.O'Coigligh looked very briefly at the file and told Matron that it seemed to be in order. He explained his situation to the Inquiry and told us that he had absolutely no idea that there was any problem at that time and he additionally felt quite intimidated by Dr. Neary.

9.10   On October 23rd. 1998, M.D. the Director of Nursing, who had now been made aware of the 2 recent hysterectomy cases, came down to the Maternity Unit seeking to view the relevant patient files. She did not feel welcome and her questioning was treated defensively. Ciara, the midwife who had expressed her concerns to the Matron the night before brought the two charts to M.D. but one of the histology reports was missing. The charts had remained on Ciara's desk overnight. Fortunately, a copy was obtained from the pathology department and M.D. was able to acquaint herself with the details. Ciara recounted her concerns to M.D. and told her of her attempt to raise the issue with Prof. C.B.. She was assured that something would be done this time.

9.11 Later that day, while M.D. was relating what she had learned in the Maternity Unit to the Medical Director Mr. Lennon, they received a phone call from the CEO of the Health Board informing them of what he had just learned from Mr. Gary Byrne, the Health Board solicitor. The following Tuesday, Dr. Neary was asked to take administrative leave.

9.12 M.D., who was the Director of Nursing since 1996, had never been made aware that there was a problem with peripartum hysterectomies. The data that she received from the unit for the previous year revealed only 1 such operation. None of her predecessors, whether sisters of the MMMs or lay Directors of Nursing, were ever notified officially of the numbers. We interviewed all of these officeholders. Their evidence confirmed that this was a very isolated Maternity Unit, which kept its own counsel and did not integrate with the general hospital. Any concerns were kept to themselves especially after the arrival of the Director of Nursing M.D. in 1996.

9.13 When asked by the Inquiry how the unit reacted to the news that something was indeed done this time, Ciara felt that her colleagues were shocked at the news that Dr. Neary was under investigation but that many were quietly relieved that the matter had been brought to a head and was now out in the open. Some others were less pleased and continued to defend Dr. Neary's practices. Several midwives felt that Ciara was identified as the whistleblower and to some extent victimised.

10 THE PATHOLOGISTS

10.1 The senior and very first of the pathologists, now retired (1993), had been the sole pathologist since the foundation of the hospital until 1981. He was one of the original 4 consultants in the hospital. He was there with the late Dr. Connolly in the early days and held him in the highest esteem. He worked as a pathologist at a time when maternal deaths were annual occurrences and he was aware that hysterectomy following birth was a life saving procedure.

10.2 His previous experience, working as a pathologist in Bath in the 1950s, was that peripartum hysterectomy was a not uncommon occurrence. He also believed that *"compassionate"* hysterectomies were carried out from time to time in Ireland when another pregnancy was dangerous for the mother. Tubal ligation was not an available option in Catholic hospitals, and thus hysterectomy was 'an Irish solution to an Irish problem'. Nothing was said and the good judgement of the surgeon was always assumed.

10.3 He was aware of the prohibition of any contraceptive therapy at the hospital at that time. This tacit 'turning a blind eye' to what was assumed to be a humane practice may have laid the ground in the pathology department for the lack of questioning of the hysterectomies carried out at the Maternity Unit in later years. It was assumed that all hysterectomies were carried out for a valid reason. He was unaware that there were any concerns relating to the unit generally. The department was very busy, although the Maternity Unit was not a major user of pathology services.

10.4 He recalled a brief conversation when his new colleague came in 1981. The new pathologist had received a perinatal uterus specimen and remarked that he did not find anything wrong with it. The senior consultant responded *"that's Michael Neary for you"*. He told the Inquiry that if he himself received a hysterectomy specimen removed for haemorrhage and if he could find nothing wrong with it, he would think no more about it because it could have been a functional failure of the uterus that caused the haemorrhage, and there would be no evidence of that in the specimen received.

10.5 He believed that the nuns ran the hospital and that the Medical Board had no power other than to advise the nuns. The then Medical Superintendent, who was a doctor, was a member of the MMMs and sat in on every meeting of the Medical Board. He believed that everything that happened in the hospital was known by the MMMs.

10.6 He said he was unaware of the cumulative number of pregnant uteri samples received in the pathology lab. However, he accepted that with hindsight, he had an impression of perhaps more uteri than usual, but there was usually a time interval between them with several hundreds or thousands of other specimens in between.

10.7   He did not know what number would be the norm and at the time had no concerns. There was no real place for a pathologist with concerns to go, apart from a personal word with the consultant himself. He recalled regular clinico-pathological conferences with surgeons but never with the obstetricians. He had never attended a perinatal mortality conference in Drogheda. If they happened, then he had not been invited.

10.8   He was aware that Dr. Neary had a bigger practice than the other two obstetricians combined and therefore expected that his specimen rate would be higher than from the other consultants in the unit. He had no idea to what extent Dr. Neary resorted to peripartum hysterectomy but had the impression when talking to the Inquiry that the rate might have risen after he retired in 1993. He had no figures and never heard anyone mention any concerns. No one ever associated the hysterectomies with sterilisations with him, but he had his own benign suspicions that consultants cared for their patients' well being and might have to do a hysterectomy to prevent further pregnancy.

10.9   The first pathologist stated that he would never furnish a report on a uterus without measuring it and describing its condition. If there were sutures there he would comment on them. He would never report placenta accreta unless chorionic villi were present and seen to be infiltrating the myometrium. If he said there was no evidence of chorionic tissue any competent obstetrician would know that he found no evidence of placenta accreta.

10.10   Dr. Neary never consulted him about any specimen. He would report on the specimen and the written report would go to Dr. Neary and that was the end of it. He had no further function. Although they were friendly, he never discussed any specimen with him. He was unaware of the Dublin hospital rates or of the international figures. He never commented on Dr. Neary's practice other than to make the comment reported. We could not quite fathom what "that's Michael for you" meant but we do not believe that he ever considered the possibility that Dr. Neary was deliberately causing harm.

10.11   The second pathologist confirmed to the Inquiry that when he was appointed (1981) he noted healthy looking uteri arriving down from the maternity theatre.

He had worked in other large hospitals but had seen very few uteri specimens emerging from the maternity theatres. As his queries did not elicit more than *"that's Michael Neary for you"*, he was not inclined to take the matter further. His colleague had no concerns.

10.12 He explained that he was the junior consultant and shared his sessions with Louth County Hospital. He felt that he was very much the *"junior pathologist"* and not perceived as an equal consultant. He believes that he may have discussed Dr. Neary's hysterectomies with one of the senior MMMs, but could not be positive on this. It was his view that the consultant obstetricians in the Maternity Unit, which was the flagship of the hospital, were untouchable and beyond criticism. It was his view that the nuns in the hospital were aware of everything that went on in the hospital and ran it with an iron fist. He felt that any problems that he raised with MMM management were ignored and he felt powerless to effect any change in the hospital.

10.13 It was interesting to hear that Dr. Neary held very similar views on the status of consultants. Dr. Neary believed that as far as the MMMs were concerned, there were only 4 consultants, and they were the foundation consultants, Dr. Connolly, Dr. Costello, Mr. Sheehan and Dr. O'Flynn. All the others were *"assistants"* to the original consultants. Dr. Neary felt that he was treated as 'a slave' when he first arrived. He also believed that nothing happened without the knowledge and awareness of the MMMs. He believed that he was not treated with respect.

10.14 In spite of the hysterectomies, both pathologists were aware of Dr. Neary's reputation for being a hard working consultant who was *"on top of his job"*. He documented everything and kept meticulous notes. The pathologists respected his competence in early diagnosis of gynaecological tumours and in carrying out difficult gynaecological repairs.

10.15 We asked this consultant pathologist why, if he had concerns about receiving healthy uteri and had received an unsatisfactory answer, he did no more. He answered that as time went on, perhaps because of the reputation which Dr. Neary enjoyed, he came to believe that many of the patients who had undergone hysterectomy by Dr. Neary were in the high risk group, including some with previously complicated labours, high parity, unbooked or from travelling families. He came to believe that there were justifiable reasons for the hysterectomies including some that were for sterilisation reasons. He was aware of the ban on tubal ligations and believed that Dr. Neary secretly had sympathy for women who already had several children. He felt that sterilisation was the possible explanation for about a third of the hysterectomies.

10.16 This pathologist is the only consultant to admit to concerns about Dr. Neary prior to 1998. He and Dr. Neary had clashed swords professionally in the past and thus he was careful not to engage in a legally contentious situation. He came to believe that a group of women who underwent hysterectomy must have suffered serious haemorrhage. He recalled several cases of major catastrophic haemorrhage in pregnancy and accepted that there was a perception by some anaesthetists that blood supply to the hospital might be problematic.

10.17 While he had qualms about several young women who had hysterectomies he nevertheless was aware that Dr. Neary worked extremely hard and was often called out to deal with emergencies including the most difficult problematic cases in the hospital. He assumed that the hysterectomy was carried out because a dire emergency had arisen. He recalled a conversation with a former anaesthetist who told him that if he saw patients bleeding following delivery, he only relaxed when the uterus was out and the bleeding stopped. This confirmed his belief that many of the hysterectomies, which were carried out were necessary and as a result of dire emergencies and that Dr. Neary was supported by the anaesthetists who observed him at work.

10.18 The pathologist often met Dr. Neary coming out of the hospital looking absolutely exhausted having spent the entire night in the unit. He felt that unless he was standing over Dr. Neary's shoulder, he could not, as a pathologist, challenge a man who was leading up the flagship unit of the hospital and who appeared to be working *"himself into the ground"*.

10.19 With the benefit of hindsight, the pathologist now sees that things were not right, especially in relation to younger patients. He was, however, unaware of the extent of the hysterectomies as he carried out histology every second week and thus was unaware of what was happening on the week when he was not occupied with histology. No one ever said that they had concerns about the number of hysterectomies carried out at the unit. He explained that the pathology department was overworked, under-resourced and understaffed. He never knew that peripartum hysterectomies were carried out by other obstetricians to any extent until informed by the Inquiry. He also reminded us that in Ireland, families wished autopsies to be performed quickly, putting further pressure on stretched services. He added that it was easier to get an autopsy in Drogheda or Dundalk than an admission to hospital.

10.20 When the foundation pathologist retired in 1993, he was the only consultant pathologist for 500 acute hospital beds in Drogheda and Dundalk, together with outpatient procedures and GP requests for tests. The pathology department was responsible for all histology, microbiology and haematology testing and reporting. They were generalists and did not have the benefit of referring to specialist areas of pathology within the department but could and did seek a second opinion in specialist areas of pathology elsewhere if required. When the second consultant's contract was renewed in January 1998, he estimated that he had worked 7 years overtime in a 16 year period.

10.21 In 1998, a new consultant pathologist was appointed to the hospital after a period of 5 years, during which time the position had been filled by a series of locums. This new pathologist had previously worked at a large general hospital in the UK, which included a busy maternity wing. In his 8 years working there, he had never come across a peripartum hysterectomy. He was surprised to see several such operations in the first 9 months working at the Lourdes. When he saw the first such specimen, he expressed surprise to the technician assisting him who said, *"you see a few of those here"*. He also discussed the matter with his consultant colleague. He was concerned that many of the wombs he examined appeared healthy. He was also concerned to see a healthy looking ovary attached to some of the wombs. He could not understand why the practices at the Lourdes Maternity Unit were so different from elsewhere, and resolved to speak to Dr. Neary about the matter at a conference in Galway during mid-October. As he approached Dr. Neary to raise his concerns, another colleague came up to speak to Dr. Neary thus removing the opportunity. He deeply regretted not persisting with his concerns. As it happened, Dr. Neary was suspended a few weeks later.

11 CAUTION RE PATHOLOGY REPORTS

11.1 We have been made aware that reliance on pathology reports to confirm the clinical reason for hysterectomy is not necessarily a reliable practice. All pathologists to whom we spoke (8) confirmed that many genuine reasons for hysterectomy are simply not capable of confirmation at histology. Bleeding from an atonic uterus leaves no evidence; friable or stretched or thin lower segments of uteri may not be obvious after fixing in formalin unless the pathologist is asked specifically to identify the condition of the specimen which would be unusual. Rupture may not necessarily be visible if the surgeon has removed the uterus close to the rupture line, and haemorrhage following manual removal of adherent placenta does not necessarily leave evidence. Placenta previa is a potent cause of post partum haemorrhage but in the absence of placental adherence, there is little to find on histology. In other words, pathological examination can confirm clinical findings but cannot exclude such diagnosis.

11.2 As pathologists interviewed have advised, pathology reports must be viewed in the context of all the records of the operation, which normally show blood loss and replacement and clinical signs of severe haemorrhage. This emphasises the need for meticulous record keeping by anaesthetists.

11.3 In reviewing many scores of pathology reports from this unit with Dr. James Feeney and the pathology witnesses, we have observed that frequently there is little information in the report of the gross examination of the uterus before slides are taken for micro examination. We consider that it would have been helpful if the report had described the uterus in more detail so that a ruptured or friable uterus or a tear would have been mentioned or photographed. The lack of detail in the reports meant that Dr. Feeney was unable, for instance, to determine whether the uterine incision had been sutured or whether the subtotal hysterectomy followed the original line of the lower segment incision.

11.4   In view of the adverse publicity now associated with peripartum hysterectomy by portions of the media, we consider it wise for an obstetrician who has carried out such procedure to take the time to discuss the clinical reasons for the operation with the pathologists. We also consider it of importance that the obstetrician carrying out the hysterectomy should clearly state his clinical summary on the pathology request form.

11.5   We are told that the pathologist's function is to examine all specimens and to report on findings. If the findings do not coincide with the clinical reason given for removing the uterus, then the pathologist writes that there was no evidence of placenta accreta or fibroids or whatever. We are informed that this means no more than that on microscopic analysis of the small samples of tissue taken, there was no supportive evidence to confirm the clinical suspicion. On the other hand, histology can and does confirm findings of placental attachment even from tiny 1 cell thick slides.

11.6   All the pathologists to whom we spoke confirmed that lack of histological support also pertains to planned gynaecological hysterectomy. Many hysterectomies are carried out for dysfunctional bleeding, but there may be nothing to see on histological examination. The Dean of the Faculty of Pathologists informed the Inquiry that the purpose of a pathological examination is to seek evidence of disease or condition, so that appropriate treatments can be set in place by the surgeon or physician. Histology is not intended to police a surgeon's activity, or to confirm a diagnosis. Frequently, the histological examination will confirm the clinician's diagnosis, but this is not the purpose of seeking a pathology report.

11.7   The senior pathologist recently contacted the Inquiry with a very telling experience. He had carried out an examination of a uterus which had a gaping transverse defect with a suture in its right margin. He presumed this to be the re-opened surgical incision. He took a large number of blocks and found a handful of chorionic villi in a small number of the blocks. He concluded that his findings were consistent with morbidly adherent placenta. The clinical situation, however, was dramatically different. What he believed to be an incision was in fact a rupture and the patient received 14 units of blood, cryoprecipitate, platelets and plasma. The incident was related to illustrate how insignificant pathological features can be in a dramatic life-threatening clinical emergency. This confirms what the Inquiry has already found in relation to caution in relying on pathology reports to confirm a clinical diagnosis.

12   LANGUAGE OF PATHOLOGY REPORTS

12.1   The very non-specific and vague nature of the language generally used in the pathology reports may have innocently facilitated acceptance of the hysterectomies, as an uninformed person reading the reports could be forgiven for believing that some abnormality was found. The Inquiry found few differences between a pathology report that confirms the clinician's judgement, and one that finds no supportive evidence of the condition giving rise to the hysterectomy. The wordings most commonly used were:

"The lining of this uterus is very vascular and contains decidual tissue, but there is no evidence of chorionic tissue or inflammation."

"This uterus is lined by a broad zone of trophoblastic tissue infiltrating the superficial myometrium."

"This uterus contains scanty fragments of decidual tissue on the inner surface, but there is no evidence of inflammation."

"The cavity of this uterus is lined by blood clot and decidual tissue. There is no evidence of chorionic tissue or infection."

"Recent pregnancy associated features endo-myometrium with several possible bleeding points identified."

"Endo-myometrium displays pregnancy associated changes. Detached mass consists of myometrium. No actual bleeding point identified."

This contrasts with reports where findings of significance are made:

"Recent pregnancy associated features endo-myometrium with several possible bleeding points identified. Implantation site shows changes consistent with placenta accreta."

We have been informed that a more useful way to report on a confirmed placenta accreta would be to outline: (1) penetration of the uterine muscle by chorionic villi; and (2) the absence of decidua. An example of such reporting, in the review of slides carried out for the Inquiry by Professor Michael Wells, reads:

"This is villous placental tissue and uterus showing an extensive implantation site with abundant non-villous trophoblast and haemorrhage. Numerous distended thin-walled vessels are seen and foreign material, which is probably suture material, is apparent. Focally, placental villi seem to be directly apposed to underlying myometrium with little or no intervening fibrinoid and no decidua.

COMMENT
The full interpretation of these changes is not possible in the absence of clinical details. The findings suggest that suturing of the placental bed has taken place prior to hysterectomy, perhaps in an attempt to arrest haemorrhage. The overall appearances suggest placenta accreta.

CONCLUSION
Placenta accreta."

12.2   The Inquiry found that placenta accreta was diagnosed as the reason for peripartum hysterectomy in about 50 cases occurring between 1960 and 2004. 7 of these occurred prior to Dr. Neary's arrival at the hospital. In those cases, the uteri were not sent for pathological examination. From 1976 on, the clinical diagnosis appeared on about 43 occasions. The diagnosis appeared to be confirmed in about 21 out of the 42 cases where histological reports were available.

12.3   A number of obstetricians from outside the Lourdes Hospital who gave evidence to the Inquiry were very sceptical at the occurrence of placenta accreta 21 times in less than 30 years in a relatively small Maternity Unit especially when for much of the time, repeat caesarean sections were less common. On the other hand, a number of obstetricians and anaesthetists who worked in the Maternity Unit gave evidence of an unusual number of torrential haemorrhages not normally experienced elsewhere, and suggested that there might be unusual features in the population of Louth/Meath. Some witnesses remarked that Dr. Neary had said to them that "*accretas*" were quite common at the IMTH.

12.4   The Inquiry engaged an independent histopathology expert to review the slides in cases where placenta accreta was diagnosed clinically, and where it had been confirmed on histology within the hospital. The Inquiry wanted to further gauge the accuracy or otherwise of the diagnosis and confirmation and to determine whether there were any unusual features with these cases. With the permission of the NEHB, the Inquiry obtained slides in the 43 cases in which placenta accreta, increta or percreta had been clinically diagnosed since 1976. These slides were reviewed by Pathlore, a laboratory in Nottingham, headed by Professor Michael Wells of Sheffield University Hospital. Professor Wells is an established expert on gynaecological pathology and the current President of the International Society of Gynaecological Pathologists. We are grateful to the two Consultant Pathologists at the Lourdes Hospital who assisted the Inquiry in the task of making available all the pathology specimen ledgers and histology reports, as well as the original histology slides.

12.5   Professor Wells was asked to review the slides, but was deliberately given no background information on the reason for the review, the clinical diagnosis, and the details of the patient or the previous histological report. He was at a further and significant disadvantage in that, unlike the original histological examination, he did not have the opportunity of a macro examination of the sample uterus.

Professor Wells's findings were:

- 3 confirmed cases of placenta accreta pre-October 1998.

- 3 confirmed cases of placenta accreta since 1998 - of which 1 was percreta and 1 increta. There was a 4th case of possible placenta accreta.

- 3 cases where there was abundant villous placental tissue, which required knowledge of the clinical circumstances to provide a full evaluation. (These could be cases of accreta).

- several samples of uterus, amniochorion and umbilical cord showing normal placentation with abundant villous placenta. His comment includes the following:

"Given the presence of umbilical cord and amniochorion, is it possible that hysterectomy has been performed without prior manual removal of the placenta?"

- 7 cases where he was unable to give an opinion because the placentation site was inadequately represented on the slides.

- He could find no histological justification for the removal of the ovaries apparent from several of the slides.

- Unusual numbers of the samples showed inflammatory changes.

12.6   Professor Wells, without any other information but the slides, correctly identified a case of secondary post-partum haemorrhage occurring fourteen days post-delivery. Of the 17 cases of placenta accreta confirmed or supported by the Pathologists in Drogheda between 1976 and1998, Professor Wells only positively corroborated 3 with a possibility of 3 others. Of the 5 cases of placenta accreta clinically diagnosed between 1998 and 2004, 4 of these cases were supported by pathologists in Drogheda but Professor Wells corroborated only 3. In the remaining 2 cases he differed in opinion, finding placenta accreta in one case where the hospital pathologist found normal placentation, and finding normal placentation in the other case where the hospital pathologist found placenta accreta.

12.7   The Inquiry was disturbed to find that placenta accreta was not confirmed in a number of cases where the obstetricians present at the operation and engaged in efforts to staunch the haemorrhage had described really massive and well documented haemorrhage associated with placental attachment. In one case, the patient had actually collapsed from blood loss and the placenta was adherent, yet the report from Professor Wells indicated *"uterus showing apparently normal implantation site together with some residual villous placenta. Normal placentation"*.

12.8   In another case where we had spoken to the patient and had reviewed her files and were aware that she underwent emergency caesarean section and delivery of a baby, Professor Wells found *"no trophoblast identified and therefore no comment can be made on placentation."*

We discussed these findings with Professor Wells. He indicated that he might have found more cases of placenta accreta if he had knowledge of the clinical circumstances, or if the slides better represented the placentation site in several cases.

From the existing hospital pathology reports, and the review undertaken by Professor Wells, it is probable that obstetricians and especially Dr. Neary diagnosed placenta accreta, increta or percreta too readily, and on most occasions this diagnosis was not confirmed. It was interesting to note that out of the 6 peripartum hysterectomy cases carried out since Dr. Neary left the unit up to the end of 2004, probably 4 cases involved varying degrees of placenta accreta.

12.9 There may have been some instances in the slides examined where the placenta was morbidly adherent, without a placenta accreta in the strict definition of that term, and therefore the diagnosis could have been clinically justified. Inadequate sampling of the placentation site in the pathology laboratory made it impossible for Professor Wells to make any finding in a number of cases so that he could not confirm that the uterus was even a gravid. A significant number of pathology reports confirming placenta accreta were written by locum consultants.

12.10 Professor Wells very fairly said that pathologists rarely see cases of obstetric hysterectomy, so histology interpretation can be quite difficult, and it very much depends on how effectively the implantation site has been sampled. In his view, he would make a diagnosis of placenta accreta only where the placental villi are apposed and infiltrate the myometrium in the absence of intervening decidua or indeed a layer of cytotrophoblast.

12.11 Perhaps, there is a difference in opinion in pathology circles on the strict definition of what constitutes placenta accreta. A review of the most recent cases of peripartum hysterectomy by Professor Wells confirms this. Certainly, in the survey we conducted amongst practicing obstetricians, the diagnosis of placenta accreta was made very often. The value of a second opinion is clearly demonstrated in those difficult cases where the uterus fails to contract, the placenta is slow to be expelled and appears ragged and massive haemorrhage ensues but yet no real placenta accreta is confirmed on histology.

12.12 The Inquiry received cogent evidence of recent studies showing a sharp rise in the incidence of hysterectomy in the presence of placenta previa and placenta accreta with repeat caesarean section. On the other hand of the 43 cases where placenta accreta was clinically diagnosed in The Lourdes Maternity Unit, only 8 cases were associated with repeat caesarean section. Certainly the literature which we have considered and the anecdotal evidence from the many obstetricians to whom we spoke suggests that the incidence of placenta accreta leading to hysterectomy was not quite so statistically rare as suggested by the Fitness to Practise Committee in their report. On the other hand, it was not quite as common as suggested by Dr. Neary. Again we are driven to the view that placenta accreta is not seen as often in countries with relatively few repeat caesarean sections and thus perceptions of what constitutes morbidly adherent placenta differs significantly.

12.13 Professor Wells thought it unusual that there was no audit in the Maternity Unit as the whole purpose of audit and of reading reports and discussing them is to effect the future management of other cases. If there had been any kind of an audit, perhaps the management of post partum haemorrhage might have been identified. Professor Wells was not aware that the hospital had produced annual reports up to 1984 when he made his remarks. The publication of annual reports is of course one of the best forms of audit.

12.14 His reports confirm the importance of seeing and being made aware of the clinical history in order to furnish a meaningful pathology report. The reports suggest that placenta accreta/increta/percreta properly so-called was probably no more common in the Lourdes Hospital catchment area than other parts of the State. The Inquiry believes that it is possible that on some occasions the diagnosis of placenta accreta could have been used to mask an indirect sterilisation.

12.15   The review by a recognised expert in gynaecological pathology demonstrates the difficulty in relying on pathology reports as the sole source of determining whether a peripartum hysterectomy was carried out in appropriate circumstances. The pathologists in the Lourdes Hospital themselves had differing views of whether they would always expect to see chorionic villi in order to diagnose placenta accreta.

12.16   Although we found little evidence to confirm that the pathology reports were relied upon by any practitioners in the unit, the frequent diagnosis and confirmation of placental attachment may have caused midwives and anaesthetists to believe that there were good reasons for the hysterectomies which were carried out thus contributing to the lack of comment. Perhaps now when a histopathologist makes a conclusion that findings are consistent with placenta accreta it would be an idea to state how he arrived at that conclusion. This would certainly have the effect of clarifying the findings to all readers of the report.

12.17   An extraordinary lack of communication existed in the pathology department, which seemed to shadow the similar lack of discussion and communication between consultants in the Maternity Unit. The Medical Council has already made findings regarding the lack of communication between Dr. Neary and the pathology department. Very dramatic events that occurred when colleagues were not on duty were not discussed. Thus a hysterectomy specimen from the Maternity Unit examined by one of the pathologists may not have been discussed with the other colleagues.

12.18   The lack of communication is demonstrated by one instance where one of the pathologists first became aware of a maternal death when he saw his colleagues emerging from the coroner's court on the 9 o'clock national news.

This predicates no discussion of the maternal death, which fortunately is a very rare event, no discussion of the autopsy findings and no discussion of the preparations for the court appearance and all this in a laboratory with at most, 2 pathologists. One of the pathologists only learned of a maternal death in 1997 from the Inquiry. He received no information on this very tragic occurrence from the locum consultant. These incidents confirm that there were no interdisciplinary meeting between anaesthetists, obstetricians and pathologists during that time. The practice of the pathologists working at histopathology on a week on week off basis does not lend itself to appropriate communication and a full appreciation of events as they occur in the absence of regular meetings with exchange of information.

12.19   Several witnesses told us that there was no mechanism in place within or outside the hospital whereby colleagues could talk to each other about individual practices, share information or to make formal complaints. This applied particularly to the pathology department where regular meetings and exchange of views did not occur. Meetings between laboratory scientists and pathologists to discuss the unusual number of gravid uteri could have alerted the department to the numbers coming down each year. It is not appropriate that a busy acute services hospital with a sizeable Maternity Unit should have operated for so long with only 2 pathologists and no haematologist and no microbiologist.

13   THE ANAESTHETISTS

13.1   Many patients asked why the anaesthetists, who were the only other consultants present when hysterectomy was carried out, remained silent for so many procedures over so many years. Many doctors asked the same question. We spoke to all the consultant anaesthetists employed at the hospital when Dr. Neary worked there and to some of the consultants who have come to work there since. We also spoke to many of the junior trainee anaesthetists who were on duty when peripartum hysterectomy was carried out.

13.2   Dr. Marie Sheehan was the original anaesthetist in the Maternity Unit. She was married to the foundation surgeon and was working in the unit for many years before Dr. Neary took up his position in 1974. She retired in 1982 and has since died. If she had made any complaints regarding Dr. Neary's hysterectomies we would, we believe, have heard some evidence to corroborate this. We have observed her signature and her writing on several charts where Dr. Neary carried out hysterectomy and must therefore assume that she did not have concerns.[15]

13.3 As we said earlier in the report, in the 1970s the rate at the unit was probably not so out of line with national norms as to cause concern although the changing profile of many of the patients was remarkably different after Dr. Neary took up his post. As against that, there were no maternal deaths on Dr. Neary's watch although he took over the bulk of the work. Dr. Sheehan must have observed Dr. Neary at work and should surely have noticed that some of his patients were young and of low parity. She should have observed that while some of the hysterectomies were undoubtedly necessary, that nevertheless Dr. Neary had a very low tolerance for haemorrhage. She had after all, worked with Dr. Connolly and Dr. O'Brien and also with registrars who carried out caesarean section and she could make comparisons. In addition she was married to one of the revered first four "foundation consultants" and would have had his ear and that of Dr. Connolly. We received no evidence to suggest that she raised any concerns about Dr. Neary.

13.4 **BLOOD TRANSFUSIONS AND ANAESTHETICS**

As both Dr. Connolly and Dr. Sheehan are deceased their evidence of Dr. Neary's management of peripartum haemorrhage was not available. The Inquiry therefore obtained records of all blood ordered or used in the Maternity Unit from 1974. It will be recalled that the maternity theatre register for the period up to late 1991 is not available. That register was not available to determine the number of caesarean sections carried out and, much more importantly, by whom and who assisted. If this register had been available to us, the Inquiry would have known which theatre nurses and midwives were on

---

[15] One of the MMMs, formerly a doctor, told the Inquiry of a conversation she had had with her great friend Marie Sheehan shortly after the revelations of Dr. Neary's high rate of peripartum hysterectomies were made in late 1998 and 1999. This witness recalled that Dr. Sheehan said *"he was afraid of blood loss," "he panicked."* Dr. Sheehan died in 2000. This witness added that Dr. Sheehan found it very hard to believe the allegations against Dr. Neary.

duty in theatre in the early days, what sections became hysterectomies and which anaesthetist was on duty. We would also have been able to determine whether the hysterectomies followed elective or planned caesarean section or whether the patient was a public or private patient.

13.5   The blood records kept and stored in the pathology department by the haemovigilance department are meticulously maintained and, as far as we could ascertain, they provide a complete record of blood used in the unit. This record demonstrates changing practices in relation to the treatment of haemorrhage. In the first few years that Dr. Neary was working in the unit caesarean sections were relatively infrequent. He ordered blood and used it when there was haemorrhage. His first two patients who had peripartum hysterectomies received 6 and 9 units of blood before they underwent hysterectomy. Several patients had very substantial blood replacement without hysterectomy – more than 9 units and as much as 20 units. By 1976, Dr. Neary had assisted at 2 haemorrhages, which ended in hysterectomy. He carried out 3 hysterectomies after very significant blood replacement and Dr. Connolly had carried out 1 hysterectomy.

13.6   The blood records for 1978/1979 still show a pattern of significant replacement blood ordered and used. The major difference is that most haemorrhages now ended in hysterectomy and they are associated with caesarean section. 19 serious haemorrhages are recorded. Dr. Neary dealt with about 16 of the emergencies and 10 ended up with hysterectomy. Dr. Connolly was involved in 5 or 6 cases of massive haemorrhage of which 4 ended in hysterectomy in the same period.

13.7   **WAS MATERNAL DEATH AN INFLUENCE?**
The pattern of ordering and using blood continued in 1980 and 1981. Dr. Neary seems to have dealt with most of the serious cases of haemorrhage although the number of cases in which more than 6 units of blood were ordered and used fell. In July 1982 a patient underwent an emergency caesarean section; 9 units of blood were ordered, only 2 units were used and the patient is recorded as a maternal death. Searches through the annual reports indicate that the patient was multiparous and died from an amniotic

fluid embolism, which followed an emergency caesarean section after a surgical induction and almost 24 hours of oxytocin drip. She was not one of Dr. Neary's patients.

13.8   The following year another patient died following emergency caesarean section. Again the cause of death was amniotic fluid embolism. Neither of the maternal deaths were Dr. Neary's patients. One can only imagine the distress to all involved in the treatment of those two women. A maternal death is obviously the very worst nightmare for anyone in the practice of midwifery and obstetrics. It would be understandable if emergencies were treated defensively after those two maternal deaths. In 1984 there was yet another maternal death. This time the patient, who was extremely young, developed a serious medical condition and died in the general hospital.

13.9   The Inquiry probed Dr. Neary to establish whether he witnessed any maternal death attributed to delay in carrying out hysterectomy. Dr. Neary did not admit to any such event and was slow to comment on any colleague's cases. He did say that he assisted Dr. Connolly in theatre a lot towards the end of his tenure. He explained he did this because Dr. Connolly had developed *"a touch of arthritis and had difficulty with tight sutures"*. Another witness told us that it was believed that Dr. Neary had come in to assist Dr. Connolly during a procedure where there had been a maternal death in 1982. The records do not confirm his presence at this death and this was confirmed by the anaesthetist present in the theatre at this maternal death.

13.10   We believe that these maternal deaths had a profound effect on Dr. Neary and all practitioners in the unit. Each of the maternal deaths occurred with a consultant anaesthetist in the theatre. This may explain the reminder to us on several occasions that *"no mother died"* with Dr. Neary. Although Dr. Neary had the heaviest workload, he was not involved in the management and care of any of the patients who died. Perhaps because of this, more trust and reliance may have been placed in his ability than perhaps an analysis of the adverse outcomes merited.

13.11 The Inquiry has been furnished with blood records for serious haemorrhage when at least 6 units of blood were ordered. After 1982, most hysterectomies carried out by Dr. Neary are not recorded in the blood book records. This means that fewer than 6 units of blood were ordered. As the years went by, far fewer major haemorrhages treated by blood replacement are recorded. The rates of caesarean section in the meanwhile, in common with the rest of the western world, rose incrementally. It is unfortunate that no one, and especially no anaesthetist, voiced any concerns regarding the now obvious practice of resort to hysterectomy without significant or any blood replacement.

13.12 THE OLD MATERNITY HOSPITAL

The two anaesthetists who worked with Dr. Neary in the late '70s and early '80s both expressed full confidence in his ability as a surgeon and as an obstetrician. Both anaesthetists described how they were conservative in relation to the use of blood saying that mothers are generally healthy, have increased blood volumes when pregnant and can withstand haemorrhage up to 1500mls. without distress or changes in pulse rate or blood pressure. They saw absolutely nothing to alarm them in relation to Dr. Neary's practice and were very happy to work with him. They both drew a picture of an extremely caring, concerned, busy and well informed obstetrician.

13.13 One of the anaesthetists described their work schedules as cruel. Until 1991 the maternity hospital was 300 metres away from the general hospital. Anaesthetists, surgical nurses and personnel with blood supplies had to travel from one building to the other in all weather. The anaesthetists who travelled over for caesarean sections were not dedicated to the maternity hospital and were required in the general hospital to cover the other theatres and intensive care unit. They did their work in the maternity theatre and then left to return to the general hospital.

13.14 The anaesthetists worked at best on a 1:3 rota and a 1:2 whenever one colleague was ill, on holiday or attending meetings or courses. They had no senior registrars in anaesthesia until after Dr. Neary left the unit. There were no anaesthetic nurses until 1998. Their equipment was frequently outmoded and they were extremely overworked. One of the anaesthetists said that after the Health Board took over the hospital they had more staff, more equipment and more support.

13.15 Asked why the threshold for carrying out caesarean hysterectomy seemed so low, we heard that the doctors were very overworked and that there was a lot of pressure and probably chronic fatigue. They were expected to work at night and be available the next day. Nowadays if anaesthetists are in all night, they have most of the next day off, since there are more consultants.

13.16 Anaesthetists take responsibility for ordering blood and blood products without consulting the surgeon. It is part of their job to keep the patient stable during and after the operation. The anaesthetists told us that Dr. Neary had a strong personality and would make a decision to proceed to hysterectomy without consulting his anaesthetic colleague. It was unheard of for an anaesthetist to challenge a surgeon. Most of the anaesthetists told us that they would usually ask the reason why Dr. Neary was carrying out the hysterectomy. If an obstetrician said an atonic uterus had to come out, they would not question his judgement.

13.17 Asked if this acceptance of diagnosis was from respect for the obstetrician or lack of training, one anaesthetist said that she had no training in obstetrics other than as a trainee doctor for some four weeks. She said that the rest of her experience in this regard was in the Lourdes Hospital and she had no exposure to obstetric anaesthesia in any other hospital or Maternity Unit. Her view was that as the obstetrician is trained in his specialty, she accepted his diagnosis. The anaesthetists did not seem to attach the same importance to the stable condition of the patient at the time of decision to carry out a hysterectomy as the Fitness to Practise Committee of the Medical Council. They described how colloids and fluids artificially maintain blood volumes and many women who are losing large amounts of blood have stable pulse and blood pressure readings.

13.18 This anaesthetist rarely worked with Dr. Connolly, as his preferred anaesthetist was the late Dr. Sheehan. She worked with all the obstetricians.

She found Dr. O'Brien to be a man of measured words and accepted that many people were nervous of him and that some people found him difficult to work with. She was his preferred anaesthetist at his elective surgery. She was also Dr. Neary's preferred anaesthetist for his elective lists. She found Dr. Neary to be a breath of fresh air. He had energy and was prepared to talk and had more time. He had an air of confidence and leadership. He didn't panic. Asked if this changed to arrogance over the years, she said she didn't notice any change in his manner. He remained the same. If asked questions by nurses or doctors he generally answered and was pleasant to work with. On the other hand questioning his decisions might not be welcome.

Asked if Dr. Neary would ask, *"What's happening at your end?"* she answered that Dr. Neary certainly didn't consult over the decision to go to hysterectomy. He wouldn't have consulted over blood loss either. She had been on cases with him where there were heavy bleeds and where the patient was stabilised without resort to hysterectomy.

13.19 Another anaesthetist who had considerable experience of obstetric anaesthesia before he came to the unit was surprised that the records indicated his presence at a large number of the hysterectomies. He was adamant that there was very significant blood loss at every case at which he was present where a hysterectomy was carried out, and that Dr. Neary had done the right thing. He believed that if a significant amount of syntocinon failed to contract the uterus and a large dose of ergometrine did not work, nothing would stop the bleeding. He had observed new methods of staunching haemorrhage applied and had no faith in any of the procedures. He believed that haemorrhage was more prevalent in this Maternity Unit than in other hospitals where he had worked. He was personally very slow to give blood, as he was aware of the increasing dangers inherent in blood transfusion. He felt that healthy mothers rarely required blood transfusions and they could make up for blood loss with iron supplements.

13.20 He had no idea what an acceptable figure for the rate of hysterectomy was and whether the rate at this unit exceeded the accepted norm. He was quite shocked to hear that rates in other provincial hospitals were low compared to the Lourdes rate. He did not argue with the figures and was clearly perturbed by the information. He suggested that we investigate the incidence of haemorrhage in the mothers presenting for section and query the treatment of the patients in the labour ward with inductions and the routine use of oxytocics that might be the cause of the excessive bleeding at section. He reiterated his confidence in Dr. Neary's skills as a surgeon but in the face of the figures, which were presented to him, he questioned Dr. Neary's judgement.

13.21　The anaesthetist who took up the position as third consultant had very similar views on her experience of Dr. Neary. He was a safe pair of hands. He was in control, he did not panic, and he knew what to do in every emergency. He came in to assist many of the registrars who had found themselves in difficulty. She was strongly of the view that nothing she observed in theatre alerted her to any problems regarding caesarean hysterectomy or Dr. Neary's technique. The anaesthetists were always happy when Dr. Neary was on duty.

13.22 THE NEW MATERNITY UNIT OPENED IN 1990

The Inquiry was intrigued as to why, in the new Maternity Unit with new equipment and a modern operating theatre and easier access to blood and blood products, anaesthetists and specialist surgeons, the caesarean hysterectomy rate rose so dramatically from about 1991. To put the figures into perspective:

- in 1989 there were 6 peripartum hysterectomies,
- in 1990 there were 3 peripartum hysterectomies
- in 1991 there were 12 peripartum hysterectomies
- in 1992 there were 8 peripartum hysterectomies
- in 1993 there were 15 peripartum hysterectomies

13.23　There was no explanation forthcoming from the anaesthetists and clearly no person expressed alarm, concern or curiosity. One of the senior anaesthetists wondered if perhaps Dr. Neary had difficulty coping with haemorrhage when spinal or regional block anaesthesia was used. It was suggested that a patient cannot recover as well from these if they have a bleed at caesarean section under regional block. The anaesthesia is effective from the chest down, but if there is a major post partum haemorrhage the peripheral blood vessels in the limbs tend to close down thus the body cannot compensate for blood loss as well. She described how Dr. Neary was –

"always very careful to make sure that any bleeding had stopped and he used to often spend a long time making sure and after the patients were given a regional anaesthetic he was not able to spend so long doing the operation – partly because the block might wear off before the operation was finished and partly because the patient was awake and listening to all the conversation going on and he was also aware, as was I, that patients who were having a spinal or epidural would not be able to compensate as well for any significant bleeding"

13.24 When asked to explain this, she said:

"It affects the tone in the blood vessels in the lower part of – well from here down – so that if you get major bleeding one of the compensatory mechanisms is for your peripheral – your blood vessels in your limbs to close down and that cannot happen in the area that's affected by the spinal or epidural block."

The effect she felt was that as Dr. Neary was a slow worker the change might have an effect on his technique. This theory was put to another anaesthetist who had limited experience of working with Dr. Neary. She explained -

"The epidural and spinal local anaesthetic numbs the sympathetic nerves as well as the motor and sensory nerves – the sympathetic nerves keep tone in your blood vessels so they are nice and taut – they take away the tone, they dilate right up so your blood pressure drops. If you lose blood your sympathetic tone increases so you constrict down but having had a sympathetic block your vessels can't do that so you don't compensate as well for blood loss.

You are less likely to compensate – it won't affect clotting but it just means that instead your body is unable to make the physiological response it wants to make to blood loss – you will tolerate loss of blood less easily – but it doesn't affect blood loss.

We give Ephedrine and Phenolron to keep the tone up...... If you had a case say a placenta previa where you are expecting a lot of blood loss you wouldn't give a spinal – you'd give a general anaesthetic – because the body will handle the blood loss a lot better under GA than under spinal."

13.25 We were told that all the anaesthetists liked working with Dr. Neary, as he was a *"clean worker"*. He liked his patients *"dry."* He tolerated very little bleeding and was assiduous in tying and clamping every little bleeder. His patients were never haemodynamically compromised. He came in frequently to check on his patients before an operation and he stayed with them afterwards. His patients who had undergone hysterectomy recovered quickly, did not spend time in ICU, did not suffer from kidney failure and generally caused them no serious concerns. They all pointed out *"no mother died".*

13.26 These anaesthetists were impressed that many nurses, midwives and doctors chose Dr. Neary as their obstetrician. Many of the nuns went to him for gynaecological problems. Even though one of the anaesthetists was very involved in examining in anaesthetics exams and was active in the Institute of Anaesthetics, she saw nothing to worry about in the treatment of peripartum haemorrhage in the unit. She was not aware of the numbers and was unaware that they were excessive.

13.27 In 1996 several new consultants were appointed to the hospital staff. They were the first new consultants appointed since 1983. Sadly, none of the new consultants had any worries about Dr. Neary and were generally unaware that anything about his practice warranted concern. The newest anaesthetist had assisted at 4 peripartum hysterectomies in the 2 years before Dr. Neary was suspended. She had observed that he was highly regarded as an obstetrician and surgeon. She accepted what her peers told her without question.

13.28 This anaesthetist described how when she joined the unit she was told of what a wonderful obstetrician Dr. Neary was. Everyone seemed to have such faith in him and so she followed along in that belief. He seemed confident and decisive. She reported that following conversations with a junior colleague who was on a 6 month period of training, she began to review her assessment and now feels in retrospect that his technique must have been flawed somewhere. His constant touching, dabbing and checking may have provoked bleeding. She wondered if perhaps he was *"doing something funny like extending the uterine incision too far or doing something odd because no one else seemed to have the same problems"*.

13.29 She had no real explanation why it took so long for her colleagues to have developed some insight into Dr. Neary's practices. She suggested that perhaps it was easy for any anaesthetists with no obstetric training to accept as normal what was deemed normal in the system to which they came. As an example of how routinely caesarean hysterectomy was treated in the unit she recounted that a junior anaesthetist told her that he was talking to the Anaesthetic Nurse about something that had been on the television the night before and *"the next thing was someone with a bucket walked past and that was the uterus gone so there'd been no question of crisis or whatever. I mean as far as he was concerned, he was so relaxed he was discussing the television programme"*.

13.30 The suggestion was that if in the theatre, everyone treated hysterectomy as routine and devoid of drama, a new anaesthetist would accept it as the norm. She was not there long enough to become totally accustomed to the procedures but she did not have serious misgivings until her junior colleagues said, *"this should not be happening. This does not happen in the Coombe"*.

13.31 This anaesthetist had read the transcripts from the Medical Council Fitness to Practise Committee hearings and on the basis of what she read on the transcripts she considers that Dr. Neary's training was poor. If, as he said, he was operating on complicated cancer cases while he was in Portsmouth only 4 years after qualifying, there had to be something wrong. He would only have been a third year SHO when he arrived in Portsmouth and should not have been doing complicated cancer surgery at that stage.

13.32 A number of witnesses involved in the examining and training of doctors on the specialist training programme have made similar observations of Dr. Neary's training. He may have been academically bright and confident as a surgeon but his training lacked the degree of supervision to identify judgement flaws. Training should include development of judgement and the recognition of the limits of one's competence. They have observed that his period of training was unusually short. He was in training as an obstetrician/gynaecologist for 7 years whereas the usual training is closer to 10 years. The Inquiry's investigations of Dr. Neary's training in Portsmouth and his own testimony to the Inquiry and to the Medical Council reveal that during a crucial part of his training, his supervisors were absent due to extended illness.

13.33 The newer Anaesthetist said that while people who worked with Dr. Neary may come forward now and criticise him, they all thought he was wonderful when she first came to the unit in 1996. There was nobody criticising him then. There was real shock and disbelief when he was suspended. This was followed by dismay when the numbers of hysterectomies became talked about. At the end of the day, she felt that there was no arguing with numbers. Individual cases could be defended but not the numbers. It was becoming more difficult for supporters and friends to believe that he would be vindicated. She personally did not believe that the prohibition on tubal ligation played a role in the period during which she worked there in the late '90s but accepted that it may have played a role in not questioning procedures in the past. She accepted that people would not be inclined to ask questions if they felt that a doctor was carrying out a compassionate sterilisation in the past. If she felt that any obstetrician was doing anything questionable now, she would go straight to the manager of the hospital.

13.34 We interviewed a young trainee anaesthetist who had spent 6 months working at the Lourdes Hospital in 1998. She had spent the previous 6 months at the Coombe Hospital. She described her experience. She was in theatre with Dr. Neary who had been called in to carry out a manual removal of the placenta following a normal delivery. She gave the patient a light spinal anaesthetic to facilitate the manual removal. She heard Dr. Neary say that it was not coming out and that he would have to do a hysterectomy. She was surprised at the rapid decision never having seen a peripartum hysterectomy carried out in the Coombe Hospital where 8,000 babies were delivered in an average year.

13.35 She reasoned that there was no major blood loss, the patient was stable so why did he not try a little more, was there not some thing else less drastic that he could do. However, she was not an obstetrician and while she was surprised, she was aware of his good reputation and said nothing. She told us that Dr. Neary seemed calm. He spoke to the new mother and told her what he intended to do. While she felt that no full explanations were given to the patient, she felt that the patient did not really question it either. There was no discussion or debate between Dr. Neary and the patient nor was there anything remarkable with the body language of any of the nurses in the theatre. She felt that while she was very surprised at what he was doing, it seemed to be just routine with everyone else.

13.36 The next case, which caused her concern, occurred a few months later. She was on duty with Dr. Neary for a caesarean section on a young mother. The patient had had a spinal anaesthetic so she was awake. Shortly after the delivery Dr. Neary said *"she is bleeding a lot"*. The anaesthetist indicated that the patient was stable and that she had no concerns regarding her condition. Within a very short period of time Dr. Neary asked for a hysterectomy set. The trainee anaesthetist informed the Inquiry that she was flabbergasted and said *"are you sure, she's quite stable she doesn't even need blood"*. She described how she was completely ignored but what struck her was the fact that he asked for a hysterectomy set and *"it was as if he was just asking for another scalpel or something very routine"*.

13.37 Dr. Neary explained to her that the patient had a placenta accreta. She was aware that placenta accreta was something that was very rare. She had not come across it but had read about it in textbooks and then accepted it as a valid reason. Nevertheless it struck her that he was resorting to hysterectomy very quickly especially in a young woman. She would never normally question a surgeon. She was so concerned that she left the patient and went to the phone, which was just at the door of the theatre and rang a consultant colleague. She relayed her concerns and asked if there was anything she could or should do but by the time she got off the phone Dr. Neary had practically finished the operation.

13.38   She felt that no one else in the theatre supported her concerns. When asked about the attitude of the nurse who had fetched the hysterectomy clamps she felt that *"it was a routine thing and you know my involvement was just basically – you know my opinion wasn't taken into account."*

13.39   The young anaesthetist recounted that she really was quite disturbed by what she had witnessed and wondered if she could have done more to stop Dr. Neary. She found that he was quite assured that he was doing the right thing and that basically who was she a trainee to question him. She spoke to some of the nurses and to others in the hospital about her experiences but there seemed to be no concern. She spoke again to her consultant anaesthetic colleague about her concerns the following day. They had a discussion about the hysterectomies and she learned that the two hysterectomies which she had witnessed were not the only ones that had been carried out. She knew that a caesarean or peripartum hysterectomy was very unusual, that she had previously seen lots of people bleeding who did not have hysterectomies and expressed her shock at what she had seen. She also mentioned her experience in the Lourdes to a couple of other anaesthetic consultants and they were horrified. She was very pleased that an Inquiry was being held and had no idea of the extent of the practice until recently.

13.40   Another matter which caused this trainee anaesthetist concerns was the widespread use of midline rather than the Pfannenstiel (bikini line) incisions for caesarean section. She questioned the various obstetric registrars about it and they said well that's the way we do it or that's the way we were taught in this department. She considered it *"strange, unnecessary and a bit uncaring to give somebody a big scar and more pain when it wasn't necessary".* The obstetricians obviously knew how to do the more modern incision as she was actually present in certain instances where the patients requested a bikini line incision and were given it. She was concerned that the junior doctors had been trained to use midline incisions which were not used routinely anywhere else.

13.41 This young trainee was instrumental in causing the most recently appointed consultant anaesthetist to review her assessment of Dr. Neary. She told us that it was to her shame that she had assisted at 4 hysterectomies in 18 months between 1996 and 1998 without having concerns and it took a junior colleague to point out to her that hysterectomies are not performed so routinely in other Maternity Units.

13.42 In probing the anaesthetists in turn as to their role as consultants in the theatre where the peripartum hysterectomies were carried out, the following answers were common to most of the anaesthetists.

- *"The numbers shocked them, as they had no idea that the operation was carried out with such frequency.*

- *They did not have access to any cumulative figures.*

- *They never attended at any multidisciplinary meeting with the obstetricians.*

- *They had no expertise in obstetrics and they had no comparative figures from any other units.*

- *They were extremely overworked."*

13.43 It seemed that by the 1990s the accepted procedure for treatment of severe peripartum haemorrhage by Dr. Neary in theatre was - fluids to keep up blood volumes, syntocinon infusion and ergometrine administered by the anaesthetists, compression and packing of the uterus by Dr. Neary if the uterus failed to contract and then hysterectomy if the bleeding continued.

Hysterectomy was a haemorrhage preventative rather than a last resort. Dr. Neary's phobia for brisk bleeding prevented him from having any faith in blood replacement. Before any of his patients became ill from haemorrhage or perceived haemorrhage, the hysterectomy was performed.

13.44 All three of the anaesthetists who were there for many years expressed the view that some of the hysterectomies carried out at caesarean section were sterilisation procedures. In only one or two of the cases did the obstetrician inform them in advance that a planned hysterectomy would be carried out. They were aware that tubal ligations were prohibited. They did not ask questions. In all the other cases they felt that the hysterectomies followed on haemorrhage. He practised an extreme form of defensive medicine.

13.45 The Inquiry accepts that the anaesthetists are not deliberately protecting Dr. Neary and accepts that their silence was born from lack of knowledge and training in obstetrical norms. There were times however when the Inquiry felt that their explanations presented a picture of a robotic presence in theatre with no capacity for inquiry or the seeking of outside validation. It is regrettable that none of the anaesthetists who worked regularly with Dr. Neary took the time to make a phone call to a colleague in Dublin to enquire as to the hysterectomy rate in that hospital. We accept that the three anaesthetists who had worked with him over a very considerable time admired his skill and his ability to cope in a crisis and thus accepted without question his reasons for the operations. In doctors of consultant status the lack of insight or curiosity or critical faculty is troubling. Some of the anaesthetists who had a great deal of experience of working with Dr. Neary gave the impression that eventually, the Inquiry would find a legitimate reason for why so many hysterectomies were carried out.

14 JUNIOR DOCTORS

14.1 It was neither realistic nor practical to track down and speak to all the junior doctors who had worked with Dr. Neary over the 25 year period in question. It was hoped that any of those doctors who had anything relevant to say would contact the Inquiry. As no such contact was made we concentrated on those doctors still in the State who had assisted at peripartum hysterectomy or carried out the operation as locum consultants while working at the Lourdes Hospital. All of the registrars were non-nationals. Some of the SHOs were Irish. There were only 2 registrars to the 3 consultants even in the late 90s. They worked on a rota rather than with a particular consultant.

14.2   They all described Dr. Neary as easy to work with in that he was usually in good humour. He regularly helped out any registrar who was in trouble and was called in by Dr. Lynch. The junior doctors met each other regularly as a group for tutorials but never discussed any concerns with Dr. Neary's surgery. He was friendly, confident and competent. Some Irish doctors felt that he was a little crude in speech and not respectful enough in sensitive situations. This was not commented upon by non-nationals. All observed that he was well liked by patients and midwives. If the junior doctors had any criticisms it was about the lack of structured teaching from the consultants, the difficulties they had with one of the consultant's personality, the lack of audit meetings, and the lack of communication between the consultants. Some doctors gave the impression of consultants who did not really like or respect each other. Many comments made by the junior doctors are not relevant to the Terms of Reference but reinforce our belief in the value of continuing medical development and audit. Several consultants used methods, which they felt were from another era. Lack of communication was a common observation.

14.3   All the doctors who spoke to us and who had spent part of their training in the Maternity Unit believed that Dr. Neary was doing most of the work, that he was always available and he was kind to them and to patients. He was described as a careful neat surgeon; he preached constantly of the dangers of bleeding and the dangers of losing a patient. Every bleeder had to be tied off; he never let coagulation problems develop. His suturing was a little different and he used a lot of sutures. They admired his skill especially in gynaecology. All the non-nationals felt that Dr. Neary did his best to teach during rounds and was caring. He seemed to have demons about two subjects, the MMMs and litigation. He talked incessantly on those two subjects. Although talkative, he was not easy to engage in an exchange of clinical views. It was his way of doing things or no way.

14.4   Some registrars who had been exposed to obstetric practice in other Irish hospitals believed that Dr. Neary moved to hysterectomy too quickly in postpartum haemorrhage but they were afraid to discuss anything openly. They spoke in whispers to some of their colleagues about the high rate of both caesarean section and hysterectomy. They recognised that a few of the midwives shared their concerns and they would talk to them but mostly they were careful not to be heard criticising or questioning.

14.5   Many of them who had been used to using Pfannenstiel incisions for caesarean sections began to use vertical or midline incisions as two out of three of the consultants regularly operated that way and they wanted to "stay in" with the consultants. Some felt that a lot of caesarean sections were carried out on private patients with whom they would have had very little contact. Non-national SHOs and registrars feared jeopardising their job prospects if the midwives or consultants perceived that they were making trouble. There was acute competition for training posts even within their own countrymen and more so between different races. Thus, Egyptians, Libyans, Sudanese, Pakistanis and Indians competed for scarce jobs. Many were prepared to work as supernumeries (unpaid) or SHOs even after 10 years in training in Saudi or Egyptian hospitals to have an opportunity to sit for their RCOG examinations. Their visas to remain in Ireland were dependent on occupying a post in training. They were therefore unlikely to criticise. They accepted unsupervised training, the lack of meetings and the lack of structured teaching. They accepted that the only teaching on offer in the Lourdes was to follow the consultant around on ward rounds - if permitted - and being told what way that particular consultant did things. There was no reviewing of unexpected or adverse outcomes, no identifying of best practice and no comparisons. They relied totally on references from a consultant to be kept on in training. If they stayed on, they had to compete at job interviews where they were interviewed by the consultants with whom they were working. Dr. Neary was the dominant consultant at interviews. Dr. Neary decided how things were done. No one questioned any of the consultants. They were here to pass their exams which they were eligible to sit only if working in an approved teaching hospital.

14.6   One doctor described how he and others had to go to Belfast to compensate for deficiencies in their training relating to family planning and the use of HRT. He was astounded to find that in Belfast, the consultant who had been on call the night before would be there in the morning discussing with the day team what they had done during the night and facilitating the change over of staff. He felt that these handover sessions were the best teaching session he had ever had. They had regular meetings and discussion with regular audit meetings.

14.7   The junior doctors who worked on in the hospital after Dr. Neary left were pleased at the changes introduced soon after by senior midwives and the remaining consultants. For the first time, protocols were discussed and the reason for caesarean section was reviewed.

14.8   The Irish doctors who worked in the unit and who have gone on to become consultants or GPs were more critical of their time there. They described how different the three obstetricians were and how there was no collegiality or unity of approach between them. Each consultant had a personal approach in relation to a whole range of obstetric emergencies. Frequently the approaches did not coincide. One doctor believed that there was no sense of a department working together to provide a service but rather three consultants who covered for each other. The SHOs were attached to all three of them. They described the different attitudes of the consultants – Dr. Neary never left the place, he was always there; as soon as Dr. O'Brien was finished he would go without a word to anyone; and Dr. Connolly would come in, do what he had to do and go. Dr. Lynch was professional. He did his work quickly and left. None of the Irish junior doctors had any idea that the hysterectomy rate was high or that Dr. Neary's practices could lead to his being struck off. Their comments were confined to the dysfunction of the unit due to the personality of the individual consultants.

14.9   The ethos of the hospital was that consultants were respected. Respect was number one on the agenda and that came before anything else. You could question as to facts – surgical or medical facts or knowledge – but you certainly wouldn't be able to question the handling and the management of a patient. The nuns had created an aura of unquestioning respect around the foundation consultants who were revered. This attitude to consultants made its way in a watered down version to later consultants but the attitude of not questioning was established.

14.10 Not one doctor to whom we spoke had any recollection of any meeting or presentation arising from the annual reports. They never saw the reports. While other departments in the hospital had regular meetings and teaching sessions there were none in the Maternity Unit. The midwives and junior doctors were sometimes invited to midwifery student lectures but there was no questioning after the presentation. Most junior doctors had no relationship with the Matron or her assistant and most of them did not recall their names. They had no feeling that the consultants treated them as important people. The Irish junior doctors had more tales to tell of serious relationship breakdowns with the consultants than the non-nationals. No one said anything which would indicate an awareness of unusual practices in the Maternity Unit. Most of the non-nationals were extremely reticent to admit any knowledge of sterilisation. Several junior doctors found that, while Dr. Neary claimed to be very up to date on obstetric literature, he followed several outmoded practices. He was inclined to follow certain procedures because of personal experience rather than from evidence based trials.

14.11 In spite of extensive interviews with junior and non-consultant doctors we found little evidence that any of these witnesses observed anything seriously wrong with Dr. Neary's practices. One or two more experienced registrars did have some concerns but were unwilling to jeopardise their career prospects by saying anything critical regarding consultants in their host country.[16]

15 HOW DOES SUCH AN UNQUESTIONING CULTURE EVOLVE? HOW DID IT CONTINUE FOR SO LONG?

15.1 When Dr. Neary first took up his post as consultant obstetrician in April 1974 at age 31 he joined a hospital founded, owned and managed by the Medical Missionaries of Mary. He knew and accepted that they practised Catholic

---

[16] One doctor recounted experience of working in several Irish provincial hospitals where he described the behaviour of consultants there as akin to third world despots.

rules on family planning in their maternity hospital and that they had great respect for hierarchical authority. Dr. Neary said that he was happy to work in such an ethos after his experience of legal abortions in England. The relevance of the ethos of the hospital to the Inquiry is well stated by a senior member of a medical training body -

"there are other issues that you can't really put your finger on when you talk about cultures in a hospital and values in a hospital and when you look at the role being played by Religious Orders in running institutions – they were very respectful of authorities and clinical authorities in particular that were represented through the various consultants and there was very much a non-questioning-- that you find this deference and respect that didn't allow a lot of questioning to happen – and good service – everybody was looked up to but there was I would say there was a culture there that needs to be appreciated"

15.2 The role of the strict ethos prior to and post the Papal encyclical Humanae Vitae on obstetric practices in this hospital cannot be overstated. Natural methods of family planning were encouraged and all other methods forbidden. Advice on *"artificial methods"* of family planning was forbidden. Tubal ligation was forbidden.

15.3 Dr. Neary has told us that Dr. Connolly advised him of the position in relation to sterilisation and explained as follows: *"Tubal ligations and contraception were absolutely forbidden but if he was worried that a uterus might rupture during a subsequent pregnancy because of what he observed at caesarean section, then neither he nor the MMMs would have any objection or problem if a hysterectomy was performed".* He told us that Dr. Connolly (who died in 2000) was totally against any artificial contraception and had admonished him and threatened to eject him for having a sample of the contraceptive pill in his offices in Fair Street, which he rented from Dr. Connolly.

15.4 He said that Dr. Connolly was a firm believer in carrying out symphysiotomies in the hopes of avoiding caesarean section and in this was influenced by Dr. Arthur Barry, the former Master of Holles Street Maternity Hospital. We found evidence of patients who had a symphysiotomy after delivery and patients who had a symphysiotomy and caesarean section. Dr. Neary disapproved strongly of this operation and never carried one out. Shortly after Dr. Connolly retired in 1982, the practice ceased.

15.5 One of the first witnesses who attended the Inquiry was a former patient of Dr. Connolly, and her evidence vividly demonstrated the extent to which his attitude influenced Dr. Neary. She had severe post partum bleeding which ended in hysterectomy. When Dr. Connolly was explaining the operation to her afterwards, he used the expression *"if the hysterectomy was not carried out, you would have been going home in a box"*. She wondered if Dr. Neary who used this expression frequently, had learned it from Dr. Connolly.

15.6 Dr. Neary was very aware from his first day at the hospital that a strict Catholic code applied. The MMMs occupied almost all the key positions in both the Maternity and the general hospitals at the time. There were MMM doctors in training and many of the midwifery students were MMMs. He believes that Dr. Connolly was trained in Drogheda by an MMM who was a surgeon. The MMMs ran a tightly controlled hospital in accordance with their ethos. Perhaps Dr. Neary did not fully appreciate what was encompassed by this ethos. Working in a Catholic hospital meant more than no abortions or sterilisations as contraception but included prohibition on many infertility treatments and investigations and information on modern family planning methods. It meant that women who should not become pregnant because of a medical condition were in a difficult position especially if there was nothing wrong with the condition of their uterus.

15.7 Hysterectomy as an elective obstetric procedure or as a planned gynaecological operation has a well defined history which was referred to in Term of Reference 1.

15.8 A number of obstetricians in practice in the '70s and '80s told the Inquiry that hysterectomy tended to be more frequently performed in areas where contraception was prohibited or not readily available. One of Dr. Neary's former mentors during his training in England sent us an extract from a book, which he had co-authored which confirms what we were told. The book is entitled 'Human Fertility Control Theory and Practice', author D.S. Hawkins and M.G. Elder, published by Butterworth (1979 edition).

".....hysterectomy as a primary sterilising procedure is reasonable in patients with uterine pathology such as fibromyomata, and in patients who suffer from menorrhagia or other menstrual abnormalities and who fully appreciate that the operation is quite irrevocable. It may also be appropriate in communities where pelvic inflammatory complications are common after tubal sterilisation. **The use of hysterectomy on relatively trivial gynaecological grounds is sometimes considered for sterilisation in environments where primary sterilising procedures have a religious or cultural stigma.** *[Our emphasis]*

The psychological consequences of hysterectomy must not be underestimated. It is not infrequent for women to regret having been sterilised and these patients have a chance of subsequently developing psychosomatic gynaecological symptoms.

The other arguments against hysterectomy as a primary sterilisation procedure are that it substitutes a major operation for a relatively minor one with a corresponding increase in morbidity and mortality. The failure rates of standard methods of sterilisation are so low that the advantage of eliminating sterilisation failures becomes theoretical, whilst the elimination of a chance of subsequent uterine or ovarian pathology does not in general justify the routine use of major surgery."

15.9 A document given to us by the MMMs entitled 'Ethical and Religious Directives for Catholic Health Facilities' published by the National Catholic Bishops Conference of the United States in 1971, deals with the issues of sterilisation, contraception, donor insemination and the collection of semen for artificial insemination. Article 22 states:

"Hysterectomy is permitted when it is sincerely judged to be a necessary means of removing some serious uterine pathological condition. In these

cases, the pathological condition of each patient must be considered individually and care must be taken that a hysterectomy is not performed merely as a contraceptive measure or as a routine procedure after any definite number of caesarean sections"[17].

15.10 The direction confirms that hysterectomy rather than tubal ligation was recommended for a serious pathological condition of the uterus. Much evidence was received to the effect that the prohibition on sterilisations common to any hospital with a Catholic ethos in the '60s and '70s gave rise to the performance of what have been described as **compassionate hysterectomies** performed on women with obstetric or socio-economic problems. In other words, the threshold for performing such procedures was fairly low and an obstetric reason was made on the operation note. For instance, the surgeon might report placenta accreta or scar adherence. The uterus was not sent for histology. The surgeon had exercised his clinical judgement and no one was prepared to question or criticise the bending of a harsh rule to the benefit of the patient. It was an unspoken Irish solution to an Irish question.

15.11 Dr. Neary was of the view that a climate of resort to hysterectomy at a fairly low threshold was well established when he arrived at the hospital in early 1974 and he believed that Dr. Connolly probably carried out compassionate hysterectomies. The number of caesarean sections was low perhaps partly due to the recourse to symphysiotomy. The perinatal death rate was high compared with the Dublin teaching hospitals but conditions were not comparable. The Inquiry reviewed all data available in the hospital to determine whether this was true and found that in the period of 1960 –1973, 31 peripartum hysterectomies had been carried out in the maternity hospital. Of those women -

- 16 had 6 or more children previously.
- 8 had 4 to 5 children previously,

---

[17] The MMMs wish to reiterate that no peripartum hysterectomies are attributable to the Catholic ethos of the hospital, nor were they aware that any secondary sterilisations ever took place.

- 2 had 3 previous children,
- 2 had 2 previous children,
- 1 had no previous pregnancies,
- 2 had no details

15.12   Of the list of 31 peripartum hysterectomies 15 were delivered by caesarean section, 13 were vaginal deliveries, most of which were instrumental deliveries, 2 followed laparotomy and 1 was unknown. The use of forceps for vaginal delivery was common. In the period of 1960-1973 there were 29979 deliveries thus giving one hysterectomy for every 967 births which considering the stillbirth and mortality figures seems acceptable. In the same period there were 1023 caesarean sections thus giving one hysterectomy for every 68 caesarean sections,

15.13   We are advised that a peripartum hysterectomy during that time period in a woman of high parity would not raise queries in any hospital. In the Lourdes Hospital, all hysterectomies following caesarean section were referred to in the Hospital's annual reports but the details were not necessarily recorded. The hysterectomies following vaginal delivery were not commented upon in the reports under a specific heading as hysterectomy following caesarean section was. Sometimes the details of these hysterectomies were found as a procedure mentioned under another heading such as atonic uterus or rupture or post partum haemorrhage.

15.14   Dr. Feeney, who assisted the Inquiry on all obstetric matters, has looked at most of the files available for the period 1960-1973 and advises that the obstetrics practised at the Maternity Unit during that period included some very extreme and challenging cases. In the same period there were 20 maternal deaths. As the Lourdes Hospital was the biggest hospital in the area, it tended to receive emergency non booked cases and to receive referred home birth emergencies and emergencies from the nearby Cottage Hospital. In examining the figures for maternal deaths it was very notable that in the first 8 years following Dr. Neary's arrival, there were no maternal deaths following post-partum haemorrhage in the hospital.

15.15 Bad luck in obstetrics is said to come in clusters and the Lourdes Maternity Hospital was no exception. The careful, conservative and assiduous Dr. O'Brien had a cluster of 3 obstetric hysterectomies in 1970. Dr. Connolly certainly had a number of failed instrumental deliveries with fresh stillbirths in the earlier years. As we have not compared these figures with those prevailing elsewhere or against any benchmark, it is not possible to comment on whether such outcomes were within acceptable limits at this Maternity Unit. It is certainly noteworthy that in the first 6 years after Dr. Neary took up his position not only were there no maternal deaths following post-partum haemorrhage, but the stillbirth and neonatal death rate fell considerably. The fall in neonatal deaths must in part be attributed to the arrival of a new paediatrician but it cannot be a coincidence that the stillbirth rate fell when Dr. Neary arrived, even though the birth rate rose. It is very probable that Dr. Neary's reputation as a competent obstetrician was deserved in the early years and more than likely served to conceal the fault lines in his practice.

15.16 We asked what experience Dr. Neary had of peripartum hysterectomy before he joined the unit. He told the Inquiry that he had assisted at 4 peripartum hysterectomies in his 2 years as senior registrar at Portsmouth. These would not have been in lieu of tubal ligation but for obstetric emergencies. He carried out his first peripartum hysterectomy at the Lourdes Hospital in 1975. Dr. Connolly had carried out one in the previous year. Dr. Neary's patient had a haemorrhage 8 days after caesarean section. There was clearly an obstetric emergency and the records show conservative measures to conserve the uterus. The case was reported in the Annual Reports. The rate thereafter followed the pattern of previous years of 2-3 hysterectomies a year at the unit. What did change was the profile of Dr. Neary's patients who were generally younger and of lower parity.

15.17 In 1978 there were 8 caesarean hysterectomies carried out – 5 by Dr. Neary and 3 by Dr. Connolly with Dr. Neary assisting at one. **In the short space of 6 years (1974–1979 inclusive), Dr. Neary had carried out 20 peripartum hysterectomies.** To put this number in perspective, in the 14 years before he came to the unit and when Dr. Feeney described the practices in the unit as somewhat at the extreme end of obstetrics, there were 31 peripartum hysterectomies. Between 1974-1979 inclusive there were 28 such operations, 20 of which were performed by Dr. Neary. **We believe that these findings go beyond bad luck or clusters.** The figures were published and disseminated openly but no one commented or questioned the figures. The crude rate of hysterectomy to delivery was now 1 hysterectomy to 579 deliveries.

15.18   Dr. Neary explained that many cases presented to him were women whose medical condition meant that further pregnancy was contraindicated. These were therefore secondary sterilisations acceptable to Dr. Connolly and the ethos of the hospital or they were for intractable bleeding. He said that from the early 1980s he referred such private patients to a colleague in Dublin for tubal ligation. He also referred patients to Newry. Some of the patients were public patients .He told us that he could not use hospital notepaper when making such referrals. He believed that the nuns had spies everywhere ready to report back to the Tripartite and to cause him to lose his job if they became aware of his practice of referring patients for tubal ligation.[18] We asked Dr. O'Brien what he did when faced with a patient who should not become pregnant again. He told us that he was not permitted to give such patients any contraceptive advice and would refer them to their GP to provide them with appropriate referrals.

15.19   Dr. Neary told the Inquiry that he would never carry out a hysterectomy as a primary contraceptive procedure. He told the Inquiry that patients frequently asked him to carry out an elective hysterectomy following caesarean section. He would say *"I will do a hysterectomy if your uterus is in poor condition but not if it looks healthy"*. Many of his patients were disappointed when he would not carry out the procedure as the uterus looked healthy. If the uterus was attenuated, thin or likely to rupture, then he would perform a hysterectomy. He would carry out the hysterectomy based on his clinical assessment and not necessarily following consultation with the patient. He was very conservative in relation to gynaecological hysterectomy for spurious reasons

---

[18] The MMMs were offended by Dr. Neary's comment that they had spies everywhere. This observation was put to Dr. Neary but he maintained his position.

and was well known for his conservative approach. If he could have advised patients on the use of effective contraception many of the hysterectomies carried out at caesarean section would have been unnecessary. Tubal ligations should have been the appropriate option for many of his patients. The lack of tubal ligations for public patients forced him to resort to caesarean hysterectomy. If he carried out a tubal ligation he would lose his job but hysterectomy for medical reasons was not a problem. He told us of a doctor who he named who would have been dismissed by the MMMs for advising contraception had it not been for his intervention.

15.20 When he first presented these responses to the Inquiry, it was felt that he was exaggerating the position about the strict Catholic ethos at the hospital. Some witnesses had previously reported that at Ethics Committee meetings, Dr. Neary and his colleague Dr. Lynch took up a very strong position on either adopting the strict application of the Catholic position or the deletion of all mention of sterilisation. They would not support a watered down version of this position, which was difficult to interpret. They wanted the situation to be black or white with no grey areas. Either they were allowed to carry out tubal ligations or they were forbidden. Their position perplexed the other members of the committee. At these ethics meetings, Dr. Neary frequently recounted the story of a young doctor who had been dismissed for counselling the use of contraception in the case of a patient advised against further pregnancy. Those witnesses were inclined to the view that as Dr. Neary never named the young doctor and as Sr. A., MMM a member of the Ethics Committee seemed unaware of his existence, then the matter was pure invention and an example of his propensity to exaggerate.

15.21 Careful perusal of the Ethics file disclosed the following letter dated 26th July 1983. It is a letter from Sr. G.,, MMM, to Sr. E. It relates to medical ethics and the training of staff in this area. the Inquiry considers this an important document.

"You will remember we discussed the two Junior Hospital Doctors who recently held posts as Obstetrical House Officers and their stand on the issue of oral contraception.

This raises some questions and I would be concerned lest we, as Religious Sisters in charge of the hospital, should be seen to fail in this area. I believe we must take a stand on this issue and should provide the necessary training and teaching by means of symposia on developments in Reproductive Science."

The letter refers to a document called *"Memorandum regarding training in Natural Family Planning".*

"The development of the contraceptive pill has brought world wide awareness of the sad fact that advances in medicine are no longer advances made for healing purposes but to interfere and cause obstruction in perfectly normal bodily function (the human reproductive process). This has resulted in much iatrogenic (medicine caused) disease, disorder, dysfunction and even fatalities. Besides this, contraceptive practice has resulted in widespread social evil – world wide – and has militated against the Christian concept of marriage and family life.

How do we, a body of religious women in the Church, dedicated to healing with a particular concern for the Christian family deal with this problem?

Do we organise regular symposia on development in Reproductive Science (a science on which natural family planning is based) for our Junior Doctors, Nurses and Midwives?

Are we seen to take a firm stand on the Church's teaching on these matters?

Do we allocate finance to provide lectures, scientific handouts, visual aids, posters, slides, and films?

Do we send members of our staff to conferences either here or overseas?

Do we have a Medical Ethics Committee?

Do we have a reputable moral theologian appointed to the hospital?

Do we have written contracts which express the obligation of medical staff to abide by the hospital's ethical moral problems?

Do we have a written Code of Ethics?

Some Facts and Experiences:

Facts:
RCOG's requirements for training Junior House Doctors must get Family Planning Training (hence the need to institute regular symposia).

Young doctors receive training in some Dublin hospitals with practicals at the Irish Family Planning Association (N.B. this body is an affiliated member of the International Planned Parenthood Federation, IPPF).

Experiences:
A young doctor is known to have offered advice to patients in Maternity on taking Oral Contraceptives.

Another Obstetrical House Officer is now about to set up Private Practice in Drogheda offering a full contraceptive service.

At a recent inspection for midwifery training one of the visiting committee, a doctor, enquired about the availability of a contraceptive birth control for patients. She remarked that it was discriminatory to promote only the natural method.

Note:
In view of the above trends it would appear that it is only a matter of time until we have doctors in our hospital with unchristian ethical values. We

need to take our stand to stem this flow of the tide. God will bless such a stand however small it may be to stem this tide.[19]

This letter confirms much of what we were told and when taken together with another incident described by Dr. Neary it helps to understand his view that the ethos of the hospital was rigid and unchanging. Dr. Neary's views were shared by all of the doctors to whom we spoke – those in training and those in consultant positions – that this was an unusual hospital as far as family planning was concerned.

15.22 When we discussed the ethos with some of the MMMs in senior positions they suggested that their stance had modified over the years and that they had come to recognise that pastoral needs had changed. Their view was that tubal ligation for medical reasons was not unreasonable and anyway they *"were not looking over the obstetrician's shoulder"*.

15.23 When this softer attitude to family planning was put to personnel in the Maternity Unit, it was treated as utter revisionism and rejected. Whatever the reality of the current more moderate stand, Dr. Neary's experience of the rigidity of the ethos was that it never modified. He described what was for him a seminal event. In 1980/1981 a patient came to him seeking a tubal ligation to be carried at the same time as caesarean section. Dr. Neary sought the views of the Matron on the matter, as he had been advised that this was a case where the tubal ligation would be seen as a medical procedure. The official Vatican position on sterilisation was that direct sterilisation where the intention was to prevent conception was prohibited but indirect sterilisation where the primary intention was to isolate a diseased organ was permitted. Dr.Neary clearly believed that this was a medically appropriate case for sterilisation. In other words this was a case of indirect sterilisation.

---

[19] The MMMs caution attaching weight to this letter as the author had a well-known propensity to write letters on such subjects. She was an extreme advocate of pro-life and the natural family planning method. She was a member of the National Association of Ovulation Method of Ireland and was a close associate of John and Lynne Billings of international repute.

15.24 The patient had consulted Dr. O'C, a professor of moral theology at Maynooth who advised that in her case, tubal ligation was permitted, as the primary intention was to prevent the death or serious ill health of the mother in a future pregnancy. This view was passed on to the MMMs who were unhappy with this advice and sought the opinion of a Bishop and a Cardinal. The Bishop disagreed with the professor of moral theology and restated the absolutist position of the Catholic Church, which would allow of no exceptions. The Cardinal advised the MMMs that they had taken the correct position in refusing to allow a tubal ligation. The patient apparently went elsewhere to have her baby and to be sterilised by tubal ligation. The Ethics Committee file confirms this position with the following advice from the Bishop –

"this is a very difficult situation. However the Church's thinking regarding this operation is very clear. It does not depend on circumstances nor on certain thinking among some theologians.

One must seek the solution outside of direct sterilisation which can only be wrong in itself. We must always recognise matters, which are wrong in themselves: example cruelty, discrimination, apartheid, sexual morality – abortion. It would be always inconsistent to attempt to find exemptions in these circumstances. If we had exceptions we would not maintain Catholic standards. No diversity of opinion can be permitted."

15.25 The Inquiry spoke at length to Dr. O'C who told us that he was saddened by the interpretation put on permitted *"indirect"* sterilisations in Catholic hospitals in the past. These sterilisations had been performed by hysterectomy instead of tubal ligation. There appeared to be an absolute horror of performing tubal ligation but an insouciant acceptance of hysterectomy, a much more invasive operation which for the patient was a major procedure with likelihood of psychological consequences. He did not recall the specifics of the particular case described in the ethics file and referred to by Dr. Neary as his advice was constantly sought on such similar hard cases in the '70s and '80s. His advice in such a case would have been that tubal ligation was the appropriate indirect sterilisation. His memory is that the debate moved on when tubal ligation as a form of contraception became available generally after 1985 in most hospitals.

15.26 Sr. E. MMM recounted this incident when interviewed in September 2004. Her colleague Sr. B. received a letter forwarded from the Matron regarding Dr. Neary's patient who was seeking a tubal ligation at the Lourdes maternity hospital. Sr. E. sought a meeting with Dr. Neary and explained that this presented an ethical matter for the hospital which was *"very Catholic and we don't do that thing here."* Dr. Neary became very angry and told her that he had consulted a professor of moral theology and he had said go ahead, that it was a special case as the lady had 5 previous sections. He threatened her with the Court of Human Rights as the woman's right to treatment was being blocked. Subsequently Prof. O'C called Sr. E. and explained why it was a special case. She became concerned that perhaps Dr. Neary would bring an action and because the hospital was under the Archdiocese, she called the Cardinal and discussed the matter with him. The Cardinal came to see her several times about the issue. Further discussions took place with Prof.O'C in person and through correspondence and further advice was sought from other theologians. The ultimate advice was that Sr. E. was correct to refuse the patient a tubal ligation. When Dr. Neary was given the news, he accepted it gracefully and the patient was never admitted to the hospital.

15.27 Sr. E. believed that the decision was right at the time because that was her training but following further training and participation at ethical meetings she became aware that a serious body of people had differing views. That was one of the reasons why an ethics committee was set up in the hospital.

15.28 Dr. Neary tells a very dramatic story of the sequel to this incident. It was his 40th Birthday and he was summoned to the convent to one of the parlours. He believed that the summons was to mark the occasion and he was touched. Instead he found that the parlour[20] contained a large gathering of senior

---

[20] Dr. Neary was made aware that the MMMs who had been interviewed by the Inquiry denied that any such meetings took place. The MMMs question the authenticity of this story. Dr. Neary was questioned again and maintained his position providing the Inquiry with further details of his memory of the meetings. Dr. Neary informed the Inquiry that following on from the meeting with the MMMs and later

figures from the MMMs who indicated that they had information of his intention to carry out a tubal ligation. He told this group of MMMs who he did not know that although he received 3-5 requests for tubal ligation every week, he always informed the patients that sterilisations were not permitted and could not be done in the hospital. He felt that the tone of the meeting was about his suspension and he was very much afraid that he would lose his job. Eventually he persuaded them that he would not carry out any tubal ligations but was nevertheless obliged subsequently to address the entire body of consultants and to reiterate his position that he had not agreed to sterilise any patient and that he upheld the ethos of the MMMs. He felt vulnerable thereafter and felt shunned by his colleagues. In June, he was summoned to a meeting with the Cardinal when it was explained to him what the consequences of performing a tubal ligation would be. The Cardinal told him that he was aware of where his siblings worked and where his nephews were at school. If he carried out any tubal ligation in the hospital, he had the power to ensure that consequences would follow for his siblings' jobs.

The Inquiry did not have the resources to confirm any aspect of this alleged meeting.

15.29 All the evidence heard and obtained from files in our custody point to a very strict interpretation of Catholic doctrine on tubal ligation in this hospital. We are inclined to adopt Prof. O'C's view that such interpretation meant that medically advised sterilisation was carried out by means of hysterectomy. This view was also referred to in the extract from *"Human Fertility Control Theory and Practice"*.

15.30 We are satisfied that Dr. Neary's fears that any observed deviation from the ethos of the MMMs would result in dismissal were well founded. It is very probable that this experience was a stark lesson to Dr. Neary and perhaps the other doctors with any connections to obstetrics in the hospital. As an example we were made aware of a pathologist who was afraid to examine

on with the Cardinal, he never again attended at any ceremony in the Lourdes Hospital when the Cardinal was present.

fallopian tubes sent from Dundalk Hospital for histology as he felt that it would breach his contract of employment with the MMMs to adhere to the Catholic ethos of the hospital. It is very probable that Dr. Neary smarted from this interference with his clinical judgement and the imposition of religious beliefs ahead of patient welfare. If he entertained any suspicions previously about the MMMs his employers, his experience following the attempt to carry out a tubal ligation seems to have fed his feelings thereafter.

15.31 We have heard so much evidence from so many Lourdes Hospital witnesses regarding sterilisations that we feel obliged to accept that hysterectomy was carried out in the Lourdes Maternity Unit where in other hospitals tubal ligation or safe methods of contraception would be advised.

15.32 When tubal ligations were first carried out in the State it was normal for the request to be reviewed by an ethics committee. Unfortunately in this hospital, there was no necessity for the obstetrician/gynaecologist to seek approval from a Board or an Ethics Committee if he wished to carry out an indirect sterilisation by hysterectomy. There was no mechanism for ensuring that secondary sterilisation was carried out reasonably. While tubal ligations were always prohibited there appeared to be no review whatsoever of the circumstance in which peripartum hysterectomy was carried out.

15.33 Many witnesses have described to us that there was no love lost between Dr. Neary and the MMMs. He is reported to have threatened to *"get"* a number of the senior sisters in management and made frequent derogatory remarks about the MMMs. Some junior doctors felt he had a serious chip on his shoulder about the nuns. Some of the sisters who were in regular contact with him through work had their difficulties with him and found him erratic, difficult and argumentative. *"You could never win an argument with him."* While some MMMs who were in senior administration had fewer difficulties, we are satisfied that Dr. Neary's relationship with his employers was not one of mutual respect and probably originated from fear and resentment following his experiences on the issue of tubal ligation. There was no evidence from any quarter to support the contention that Dr. Neary was protected by the MMMs.

15.34 Most doctors were aware of the possibility that hysterectomy might mask a compassionate sterilisation and as many were uncomfortable with the absolutism of the hospital's ethos, they turned a blind eye. Almost every consultant questioned was prepared to admit that this sometimes happened, no matter which hospital they practised in. This may well have created an atmosphere of tacit approval of the activities of the consultants and especially Dr. Neary, if it modified the application of unpopular ethics. If the MMMs did not know, then there would not be a problem.

15.35 If the MMMs did know that peripartum hysterectomy had taken place, they seemed to consider that the hysterectomy accorded with their ethos as it had to be for a medical reason. They never questioned medical practices. Unfortunately, this provided a culture of unquestioning acceptance of all hysterectomies until too many young women had been needlessly deprived of their uterus. The combined effect of respect for clinical decisions and the pushing of curiosity into a subliminal state contributed to the widespread inability to distinguish compassionate practices from really bad medicine. The Inquiry believes that this provides some explanation for why the MMMs, who were so concerned about sterilisation by way of tubal ligation, did not act despite the large numbers of peripartum hysterectomies.[21]

15.36 It is possible that after 1981 Dr. Neary felt that consulting an ethics committee in relation to tubal ligations for therapeutic purposes was a waste of time and he continued to carry out hysterectomies wherever he felt that another pregnancy would compromise the patient. In other words he followed the advice given to him by Dr. Connolly when he arrived in the hospital first. If the advice was right in Dr. Connolly's time it continued to be right and kept him out of trouble. Dr. Neary's own evidence ranged from stating that 75% of hysterectomies carried out were attributable to the unavailability of tubal

---

[21] The MMMs state that they were unaware of the number of hysterectomies and have reminded the Inquiry that the primary ethos of the MMMs is to protect the mother and child. Under no circumstances would the MMMs have acquiesced in unnecessary peripartum hysterectomies

ligations to the assertion that he had never carried out a sterilisation and he referred patients to Dublin and Newry for tubal ligation. The Inquiry contacted the doctors he named and confirmed that this evidence of referrals was accurate.

15.37 The Inquiry rejects the evidence that 75% of hysterectomies were attributable to the ethos of the hospital. Researching the numbers and speaking to many of Dr. Neary's former patients reveals that the number of patients who fit into the category of damaged uterus fell steadily as family size shrunk especially in the 1990s. Many of Dr. Neary's patients were of low parity having their first or second caesarean section unlike the majority of patients who are found on Dr.Lynch's list of caesarean hysterectomy. While evidence suggests that hysterectomy for contraceptive purposes was still resorted to in the 1990s the Inquiry is nevertheless convinced that the prevailing insular atmosphere of the unit which never questioned, reviewed or audited outcomes, allowed hysterectomies for perceived haemorrhage to continue at unacceptable rates throughout the last 10 years of Dr. Neary's practice.

15.38 The strict ethos may have contributed to the acceptance of high numbers of hysterectomies in the past but the acceptance should not have extended to the extraordinary numbers in the 1990s. At this stage it was obvious that families were being planned and tubal ligation was available in other hospitals in the North East region. It may well be that the history of openly accepting hysterectomy as normal in the past set the scene for the continued acceptance of the procedure until it came under scrutiny in October 1998. Unfortunately, if the habit of turning a blind eye or never questioning is combined with a lack of audit, it permits systemic malpractice to go unobserved. The unusual slowly become the norm. This happened in this Maternity Unit.

15.39 There has been no evidence to suggest that those who questioned were weeded out or punished or not listened to. With the exception of Matron of the Maternity Unit in or about 1980, there was no evidence that anyone questioned the figures of peripartum hysterectomy in the unit at all until at the earliest 1996. There was no evidence whatsoever that Dr. Neary was protected by the MMMs, by the midwives or his consultant colleagues.

15.40 The religious ethos and the hierarchical system must not be judged harshly and must be seen in the context of the times. Family planning was seen as a moral issue in much of rural and provincial Ireland until perhaps the mid '80s. There were many people who believed that artificial, as opposed to natural, methods of family planning were somehow wrong and damaging to society generally. It is difficult now to remember the not too distant past when many couples had to break the law in accessing contraception from the very few Irish Family Planning Clinics set up in 1969 or personally importing condoms from the UK or the North of Ireland. The Magee judgement is illustrative of where we were in 1973. Chief Justice William Fitzgerald in a minority decision said the following:

"One must naturally be sympathetic with the plaintiff in the dilemma in which she finds herself and which is attributable to her own physical health. It surely, however, must be recognised that the physical and mental health of either spouse in a marriage may effectively preclude a pregnancy either temporarily or, in some instances, permanently. Having regard to the provision in the Constitution prohibiting divorce, the physical or mental illness of one spouse necessarily has its repercussions on both, perhaps for their joint lives. These appear to me to be natural hazards which must be faced by married couples with such fortitude as they can summon to their assistance. In my opinion, the plaintiff has failed to establish a case entitling her to the relief claimed, and this appeal should be dismissed."

15.41 The Chief Justice and the President of The High Court did not recognise the right of a married woman with a serious medical condition to import a diaphragm contraceptive that could not legally be imported into the country. This thinking merely reflected the moral code of the majority of citizens of Ireland at the time and should be borne in mind when remarks are made about the events which occurred at the Lourdes Hospital in the '70s and '80s. It is simply unfair to impose the freedoms of today, achieved by years of slow incremental steps brought about by the women's movement, court actions, legislation and social evolution, onto the majority Catholic mores of yesteryears. It may be difficult to remember that three attempts to introduce legislation legalising contraception were defeated in the early and mid '70s. A booklet distributed by the IFPA was banned by the Censorship Board, although the prosecution of the publishers subsequently failed. The MMMs should not be criticised but their ethos understood in the context of the times.

15.42 Prior to 1979, all contraception was prohibited under the Criminal Law (Amendment) Act of 1935. The exception was the anovulatory pill, which was launched after the passing of the Act and thus not caught by the wording. Nevertheless it was imported under licence and prescribed as a cycle regulator and thus permitted as a medicine. A great number of prescriptions for the cure of irregular cycles were written. Again, an official blind eye was turned and we had yet another Irish solution to an Irish problem. The following article was found on the Ethics Committee file furnished to us by the MMMs and is a reminder of how life was in the period leading up to the decriminalisation of the import of contraceptives in 1979 and the amendment and liberalising of the distribution and availability of contraceptives in 1985. POSITION PAPER 68, which deals with the proposed legislation to decriminalise contraception following the Magee decision in summing up says:

"Catholic doctors, nurses, chemists and others who may be asked for assistance in the provision of contraceptives must, if they follow the teaching of the Church, refuse to prescribe, dispense or provide any assistance in the provision of contraceptives. It is doubly wrong to be involved in any way in the provision of possibly abortifacient "contraceptives". In regard to pills which are for medical use as well as contraceptive use, those who know they are wanted for contraceptive use (doctors and nurses will presumably know this) may not accede to a request to be involved in providing contraception; those who do not know which use will be made of them (chemists in particular) should not sell them unless they have some kind of assurance that they are to be used

for strictly medical ailments, for the subterfuge that they are not really contraceptives is wearing exceedingly thin."

15.43 Another document included in the Ethics file is a statement of the medico-moral code of the Catholic hospital which inter alia states that -

"the total good of the patient, which includes his spiritual as well as his bodily welfare, is the primary concern of those entrusted with the Catholic health facility. So important is this, in fact, that if an institution could not fulfil its basic mission in this regard, it would have no justification for continuing its existence as a Catholic health facility".

15.44 In writing this report, the Inquiry is aware that religion and medical care, especially in the area of women's fertility, are very involved in personal sensitivities and changing public mores. What is unacceptable now may have been perfectly acceptable in the past. One very eminent gynaecologist told us of the inappropriateness of mixing personally held beliefs with the medical needs of one's patients. Perhaps in a more conservative Ireland this was not fully appreciated.

16 THE MMMs

16.1 We found no evidence that the MMMs ever perceived that Dr. Neary was doing anything to harm patients. If any of the sisters had qualms about the rate, such doubts were assuaged when a former member of staff married to a doctor had a hysterectomy following the birth by caesarean section of her first baby. If that doctor or nurse, they reasoned, had no problem with the operation, well who were they to question the need for such procedure in a young mother. They were aware that hysterectomy following birth was necessary when haemorrhage could not be stopped. It has to be said however that almost every MMM interviewed stated that she had no knowledge of the peripartum hysterectomy rate. Several of the MMMs engaged in midwifery had vivid memories of mothers who had exsanguinated and felt that hysterectomy was a price all women were prepared to pay in such a situation. We heard several descriptions of mothers who had died because hysterectomy was not available.

16.2   The sisters evoked our sympathy. They belonged to an Order which obeyed the rules. They believed in hierarchy and saw their place in that hierarchy. They were individually subservient within the Order and the Order was subservient to the bishops and cardinals. They sought guidance and followed the advice received. They sincerely believed that what they were doing was right. They chose consultants who agreed to be bound by their ethos and they believed that a clinical decision should not be questioned and trained the nurses in the same way. Consultants were at the top of the hierarchy in the clinical management of their patients.

16.3   The MMMs had given their lives to the training of nurses and doctors for the missions in the developing countries of the world. Many of them have worked in medicine in trying and dangerous conditions in war torn countries in Africa. They found it difficult and perhaps painful to see their flagship hospital in Drogheda the subject of an Inquiry and the object of so much media comment. Although most of the senior members of the Order in Drogheda presented as exceptionally competent, capable no nonsense women, their training as nurses was that they did not question a consultant in how he carried out his work. Consultants were from time to time questioned and if necessary reprimanded on the occasions when patients complained. No patient as far as we could ascertain ever complained about Dr. Neary's clinical treatment until 1998 when the MMMs were no longer the owners of the hospital. The complaints related to rudeness, abruptness or shouting at midwives or patients and were not confined to Dr. Neary.

16.4   As mentioned previously, some of the MMMs got on with Dr. Neary and enjoyed his strong personality. Others left him alone being a little intimidated by his erratic moods and occasional displays of temper. They admired his dedication to his patients and were aware of his popularity with patients and midwives. They left him to get on with his work and had no concerns regarding his clinical practices. They did not look over his shoulder in theatre. One senior MMM did not believe anyone would have informed her if they had suspicions that Dr. Neary was carrying out sterilisation by hysterectomy or for any other reason, as it would be a breach of patient confidentiality and wrong for her to receive such information.

16.5　Lack of transparency was another feature, which contributed to the isolation of the Maternity Unit. Transparency and accountability are features of administration which were not apparent in the management style of the hospital. There appeared to be very little involvement between the MMMs and the consultants after Dr. Connolly retired. There was no evidence of any shared involvement between the MMMs, the Matron of the Maternity Unit and the senior midwives and the consultants in the management of the Maternity Unit. There was little to suggest that the different levels of hierarchy ever sat down together to discuss issues of concern. There was little to suggest the existence of informed communication systems.　Layers of hierarchy ran in parallel lines.

17　CONCLUSIONS

17.1　The numbers of caesarean hysterectomies carried out by Dr. Neary in the late 1970s caused the Matron some concern. She spoke to his colleagues to express her concerns. She was not heeded although Dr. Connolly very perceptively observed that he was *"afraid of haemorrhage"*. No one acted on this fear or appreciated that his fear might actually harm patients. The Matron was afraid to speak out further as she believed Dr. Neary's practices had been reviewed and found acceptable.

17.2　A temporary MMM midwifery tutor had concerns at the same time. Her concerns may have been partially that Dr. Neary was carrying out sterilisations. She did not bring her concerns to the MMMs or to any person in authority.

17.3　Many of the hysterectomies were accepted as sterilisations even though Dr. Neary said that the patient was haemorrhaging.

17.4　No other person had any concerns until the late 1990s when hysterectomy was carried out on a number of young women of low parity.

17.5   Dr. Neary's air of competence and confidence in the theatre masked any further appreciation of his fear of haemorrhage from his colleagues. Dr. Neary's competence in other areas of obstetrics and gynaecology concealed his defensive practices in carrying out hysterectomy when faced with a particular type of bleeding.

TERM 4

To inquire into what, if any, review and consultation took place, either within the hospital, or externally following peripartum hysterectomy.

1. The Inquiry has determined that every peripartum hysterectomy performed during the period relevant to this Inquiry was recorded, on a day report, either to the Matron of the Maternity Unit, or to her deputy

2. The Labour Ward Superintendent or one of the seven labour ward sisters prepared the day report. Originally this officeholder was an MMM, but since the 1980s, the Labour Ward Superintendent has been a lay midwife. The day report was a report of all activity in the unit and not confined to peripartum hysterectomy. It was produced twice daily.

3. Peripartum hysterectomy was recorded and treated as any other operation carried out in the maternity theatre. All deliveries and surgical procedures on the labour ward were recorded in Day Books to facilitate hand over when the shift of midwives changed. The Matron and her assistant, the Labour Ward Superintendent and the labour ward sisters were all senior members of nursing staff who were aware of every hysterectomy that took place in the Maternity Unit on their shift. The significance of peripartum hysterectomy as an adverse outcome was appreciated if the woman was young or had very few children but there was no realisation that that the rate in the Maternity Unit was different. Before 1997 it was not included as an item on the daily statistics kept on the labour ward.

4. Until 1986 any emergency caesarean section or examination under anaesthetic involved theatre nurses walking over from the general hospital – which was five minutes away - to assist in the operating room. If the hysterectomy followed a postpartum haemorrhage, the patient was transferred between the two hospitals by ambulance and the operation was carried out in the general hospital with regular theatre staff.

5. It is reasonable to assume that the theatre sister who had to make arrangements to release theatre nurses to the maternity hospital would have been aware of every hysterectomy that followed a caesarean section or uterine rupture. We were unable to interview the former gynaecology theatre sister, as she was not prepared to be interviewed. The gynaecology ward sister was unwilling to speak to the Inquiry as she told us she was not well. They are the only two nurses who were not willing to be interviewed.

6. In 1986 several of the midwives were trained to assist at caesarean section and there was no longer a need to contact theatre nurses in the general hospital. Other hands therefore had to be called to manage the labour ward to replace those midwives who had been borrowed for theatre. If the caesarean section or procedure under anaesthesia turned into a hysterectomy, then obviously, the theatre nurses were delayed in returning to their duties. The notification to the matron or her administrative assistant appeared to be an organisational and staffing issue. The day reports did not give any appearance of noting peripartum hysterectomy as an adverse outcome. No consequences followed peripartum hysterectomy from the matron's point of view. Her day reports were stored in her office. The matron in the general hospital was not specifically notified. No information in relation to peripartum hysterectomy was forwarded to any outside body or authority. There was no obligation or process to report such a procedure.

7. As midwives spent more time in theatre away from the labour ward, more midwives were needed to take their place. More temporary contracts could be approved by the Department of Health and converted into permanent jobs. The Inquiry has formed the view that the administrative noting of peripartum hysterectomy in the Maternity Unit in 1997 was associated uniquely with human resource issues. This appears to have been the case when the operation was recorded in the daily figures.

8. The Inquiry interviewed the senior midwifery staff and could not elicit why, from 1997, caesarean hysterectomy was included as an entry in the daily figures, apart from advancing the argument that although the birth rate was falling, operations requiring midwifery assistance were rising. One of the

senior administrators in the Maternity Unit told the Inquiry that her only specific interest in statistics was:

"when we were looking for more staff I would say to the Labour Ward Sisters, 'well, you have the statistics there, can you draw a graph of the number of epidurals, the number of people that had general anaesthetics', because this impinged more on – we needed more staff because we were trying to get an Anaesthetic Nurse, to get somebody trained that could do anaesthetic, you know, and that really is the only time. But I never actually put the thing together myself and looked at it and said; you've had so many to-day and so many last month."

9. Peripartum hysterectomy was not noted on the monthly statistics in the labour ward in 1993 when the number of hysterectomies was 15 - the highest rate ever in the unit. In 1994 there were 9 hysterectomies carried out and in 1995 there were 11 such procedures. We heard no evidence from any source of any concerns during that period.

10. Before January 1997, if a peripartum hysterectomy was carried out, it was possible for the midwives who took up duty 24 hours later to be unaware that such a procedure had taken place, as a new day sheet would have been opened. There was no notification of the event. There was no meeting in the Unit to discuss whether anything could have been done to avoid the operation, or if any procedure could be improved if the same circumstances giving rise to the hysterectomy occurred in the future.

11. As far as we could ascertain, there was no formal discussion between the consultants about why the procedure was necessary or whether anything could be learned from the experience. Peripartum hysterectomy was treated as a variation of a normal delivery. It was assumed the procedure was carried out for a legitimate reason, and work went on. Three obstetric consultants who spoke to the Inquiry were unaware of their colleagues' activities in theatre. There was no system to discuss adverse or unexpected

outcomes, although it was open to every consultant to refer to the theatre register, which was supposed to record every procedure.

12. For the most part, the peripartum hysterectomies were well spread out through the 1980s, although from time to time there were clusters of 3 such procedures. For instance, 3 peripartum hysterectomies were carried out between the 1st and 11th.October 1980. 2 of these operations were carried out in one day by two different surgeons. In all 3 cases, blood was requested and used. The minimum transfusion was 8 units, and in 1 case 12 units were transfused. While the charts are missing in 2 out of these 3 cases, secondary documents indicate ruptured uterus in 2 of those cases. The alarming looking figures can thus be legitimately explained in 2 cases and probably go a long way towards explaining the belief that the hysterectomies were always carried out for good reasons in the face of major obstetrical emergency. All the cases were reported in the annual reports, with the caveat that the annual reports were not actually printed or disseminated for some years after the events.

13. Dr. O'Brien does not have any recollection of any discussion or analysis following any peripartum hysterectomy. Dr. Neary told the Inquiry that, from the time of his arrival in April 1974, he was responsible for producing the biennial report and sending statistics to the RCOG in London and the Institute of Obstetricians and Gynaecologists in Dublin. As a consequence, he was very familiar with statistics for all procedures in the Maternity Unit. He told us that he and Dr. Connolly had many discussions about the caesarean section rate, the maternal mortality rate, the caesarean hysterectomy rate and symphysiotomy. He did not tell us about any analysis or discussion regarding each specific peripartum hysterectomy.

14. Dr. Neary had trained in a hospital where formal discussions on adverse outcomes took place. In particular, Dr. Neary told the Inquiry that during the 3 years that he spent in Portsmouth, he assisted as senior registrar in theatre with different consultants on 4 different occasions for caesarean hysterectomies. The 4 cases were discussed at a half-day clinical meeting. There is no evidence that clinical meetings took place regarding any such procedures during the period that Dr. Neary was a consultant in the Maternity Unit of the Lourdes Hospital.

15. Dr. Neary told the Inquiry that informal discussions took place after emergency caesarean hysterectomy in the Lourdes. When pressed, he agreed that these might take the form of his giving reasons to the Labour Ward Superintendent or to the Matron or her deputy for why the hysterectomy had to be performed. The senior ward sisters and the anaesthetists confirmed that reasons were generally sought by them and provided by Dr. Neary. Dr.Neary's reasons were never questioned. Very few witnesses seemed to have recollections relating to hysterectomies carried out by the other obstetricians or registrars, and they were shocked to hear that there were so many. We heard no evidence to believe that the reporting procedure differed for those hysterectomies.

16. We would have welcomed an opportunity to discuss many questions with Dr. Finian Lynch, the consultant who replaced Dr. Connolly in 1982. We obtained written responses to questions posed to Dr. Lynch. From his responses we learned that until the controversy about the number of caesarean hysterectomies in the Lourdes Hospital emerged in late 1998, he was not particularly conscious of the rate, nor of any issues with regard to the rate of caesarean hysterectomy at the hospital. He stated that the information available on the rate of these procedures was extremely limited. Following his appointment as a Consultant Obstetrician/Gynaecologist at the Lourdes Hospital in 1982, he requested that an appropriate IT system be installed to ensure the accuracy of all the data and information available to the medical staff. Such a system has still not been installed. Annual Clinical Reports were prepared which provided useful statistical information. When it was his turn as newest consultant to prepare the annual reports he refused to participate until a computerised database of procedures was in use. It was Dr. Lynch's belief that the last such report was completed in 1984. He stated that as there was no adequate statistical information available to him or his colleagues from that time onwards, there were no comparisons of the Lourdes Hospital and the three Dublin maternity hospitals with regard to peripartum hysterectomy. In Dr. Lynch's experience, there was no material difference between the treatment of postpartum haemorrhage at the Lourdes Hospital and elsewhere.

17. Dr. Lynch stated that there was no specific protocol for calling for assistance in a situation where it seemed that hysterectomy was likely. There was a general understanding that if assistance was needed, it would be available either from obstetricians, surgeons or anaesthetists as necessary. No person ever commented to Dr. Lynch about the rate of peripartum hysterectomy in the unit. There were no formal meetings to discuss any operation, neither was there any forum for discussing any concerns. The Lourdes Hospital never compared its peripartum hysterectomy rate with that of the three Dublin maternity hospitals. He was not necessarily aware when Dr. Neary performed a post partum hysterectomy, although sometimes he was informed anecdotally by the Matron or Dr. Neary on an informal basis. From time to time, he called in Dr. Neary to assist in theatre, and he recalled being called in by his colleagues to assist them.

18. The remaining consultant in the unit was Dr. Seosamh O'Coigligh who joined the unit in October 1997 as a consultant on probation for 12 months to replace Dr. O'Brien who retired in 1996. Dr.O'Coigligh had never carried out or assisted at a peripartum hysterectomy before he took up his post in Drogheda. In his first year there he remarked that there were no meetings, either with his colleagues or as clinical pathological conferences. He found this odd. The first hysterectomy he carried out was for a completely ruptured and disintegrated uterus. He heard no feedback from his colleagues following this hysterectomy nor was he asked to present his findings. If any comment was made, it might have been in sympathy, saying that *"this sort of thing eventually happens to all of us"*. He had no recollection of any query from the Matron or the Labour Ward Superintendent as to why the hysterectomy was necessary. No person appeared to have any interest in the operation, nor was Dr.O'Coigligh obliged to notify any person.

19. When he carried out a second hysterectomy later that year, his initial reaction was that he could not believe that he was doing another caesarean hysterectomy within a year of having done the first one. He does not recall sitting down with his colleagues and having a meeting with them or anybody about it.

20. The Inquiry appreciates that adverse and unexpected outcomes are part and parcel of everyday hospital life. One of the objects of clinical audit is to identify those outcomes that were both unexpected and avoidable, and to minimise their recurrence. The steps taken to analyse the event into the 'why and how' it occurred, and the sharing of that knowledge is an essential part of good medical practice. The modern version and language for this long accepted practice is now known as 'risk management' and 'clinical governance', which have at their heart the need to identify best practice and to avoid harm to patients.

21. The culture in the Lourdes Maternity Unit was one of recording and acceptance. There was no discussion or analysis. There was no identifiable intent to deceive in this lack of analysis. Comparisons with other hospitals were not made. Best practice was left to each individual consultant to identify and apply without any review or audit. This seems to be *"the way things were done."* If a consultant did something, then it was automatically accepted as right. One consultant never reviewed or queried another colleague's decisions or procedures. Strange as this may seem, the preponderance of the evidence that we received indicates that small units like the Lourdes Maternity Unit frequently operated in this way, as the alternative was perceived to create unworkable tension. It appeared to the Inquiry that, for the most part, the ability and integrity of individual consultants in outlying hospitals is what keeps a reasonable health service afloat. Prior to the shocking revelations from the Bristol Inquiry and the consequent recognition of the need for clinical governance, once appointed and if not suspended, a consultant worked without any assessment of performance or assessment until retirement.

22. Dr. Neary told the Inquiry that no maternity hospital in Ireland had weekly meetings to discuss unusual or adverse outcomes in the 1970s, 1980s or early 1990s. He says that it was only in 1998 that the idea of weekly or monthly meetings to discuss adverse or unusual outcomes was introduced in the Lourdes Maternity Unit. Contrary to what Dr. Neary stated, we heard evidence that weekly or monthly discussions on outcomes were a feature of practice in the Dublin maternity hospitals for as long as any of the witnesses who assisted the Inquiry could recall. Some eminent practitioners recalled

occasions from the early days of training in their specialty, when their own adverse outcomes were discussed in an anonymous format, and where the pain of the discussions still lingers to the present day, but the lessons were learned. We were aware that in some similar sized units as the Lourdes Maternity that the individual personalities of the consultants ensured constant review and discussion of throughput and outcomes. The Inquiry could not agree with Dr. Neary about other hospitals but accepts that it was certainly true that there were no meetings to discuss activity and outcomes with the consultants of this unit.

23. The Lourdes Maternity Unit was recognised as a training hospital for Obstetrics and Gynaecology. We could find no good reason therefore why as a training hospital regular meetings and discussions on adverse or unusual outcomes did not take place. We could find no good reason why subjects were not identified for audit and audit carried out. The suspicion is that as there had been no such meetings in the past, then there was no inclination to introduce any change. When Dr. Connolly retired in 1982 there was no overall leader to give direction to the maternity hospital.

24. We found no evidence to suggest that any discussions ever took place between the pathology department and any of the obstetricians relating to any major divergence between the clinical reason given for hysterectomy and the pathology findings.

25. We found no evidence that any discussions between the anaesthetists and the obstetricians on any of the hysterectomies carried out took place. We found no evidence that anaesthetists were concerned that blood was rarely given or that the patient appeared stable at the time of hysterectomy. As outlined earlier, some of the anaesthetists always asked the reason for the hysterectomy and did not question what they were told. We found no evidence of any policy decision taken collectively by the anaesthetists to identify the situations when blood would be transfused and when it would not.

26. As outlined in a previous chapter, we had the distinct impression that where the patient's condition did not seem to present as an obstetric emergency, there was the unspoken belief that this might be a sterilisation procedure.

Thus questions were not asked. This seemed to apply to midwives, anaesthetists and pathologists. This lack of openness, seen in the context of the unchanging ethos of the hospital, provided the backdrop to the tolerance of what can only be described as rebarbative practices throughout the 1990s.

ROYAL COLLEGE OF OBSTETRICIANS AND GYNAECOLOGISTS

27. We are aware from documents furnished by the hospital management and the RCOG in London that on various occasions, representatives of the RCOG Hospital Recognition Committee visited the Maternity Unit. These visits were concerned with the recognition of hospital appointments, particularly Registrars and Senior House Officers, for training purposes. The visits were preceded by the submission to the RCOG of pro-forma statistics on activity in the unit for the previous year. Dr. Neary always completed these forms. Although various statistics were sought for gynaecological hysterectomies and tubal ligations, there were no queries for obstetric hysterectomies. In the 1985 statistics, completed by Dr. Neary preparatory to an inspection in 1986, he recorded 77 abdominal hysterectomies (gynaecological) and no tubal ligations, and in specifying the Family Planning Clinic available in the hospital stated "Natural Family Planning".

28. The inspection took place on 5th September 1986 and the "Visitors' Report and Recommendations" remarked that the unit was:

"an old converted building, not purpose-built, which gives rise to difficulties, but it copes with the workload… the wards and clinic area are cramped for space…there is no epidural service nor are there any plans to introduce them".

29. On the subject of "training" the visitors state:

"The workload in clinical experience is adequate for the present staff. The Senior House Officers rotate through obstetrics and gynaecology and share the night cover for both units. There are perinatal meetings and a Journal

Club held in the general hospital. There are no separate obstetrics meetings and teaching is limited to ward rounds and clinical situations".

30. They noted that only natural methods of family planning were taught.

31. They talked to the one Obstetric Registrar who –

"expressed the opinion that his clinical commitment was too much, leaving little time for study. He also commented that the ultrasonic scanner was not available for use of the junior staff. In discussion this was denied by the Consultant but it was noticeable that a portable scanner was not readily available. We had the impression that the Registrar was not totally happy with the situation. This isolated post lacked stimulation to study or research. Though the fault may be due partly to the lack of initiative on the Registrar's part, there did not appear to be much organised teaching".

32. The report makes no mention of the visitors having access to, or consulting, the maternity theatre register or other hospital records.

33. Following this inspection in February 1987 the RCOG gave a provisional recognition for one Registrar and four SHO training posts subject to a satisfactory report from Dr. MD. who was to re-visit the Lourdes after three months. The main concern was to observe whether structured teaching in the form of tutorials and case presentations had occurred and a better library had been provided. It had been reported to the inspectors that there were no modern books and no journals.

34. Dr. MD re-visited on 30th May 1987, and was met by all three Consultant Obstetricians and the Registrar. They emphasised that the new maternity hospital was "advanced in construction" and that:

"At least ten candidates had taken their MRCOG from Drogheda with 100% success. The hospital also had a 100% success in the Diploma in Obstetrics of the Royal College of Physicians in Ireland".

35. Dr. MD was informed that a Journal Club met to discuss current literature every Tuesday and that perinatal deaths were also discussed at the meeting, that teaching ward rounds were held every day and that a clinico-pathological conference took place once a month in rotation with medicine, surgery and other specialities. The inspector spoke privately to the registrar who stated that the teaching programme was very much improved and that he was receiving more direction from his senior colleagues. Again there is no evidence from this report that the assessor considered hospital records, or enquired into clinical practices in any detail. Following this visit the hospital received recognition for training a further five year period.

36. We know that in spite of what was reported to the inspector, no clinico-pathological conference relating to obstetrics and gynaecology ever took place. It was true that other specialities did engage in such conferences and Journal Clubs.

37. The next significant visit on behalf of the RCOG Hospital Recognition Committee was on 11th December 1992. This followed the submission of statistics for the previous year, again prepared by Dr. Neary, on a form that made no provision for the recording of peripartum hysterectomy. Included in a series of forms sent for completion was a checklist for audit in Obstetrics and Gynaecology. The title included an explanation for the form which stated

" *This constitutes a check that suitable audit mechanisms not only exist but function to a satisfactory level (audit of audit). An adequate gynaecological component should be ensured. Scrutiny of the annual report or (log) of the Hospital Audit Committee should provide most information.*"

38. Dr. Neary answered the questions by stating that he was the consultant responsible for audit and that audit of perinatal and obstetrics statistics took place twice yearly. All the other questions posed in the form were left unanswered or answered in the negative.

39. The Hospital Recognition report following the visit on 11th December is quite detailed. It is full of praise for the accommodation and equipment in the new

Maternity Unit, but notes, *"Urodynamics, assisted reproduction, minimally invasive surgery and endometrial ablation/resection are not practised."* It praised the paediatric department but noted *"the current SHOs in the obstetric department had not been given any formal instruction/training in neonatal resuscitation"*.

40. While Dr. Neary's Return indicated four clinical meetings, one perinatal meeting and one CPC per month, together with a weekly Journal Club and regular tutorials, it became clear to the visitors during interviews that *"most of the teaching in this department took place on an informal or opportunistic basis during ward rounds, clinics and theatre sessions and that very few of these meetings actually took place"*. Neither of the two registrars was interviewed. No comment was made on the lack of an audit committee or the lack of an annual report or audit log. If the untruths or exaggerations in Dr. Neary's annual return were recognised, they elicited no overt comment but were implied in the recommendations.

41. Following this visit the RCOG gave recognition to the Lourdes for two Registrars, four SHOs and one Diploma SHO with the following recommendations –

"There should be regular perinatal audit meetings with consultant staff in attendance;
A formal tutorial and meetings programme should be produced;

There should be formal instruction in neonatal resuscitation at the beginning of each six-month period;

Provision should be made for instruction in Family Planning;

SHOs should be made aware of and attend existent clinico-pathological meetings;

A rolling weekly rota seems disruptive. Thought should be given to constructing timetables which produce more even experience, better continuity of care and less frequent changes of timetables;

Regular audit meetings should be introduced; and

Junior staff should be circulated in writing concerning other hospital clinical meetings and clinico-pathological conferences."

42. From the foregoing it is apparent that the RCOG visitors were not concerned with clinical practices as such, and they do not appear to have carried out any sample inspection of theatre registers, patient charts or labour ward records. They clearly had no knowledge of the practice of peripartum hysterectomies in the Unit, the routine midline incisions for caesarean sections or the other procedures commented upon in other parts of this report. The visits were well heralded and involved lunch at Dr. Neary's house. The focus of the visits and assessments was on the suitability of the Unit for training purposes. They reported a well-equipped, spacious labour ward that was capable of providing a high standard of intrapartum care. The anaesthetic and pathology service were deemed very satisfactory. The only note of criticism was in the lack of meetings or tutorials, which did not match the details in the annual statistical form, filled in by Dr. Neary. They made no criticism on the lack of responses to the audit questions. The hospital accreditation committee made several very appropriate recommendations. They did not follow up on the recommendation that instruction in family planning be provided. They did not comment on the fact that tubal ligations were not offered. The recognition, which was clearly concerned by the lack of audit and formal teaching, did not seem to be subject to any further visit to ensure compliance with the recommendations. The report was sent to Dr. Neary and the Hospital Manager in February 1993. The RCOG has not carried out further inspections. There were no further inspections of the Maternity Unit until 2004 when The Institute of Obstetricians and Gynaecologists in Ireland carried out an inspection.

AN BORD ALTRANAIS

43. This is the statutory body responsible for nursing and midwifery in Ireland. It also approves and monitors standards of education and training. In this capacity it undertook inspection visits to the Lourdes general hospital and of the midwifery programme in the School of Midwifery. Inspections of the Maternity Unit were carried out on 24th February 1983 and 7th November 1990, with a follow up inspection report on 15th July 1991 and 20th September 1996.

44. The report of 24th February 1983 noted the difficulty for students in achieving the requisite number of deliveries (30) due to the number of private and semi-private patients in the hospital. It noted,

> *"i. total deliveries in 1982 – 2,400,*
> *ii. private – 1,300"*

45. Its other criticism was of grave overcrowding in the postnatal wards. The report recommended that these matters be attended to but that the hospital continued to be approved as a training centre. It made no mention of the practice of peripartum hysterectomy. The main concerns for approval were adherence to the approved syllabus, adequate numbers of ordinary and assisted deliveries, antenatal and postnatal care, neonatal and baby care.

46. The concerns expressed relating to inadequate numbers of deliveries attended by students were cured by Dr. Lynch's willingness to permit midwives to attend with him for private deliveries.

47. There is nothing of note in the documentation concerning the inspection in 1990 and the follow up inspection in 1991. A three day inspection was undertaken in February 1993 and it emerges from the documentation that a Midwives Education Committee was established in July 1986 to promote and encourage in-service education amongst midwives in the hospital. This committee promoted at least three study days a year and a Journal Club where midwives could discuss topics of interest. This club reportedly met every two weeks and latterly weekly, and had lectures and debates. There is

no evidence that any clinical concerns relating to consultant practice were discussed at such meetings.

48. The inspection report of 20th September 1996 was compiled from information provided from a questionnaire, by observation and assessment of inspectors, and by views expressed by staff and students. This process provided an opportunity for students and tutors to express and discuss any clinical concerns. The inspectors reported of the wards/clinical areas: *"the environment is a happy one, with lovely conditions for mothers and babies"*. Student midwives who engaged in open discussion with the examiners, reported they had *"great opportunities to learn in the clinical areas"* and that *"midwives and doctors are very approachable."*.

49. As far as we could ascertain, no comments were made by any midwives to any inspector regarding any of the unusual practices in the unit which included: vertical midline incisions for caesarean sections, routine episiotomies, rectal examinations to check the descent of the baby during labour, the use of a gynaecology chair for examinations, the routine shaving and prepping of patients for all gynaecology procedures and the high rate of caesarean hysterectomy.

THE MEDICAL COUNCIL

50. The Medical Council inspected the general hospital from time to time for suitability for the training of interns. As interns did not have any role in the Maternity Unit, the Maternity Unit was not visited by any committee of the Medical Council.

51. We found no evidence to indicate that the peripartum figures were reported anywhere within or outside the unit after 1984. There was no central data collection system that required that peripartum hysterectomy or obstetric hysterectomy should be recorded in any return of statistics. There was, and is, no national system for recording sentinel events and unexpected or unusual outcomes, although it is hoped that this will change when the National Perinatal Epidemiology Centre commences its planned activities.

REVIEW FROM OUTSIDE THE UNIT

52. We found no evidence of any queries from any of the recipients of the Maternity Unit's annual or biennial Clinical Reports regarding peripartum hysterectomy. Dr. Neary recalled that few acknowledged receipt of the report. He recalls that some obstetricians commented on the induction rate but never raised any queries relating to the caesarean hysterectomies which were always clearly indicated as an item in the table on caesarean sections. He also told us that no one ever commented on the symphysiotomy rate either.

53. We found no evidence of any review or consultation between the MMMs, owners and managers of the hospital and the obstetricians following any peripartum hysterectomy. We found no evidence of any awareness of such procedures on the part of the Department of Health, the Institute of Obstetricians and Gynaecologists in Ireland, the RCSI Medical School, the RCOG, the Public Health nurses, the local association of GPs or any other body.

There were many opportunities for medical and midwifery trainees to express concerns if they had any.[22] We have concluded that few people were aware of what constituted an acceptable peripartum hysterectomy rate and that until 1997/1998 no one questioned any of the procedures although some midwives were beginning to be uneasy from 1996 when 6 peripartum hysterectomies were carried out in January of that year.

---

[22] We recently became aware of one attempt to complain which may have discouraged others from following. Several nurses who were training in the Nursing School attached to the Lourdes Hospital described the use of a gynaecology chair for examination of patients in the gynaecology department and the routine prepping and shaving of patients for all gynaecological procedures when other hospitals had long abandoned these practices. An attempt by those students to complain to the nursing sisters resulted in the students being forced to withdraw their letter of complaint or face the threat of expulsion from the Nursing School. Some of these complainants attributed the angry reception to their letter to the consultants; others attributed the reaction to the senior sisters. We tried to speak to the gynaecology sisters who were in the hospital in 1997 when the letter was written. Some of them appeared to be unwilling to discuss the incident pleading illness and unavailability. One or two were suspicious and defensive. Others were happy to talk and agreed that what Dr. Connolly had decreed in the 50s and 60s became the established and unquestioned routine but that Dr. Neary and Dr. Lynch were "more modern" about the procedures complained of. There is no doubt that the letter was written and withdrawn.

Dr. Neary was aware of the letter and said he applauded the students' actions as he himself was affected by these routines and refused to use the gynaecology chair, which he described as a mediaeval instrument. It has been reported to us that the new consultants do not use the chair and that the procedures objected to by the students in 1997 are no longer applied.

TERM 5

TO ASCERTAIN WHETHER PERIODICAL CLINICAL REPORTS WERE PREPARED BY THE MATERNITY UNIT AT THE HOSPITAL AND, IF SO, THE PURPOSE OF THOSE REPORTS; TO WHOM THEY WERE FURNISHED; AND THE ACTION, IF ANY, WHICH WAS TAKEN ON FOOT OF THOSE REPORTS.

1   When this Inquiry commenced, it was a commonly held view that all Maternity Units in the country were obliged to present statistics and reports to the Royal College of Obstetricians and Gynaecologists in London and to the Institute of Obstetricians and Gynaecologists of Ireland, the bodies founded to regulate and educate the profession of Obstetricians and Gynaecologists. While the Maternity Units are obliged to furnish key statistics of activity to the two institutions, we were surprised to discover that no Maternity Unit has an obligation to prepare annual or periodic reports for furnishing to those two bodies nor has either of the bodies an obligation to consider the contents of any reports received, to analyse them or comment on them.

2   The Inquiry heard evidence that each of the Dublin teaching maternity hospitals produced annual reports for public presentation because of an obligation in each of their individual founding charters. Any other Maternity Unit that produces a report does so because the practitioners believe that it is good practice and are prepared to put in the work to prepare the reports in their own time.

3   Each Maternity Unit furnishes the Royal College of Obstetricians and Gynaecologists in London and the Institute of Obstetricians and Gynaecologists of Ireland with annual statistics, as distinct from reports, in order that the activity in the hospital can be assessed as adequate for post-graduate training in obstetrics and gynaecology. Until 1998, Dr. Neary filed these annual returns for the Maternity Unit at the Lourdes Hospital. However, there was no heading for peripartum hysterectomy in these statistics.

4   Clinical reports concerning the Maternity Hospital were published annually from 1952 to 1959, biennially from 1960 to 1979 and annually thereafter until

1984. No reports concerning the Maternity Unit were published covering years from 1985 to 1989. From 1989–1992 a general Hospital Annual Report was produced. This contained a very brief chapter consisting usually of one page dealing with to the Maternity Unit (Obstetrics and Gynaecology) statistics, and contained no details of any peripartum hysterectomies.

5   The Inaugural Annual Report for the General Hospital covering 1988 had no chapter dealing with the Maternity Unit. Annual reports specific to the Maternity Unit were recommenced in 2002 but the 2003 and 2004 at the time of writing have not been published.

6   Table 5A shows the Clinical Reports for the Hospital seen by the Inquiry with the relevant numbers of obstetric hysterectomies listed, as well as the figures ascertained by the Inquiry, where appropriate. The Table shows the year, the author of the report, the date the National Library have stamped the report as received by them (which the Inquiry believes is the closest known date of publication), the number of peripartum hysterectomies as evident in each available annual or bi-annual report, and the number of peripartum hysterectomies established by the Inquiry for a particular year with the operating surgeon for such procedures. Prior to 1964 there was only one Consultant, Dr.Connolly, practising in the hospital.

TABLE 5A: CLINICAL REPORTS FROM OUR LADY OF LOURDES HOSPITAL DROGHEDA

n/a = not available
* Publication = date received by the National Library
^Peripartum Hysterectomy – Inquiry = established figures according to information available

YEAR(S)	AUTHOR	PUBLICATION* NATIONAL LIBRARY	PERIPARTUM HYSTERECTOMY - REPORT	PERIPARTUM HYSTERECTOMY -INQUIRY^	Consultant Breakdown
1952	Dr.Connolly	n/a	2	n/a	Dr.C
1953	0	n/a	n/a	n/a	Dr.C
1954	Dr.Connolly	n/a	1	n/a	Dr.C
1955	Dr.Connolly	n/a	0	n/a	Dr.C
1956	Dr.Connolly	n/a	0	n/a	Dr.C
1957	Dr.Connolly	n/a	0	n/a	Dr.C
1958	Dr.Connolly	n/a	2	n/a	Dr.C
1959	Dr.Connolly	20.6.66	3	n/a	Dr.C
1960 1961	Dr.Connolly	15.2.62	2	n/a	Dr.C
1962 1963	Dr.Connolly	21.1.65	4	n/a	Dr.C
1964 1965	Dr.Connolly	n/a	3	n/a	n/a
1966 1967	Dr.O Brien	n/a	9	n/a	n/a
1968 1969	Dr.O Brien	12.8.71	3	n/a	n/a
1970				3	n/a
1971	Dr.O Brien	13.12.73	5	3	n/a
1972				1	n/a
1973	Dr.O Brien	28.10.76	2	0	n/a
1974				1	Dr.C: 1
1975	Dr.Neary	7.10.81	3	2	Dr.N: 1; Dr.C: 1
1976				5	Dr.N: 4; Dr.C: 1
1977	Dr.Neary	7.10.81	6	3	Dr.N: 3
1978				8	Dr.N: 5; Dr.C; 3
1979	Dr.Neary	8.2.82	17	9	Dr.N: 7; (1?); Dr.C: 1
1980	Dr.Neary	26.7.82	4	6	Dr.N: 5; Dr.C: 1
1981	Dr.Neary	4.11.83	7	6	Dr.N: 5; Dr.O B: 1
1982	Dr.Neary	3.9.84	1	5	Dr.N: 5;
1983	Dr.Neary	9.11.87	3	7	Dr.N: 5; Dr.L: 2
1984	Dr.Neary	9.11.87	1	2	Dr.N: 2
1985	No Report	n/a	n/a	12	Dr.N: 10; Dr.L: 2
1986	No Report	n/a	n/a	9	Dr.N: 6; Dr.L: 3
1987	No Report	n/a	n/a	8	Dr.N: 8
1988	General Hospital Report Only	n/a	n/a	7	Dr.N: 5; Dr.L: 2

1989	General Hospital Report only	n/a	n/a	6	Dr.N: 4; Dr.L: 2
1990	General Hospital Report only	n/a	n/a	3	Dr.N: 1; Dr.L: 2
1991	General			12	Dr.N: 7; Dr.L: 5
1992	Hospital Report only - biennial	n/a	n/a	8	Dr.N: 4; Dr.L: 3 Registrar: 1
1993	No Report	n/a	n/a	15	Dr.N: 9; Dr.L: 5; Dr.O B: 1
1994	No Report	n/a	n/a	9	Dr.N: 3; Dr.L: 6
1995	No Report	n/a	n/a	11	Dr.N: 7; Dr.L: 3; Registrar: 1
1996	No Report	n/a	n/a	14	Dr.N: 10; Dr.L: 1; Registrar/Locum Consultant: 3
1997	No Report	n/a	n/a	10	Dr.N: 6; Dr.L: 3; Locum Consultant: 1
1998	No Report	n/a	n/a	10	Dr.N: 7; Dr.L: 1; Dr.O'C:2
1999	No Report	n/a	n/a	0	
2000	No Report	n/a	n/a	2	Dr.L: 1; Dr.O'C: 1
2001	No Report	n/a	n/a	0	
2002	Dr.Milner	n/a	1	1	Dr.R
2003	No Report	n/a	n/a	2	Dr.O'C: 1; Dr.M; 1
2004	No Report	n/a	n/a	1	Dr.M

7   The earlier annual reports were published in tabular form with Tables set out for each obstetric event. Each report commenced with an Introduction giving a summary of the main chapters in the report with the relevant statistics, as appropriate. The individual chapter showed the relevant numbers of the particular obstetric outcome, the percentage per deliveries, maternal mortality and fetal loss. Each Table began with columns showing whether the individual case was booked or non-booked (a not unusual occurrence in earlier decades as many women were attended to by their GPs in their locality, distance and financial resources being significant issues); the chart number of the case; the age and parity of the mother and thereafter synopsised the case according to the relevant Table - which included disease, PET, haemorrhage, breech, disproportion, placental abnormalities, multiple pregnancies, inductions, caesarean sections, symphysiotomies,

craniotomies, and stillbirths/neonatal deaths. A 'Remarks' column briefly explained the individual outcome. Maternal Deaths were explained in detail.

8   In 1956 the format began to change with some Tables being replaced by summaries for less prominent events and other Tables supplemented by more detailed explanations. From 1957, the format of the Clinical Reports followed that set out in the Standard Report of the Royal College of Obstetricians and Gynaecologists to allow some comparison with other hospitals. The style of the reports changed into a narrative format rather than statistics in columns, but the high level of information remained the same. Reports commenced with a statistical summary covering admissions, mothers delivered, births and mortality rate. The reports from 1966/1977 to 1984 had a Comparative Table which compared the statistics for babies born, perinatal mortality rate, mortality rate, mothers delivered, maternal deaths and caesarean section rate for the particular years under review with the statistics from (usually 7) previous clinical reports. Clinical causes of perinatal mortality were also compared. Peripartum hysterectomy statistics were not compared.

9   The reports of the 1970s (biennial) and 1980s all followed the same pattern whereby each chapter would set out the relevant figures and percentage rate for the obstetric outcome under review. The chapter on caesarean section set out the number of cases, the incidence percent and outcome. Under 'hysterectomy at time of section', the relevant number was recorded.

10   In each chapter, following on the statistics, all cases of stillbirth and neo-natal death are set out individually in detail, recording the age, parity and medical history of the mother as well as a summary of the labour and delivery. If a post-mortem had been performed, the findings are also recorded. However, apart from Tables other outcomes were no longer recorded in detail. The chapter on caesarean section set out the relevant numbers, indications (with a separate section for primigravida), the incidence percent and outcome. Under 'hysterectomy at time of section', the relevant number was recorded but the individual cases were no longer detailed. The chapter on Ruptured Uterus outlined the relevant medical detail of each case and included a reference to hysterectomy where it occurred. In the case of post partum

haemorrhage, the numbers were set out, indicating the incidence percent and the causes, but individual cases were not detailed. In a narrative commentary on post partum haemorrhage (PPH) in the report of '1970/1971, reference to a sub total hysterectomy performed to control an atonic PPH is made. No other report seen by the Inquiry covering the 1970s and 1980s contains a narrative section on PPH or record a hysterectomy performed for PPH.

11   The reports provided valuable statistics of the numbers of live births, the complications of pregnancy and delivery, the outcomes and treatment of the still births/neonatal mortality and maternal mortality. There was no effort to conceal any procedures; for example, symphysiotomies were recorded as well as deliveries or caesarean section after previous symphysiotomies. Peripartum hysterectomies were not recorded separately unless they accorded with a medical condition which merited a special heading of reporting. Hysterectomy appeared as a complication of caesarean section or as a treatment for ruptured uterus or PPH. Thus it was easy to see how many of these operations were performed. Peripartum hysterectomies were documented openly, including the unusually high number of caesarean hysterectomies in 1978/79 when 16 such procedures were recorded as well as a further hysterectomy for ruptured uterus, totalling 17 in all.

12   There was very little of this type of detail contained in the later Obstetric/Gynaecological section of the main Hospital Reports of 1989, 1990, 91/92 where only statistics setting out the number of births (including miscarriages) - broken down into percentage inductions, forceps/ventouse and caesarean section – perinatal mortality, epidurals and scans were recorded. There was no mention of peripartum hysterectomy.

13   **PREPARATION OF THE REPORTS:**
The Inquiry was told that the first reports were prepared by the foundation obstetrician Dr. Connolly with the assistance of one or several of the MMMs who was medically trained. In 1964 Dr.Connolly handed over responsibility for collecting the statistics and preparing the report to the newly appointed Dr. O'Brien, and the custom developed that clinical reports were prepared by the most recently appointed Consultant. Dr.O' Brien was responsible for the

reports from his arrival until 1974, and thereafter they were completed by Dr.Neary from 1974 until 1984. Dr.Lynch was appointed in 1982.

14   Statistics had to be researched and compiled in the author's free time - at night or on the weekends. Statistics were established from information supplied by the main registers.

15   The main source for deliveries was the birth registers which kept a running total of mothers delivered, together with details of each birth. The theatre register was the source for caesarean sections, all obstetric surgical procedures and manual removals of placenta. Preparing the periodic reports was a lengthy and cumbersome task.

16   Each procedure had to be painstakingly counted. Individual cases requiring comment necessitated sourcing and reviewing the particular patient's chart and synopsising the case notes. Identifying the charts to be pulled was determined by the 'copy files' which were rectangular cards punched by the secretaries (or junior doctors in complicated cases) after discharge, according to what condition or treatment applied to the patient while in the hospital. Each hole punched represented a particular procedure or outcome. Thus if the number of mothers with PET (pre-eclampsia toxaemia) was sought, the cards for a certain period would be put together and a knitting needle was inserted through the hole punched for PET and the cards were shaken. The needle captured the cases of PET and the other cards fell away. Once those patients had been identified for review, their case notes would be retrieved. Without the administrative assistance of someone familiar with all the filing system, the job was impossible.

17   We have been informed that finance was always a problem in the hospital, and indeed this is borne out by minutes of Hospital Board meetings that were for the most part involved with how the money required could be sourced and raised. Staffing and other resource constraints created added difficulties for the preparation of these reports. Dr. Neary recalled that in the years in which he prepared the reports, funding was not available for him to be assisted by

secretarial or administrative staff over the weekends. He said that he had to do most reports without any assistance.

18   Although the reports were very admirably prepared, they were perhaps of reduced value or interest as they were sometimes published several years in arrears. Annual Reports for the Dublin Maternity Hospitals are published approx 10 months after the year's end for presentation at the Royal Academy of Medicine meeting in October/November of each year. The Inquiry heard conflicting evidence from various obstetric consultant witnesses that the detail recorded in the modern Dublin Hospital Reports reduced from the 1980s onwards. They believed this was related to medico legal concerns.

19   Dr.Neary told the Inquiry that, while the reports were ready once they had been typed by administrative staff in the Hospital, funding limitations delayed their publication for considerable periods. Dr. Neary's recollection of the reports for which he was responsible is that they were always published later than he would have liked. He does not recall precisely when the reports were published and cannot disagree with the National Library dates as set out in Table 5A. His recollection is that there was an intention, not always achieved, to publish their reports in and around the same time as the Dublin reports were presented. This is a good indication of an original intention to compare outcomes at the Lourdes Maternity Unit with the Dublin figures.

20   The switch from biennial to annual reports in the 1980s eased funding complications and the earlier 1980s reports seem to have been published more speedily than the later ones in the 1970s.

21   Dr.Lynch was appointed in 1982 and, according to the custom, he should have been responsible for the preparation and publication of the annual reports. We are informed that Dr.Lynch was unwilling to prepare the reports for 1983 and 1984, which were then prepared by Dr.Neary and published, he believes, in 1986, though the National Library records indicate receipt of the report in November 1987. Dr. Lynch informed the Inquiry that when he took up his position in 1982 he recommended the immediate introduction of an IT system in the Maternity Unit. He advised that such a system was vital so that

statistics could be accessed and data preserved. The IT system has still not been set up although the Inquiry was informed in June that the process is finally underway.

22   Credit is due for the not inconsiderable commitment required to compile the statistics and publish the reports at a time of very limited staffing and financial resources. Dr.Neary told the Inquiry that there was less assistance available to him when compiling the statistics than he believed was available to his predecessors. Such was the pressure on his time that, for family reasons, having brought the 1984 and 1985 reports to publication, he was not willing to continue with their production. Senior MMMs believed that they had received legal advice to discontinue the reports in their clear format. They were not published again until 2003.

23   The annual Clinical Reports from the Lourdes Hospital were made available to other maternity units, every practising obstetrician in the State, some practising obstetricians outside the State, the National Library of Ireland and the Royal College of Obstetricians and Gynaecologists in London.

24   Dr.Neary informed the Inquiry that the distribution list compiled in Dr. Connolly's time was the same list he used when he prepared the reports.

25   The Inquiry team visited the headquarters of the Royal College of Obstetricians and Gynaecologists at Regents Park in London. It was confirmed that clinical reports from the hospital dated from 1970 through 1984 were filed in its archives. On inquiry as to the reaction to the numbers of caesarean hysterectomy cases noted in the reports, we learned that these reports were received by the Royal College and were archived unread. The secretary dealing with most of the annual reports told the Inquiry that these reports would *"have been filed unread pending a hospital visit or an inquiry relating to the recognition of educational posts within the hospital itself"*.

26   An RCOG visit to the hospital occurred in 1987.   Records of this hospital visit, including the submitted delivery statistics of 1986, made no comment as to the rate of hysterectomy at caesarean section. It is not known whether the

hospital visitors had access to the archived clinical reports from previous years. Most of the visiting committee members were Irish practitioners.

27   The Inquiry considers it a matter of regret that the custom of publishing periodic reports was discontinued. They provided a method of internal comparison with previous statistics and were a method of raising awareness within the unit of its statistics compared with those of the Dublin maternity hospitals and any other maternity hospital that published in the same format. While it is disappointing to note that the reports, when published, elicited no comment on the peripartum hysterectomy figures, we observed that fairly high peripartum rates during the period before the mid 1980s may quite legitimately have been unremarkable in their time. For instance, in 1970 there were 16 "Hysterectomy with Pregnancy" cases reported in the National Maternity Hospital annual reports. There were only 282 caesarean sections carried out that year. We have already referred elsewhere to the 70 "Hysterectomy in Pregnancy" cases referred to by Dr. James Clinch during the period 1972-1977.

28   The Inquiry heard from several witnesses that the ethos of the Maternity Unit at the Lourdes Hospital was well known and that it was quite likely that what may have been remarkable in a Dublin hospital may have been regarded as unremarkable in this unit. It is perhaps for this reason that, until recently, many obstetricians to whom we spoke asked whether the high rate of caesarean hysterectomy at this particular hospital was contributed to by sterilisations.[23]

29   Undoubtedly, the cessation of periodic clinical reports and the consequent lack of comprehensive analytical statistical information was a contributory factor in the lack of awareness in the unit of the rate, as opposed to the number, of hysterectomies in the 1980s and especially in the 1990s. The Inquiry nevertheless believes that if any party working in the Maternity Unit had any real concerns about the numbers as compared with the three Dublin

---

[23] The MMMs objected to this paragraph and commented that there was no correlation between the Hospital ethos and the issue of sterilisations.

maternity hospitals, it would not have been difficult to obtain copies of the Dublin reports to make comparisons.

30 **WAS ANY ACTION TAKEN ON FOOT OF ANY REPORT?**

No action appears to have been taken on foot of the earlier reports. As previously stated, contrary to popular belief, there was no obligation on any maternity hospital to file annual reports with the RCOG or the later Institute of Obstetricians and Gynaecologists in Ireland, nor was there any obligation on the part of those institutions to read them. For the most part they were received and archived. A copy was sent to the National Library where they became public documents.

31 Dr.Neary told the Inquiry that he would receive approximately 20 letters of thanks from consultant colleagues who had received the periodic reports. They would comment about rates of inductions, caesarean sections, instrumental deliveries and maternal deaths. Dr.Neary said that there was never any comment from these colleagues about the numbers of caesarean hysterectomies or symphysiotomies.

32 Dr. C.C. from Portiuncula Hospital in Ballinasloe, Co. Galway informed the Inquiry that he had copies of the Clinical Reports from Drogheda for the years 74/75; 78/79; 1981, 1983 and 1984. He noted that he had personally underlined the numbers of caesarean hysterectomies for 1981 at 10, as he presumed he found it surprising. However, Dr. C.C. does not appear to have made any comment to the Obstetricians in the Lourdes Hospital.

33 The periodic reports for the Lourdes Hospital were printed by Cahill Printers who informed the Inquiry that older records were no longer available and they were unable to assist us as to when the reports were submitted for printing. However, when the reports were received by the National Library they were date stamped. We have used those dates in Table 5A.

34 **STATISTICAL REPORTS**

No further clinical reports were published which related exclusively to the Obstetrics Department until 2002 when a Maternity Unit Annual Report was re-introduced and prepared by Dr. Máire Milner.

35 From 1988 some annual reports were published by the General Hospital. In the Inaugural Report in 1988 no information is set out concerning the Department of Obstetrics and Gynaecology. Thereafter a one page summary was contained in the 1989 and 1990 reports, becoming a two page for the biennial report in 1991-1992. Only numbers of births (indicating percentage inductions, forceps/ventouse and caesarean sections) and perinatal mortality was recorded. The midwifery chapter in these reports records the difficulties created by staffing embargos, despite the move in 1990 to the new Maternity Hospital with a larger unit and increased uses of the facilities. There is no reference to caesarean or peripartum hysterectomies anywhere in these very truncated reports.

36 **CURRENT CLINICAL REPORTS**

The 2002 Maternity Unit report highlights the very significant changes that occurred in the maternity services in the North East. The opening of the Mosney reception centre for asylum seekers in 2000, the suspension of deliveries in Monaghan and Dundalk hospitals in 2001 and capacity strain in the Dublin Maternity Hospitals all contributed to an increased attendance in the Maternity Unit in Drogheda and consequent complexity of care required. The increase in population due to the ever-expanding commuter belt to Dublin is noted.

39 The content and format of the report has changed significantly from those published after 1984. A significant level of detail has returned. The report commences with statistical summaries for the year and, as well as setting out the traditional categories of deliveries, births and obstetric outcomes, now includes sociological data on nationality, age and parity, marital status, demographic address by county and medical outcome for the mother as well as gestational age and weight of the newborn. Trends are analysed by graph.

Obstetric outcomes including stillbirths, neonatal and maternal deaths, ruptured uterus, and caesarean hysterectomy, are explained on an individual case basis. Antenatal outpatient services, including outreach clinics in Navan and Mosney, are set out and chapters from the departments of neonatology, gynaecology, anaesthesia and midwifery are included. The caesarean hysterectomy performed in 2002 for rupture of uterine scar is explained under a separate chapter. Individual chapters including headings for accidental haemorrhage, placenta previa and postpartum haemorrhage have replaced many of the more general chapters previously included in the older reports.

40   The 2002 report indicates that the statistical data had to be collected manually from monthly statistics collated by midwifery staff and from data in the labour ward register (which was initiated in its present format in 2001). This reinforces the need for a computerised database which, to date, has not yet been installed. **Given the importance of audit and analysis, the lack of an appropriate IT system for the purpose of data collection is unacceptable in a modern Maternity Unit.**

41   The Inquiry had noted that in the preparation of the 2002 Report, statistical data already collected by specially trained personnel within the Hospital for the HIPE (Hospital In-Patient Enquiry) system was not utilised. While the national HIPE database was not instituted for the purpose of producing internal hospital reports, it nevertheless is a rich source of easily obtainable accurate statistical information. Obstetrical input will always be required for the analysis of individual patient outcomes, but access to the system's information might remove much of the current drudgery in collating statistics.

42   The national HIPE database is prepared for transmitting hospital activity and case mix to the Department of Health and Children, via the ESRI, primarily for funding purposes. The information is likely to be accurate as, to a great extent, the hospital's funding is dependant on comprehensive inputting of all inpatient diagnoses and treatments or operations.

43   The former Master of one of the Dublin hospitals informed the Inquiry that he was unaware of any Maternity Unit utilising HIPE as a resource for data

collection in the preparation of annual Clinical Reports. If there is a reason why so much hospital produced data is unavailable to its own consultants for the preparation of reports, then the reason was not clear to the Inquiry. Personnel from ESRI and the Department of Health and Children could see no valid reason why the system could not be used by individual hospitals to access their own statistics.

44   The value of HIPE as a tool was demonstrated while preparing this report. The Inquiry sought current and recent peripartum hysterectomy figures from HIPE for each maternity hospital for the years 1999–2004. These figures were compared with those furnished directly to the Inquiry by the maternity hospitals. Discrepancies were found. The figures from HIPE were higher than those furnished by the hospitals. When re-confirmation of peripartum hysterectomy figures was then sought from the hospitals, the Inquiry discovered that, in most instances, the HIPE figure was correct. For example, in the case of one Dublin hospital, the figure originally submitted for peripartum hysterectomy from 1999-2003 was 7, but the figure of 13 provided by HIPE was subsequently accepted as correct. In another case, the HIPE figure of 5 was accepted over the original hospital figure of 3. The Inquiry discovered that the HIPE figures for peripartum hysterectomy in the Lourdes Hospital for 1999-2004 were totally accurate.

45   No reports for 2003 or 2004 have been published as yet. Many of the vital hospital records were with the Inquiry since April 2004 and thus unavailable for preparing reports. During much of this period consultant numbers were depleted by ill health, family bereavement and recruitment difficulties.[24]

46   **PURPOSE OF THE FORMER REPORTS**

There was no discernable purpose for publishing the annual clinical reports. At one stage there was probably a strong desire to emulate the National Maternity Hospital and use its statistics as a comparator and measure of excellence. The hospital started with the best intentions but the preparation of the reports was not always adequately funded, leading to later and later publication, making comparisons less valid. The collection of data for the

---

[24] We have been informed that the reports are ready for printing when resources are available.

earlier reports ensured an excellent level of audit, while publication allowed for external professional review. When the threat of increased medical litigation became a reality in the late 1980s, the reports ceased. Thereafter, regrettably, no audit took place in relation to the Lourdes' statistics and no professional review, internal or external, occurred.

47   The Lourdes Hospital Reports for 1956, '57, and '58 show that a meeting of the Royal Academy of Medicine to discuss the reports of provincial hospitals (akin to the meeting of the Dublin teaching hospitals) occurred in Drogheda. Reports from St. Finbarr's Hospital, Cork, Waterford Maternity and the Lourdes were discussed. In the Introduction to the 1956 Report, Dr. Connolly notes:

"It was an event of the utmost importance to all interested in Maternity in the provinces, when the Royal Academy of Medicine, Section of Obstetrics, decided to hold a meeting in Drogheda, at which the reports of the provincial Maternity Hospitals would be discussed. The discussion, held annually, of the Dublin Maternity Hospital Reports, has been one of the important factors in keeping the standard of Obstetrics in Dublin at the high level it enjoys today. It was rightly thought that a debate, on similar lines, would be a stimulus and a help to provincial obstetrics"

The Inquiry regrets that the wisdom evident in the '50s did not continue.

48   The Inquiry heard that on one or two occasions, probably in the '70s, the few provincial hospitals that prepared annual reports presented their figures and discussed their outcomes in the same way as the Dublin hospitals under the auspices of the Royal Academy of Medicine. This custom was not continued beyond a couple of years and fell into desuetude.

49   Dr. Neary informed the Inquiry that he recalls that between 1974 and 1984 it was the custom to discuss the reports at a clinical club where paediatricians and obstetricians presented their part of the reports. He believes that all consultants in the hospital, all junior medical staff, all senior nursing and

administrative staff, were invited to attend. This was not the recollection of many of the witnesses to whom we spoke. Most witnesses told us that they either did not receive a copy of the reports or they did not read them as they were so much out of date. While most witnesses were aware that periodic reports were published, few seemed interested in the detail of the contents.

50   The founding charters of the Dublin maternity hospitals obliged them to publish annual reports. The custom is well established that the reports are presented together in a venue well publicised within the profession. The intense competition between these three hospitals is aired at an open annual meeting where the three Masters present their statistics. An outside assessor reads and analyses the three reports and comments at the annual meeting. The three Masters are then given an opportunity to defend their reports and the floor is then open for discussion.

51   The significance of openly publishing and analysing statistical outcomes in maternity hospitals cannot be over emphasised. The benefits of transparency and accountability are honest criticism or acclaim which allow evidence based protocols to be developed. It is very probable that had the excellently prepared reports of earlier times continued into the 1990s, the appalling rate of peripartum hysterectomy would have been noted and questioned. The Inquiry was constantly astounded by witness after witness who said that they simply did not *know* the rate of peripartum hysterectomy within the hospital. Concern only began to dawn due to the increasing number of young, low parity patients in the late 1990s, not because of an increased rate. None of the obstetricians who worked in the unit was aware of the rate or numbers.

TERM 6

TO INQUIRE INTO WHAT PRACTICES AND PROTOCOLS HAVE
BEEN ADOPTED AT THE MATERNITY UNIT OF THE HOSPITAL
SINCE OCTOBER 1998 OR ARISING FROM THE PUBLICATION
OF THE REPORT.

1. The immediate period following Dr. Neary's suspension was fraught and inter-professional relationships in both the Maternity Unit and the hospital were strained. Many staff had difficulty coming to terms with the situation. Trust, confidence and morale were in short supply. The working relationships between the Hospital and Health Board management were very poor.

2. When the Health Board solicitor acted immediately on concerns expressed to him by two midwives on the 22nd day of October 1998, instead of general relief that finally these concerns had been aired, there was resentment towards the "whistle blowers". We heard of comments to the effect that the whistle blowers would "never get a job in Ireland", that they would be sued for defamation and would generally come to a bad end. It would be difficult to say that there was general support for their criticisms of some of Dr. Neary's practices.

3. The Health Board protected the whistleblowers' identity by permitting the perception that they were student midwives to be circulated. The support for Dr. Neary was considerably stronger than for the several midwives who through various means had tried to raise their concerns and were known to have done so. In the meanwhile, someone familiar with the Maternity Unit's recording and storing system and who had access to the information consciously, carefully and deliberately removed many key documents and altered others. The documents were removed and entries altered with the intent of removing evidence and of creating an impression that carelessness in filing, storing and recording would be seen as the reason for key charts and records to be unobtainable. It is highly likely that a small number of charts relating to other consultants was also removed in the expectation of creating a smoke screen.

4. Perhaps some more of the clinical staff of the Maternity Unit would have been supportive of the effective inquiry into the allegations regarding Dr. Neary's

practices if the news in November 1998 that he had been exonerated by his peers, had not been circulated. This review was commissioned by Dr. Neary's union representatives in order to enable Dr. Neary to continue in his post pending a full review of his peripartum hysterectomy rate by the Institute of Obstetricians and Gynaecologists. The Terms of Reference and limitations of this initial peer review were not known. The news that Dr. Neary was exonerated did cause fear and confusion in the minds of those who had questioned his practices and gave confidence to the majority who had no concerns.

5. The later wrongful leaking of the contents of much of Mr. Michael Maresh's report on nine of Dr. Neary's recent peripartum hysterectomies exacerbated the climate of mistrust towards management and the Health Board but did nevertheless have some influence in diluting the opinion of some of Dr. Neary's strongest supporters. There was a great deal of disbelief and reluctance to accept that a popular colleague could or should be asked to withdraw from practice.

6. The Inquiry heard that because Mr Maresh was British, there was suspicion as to his qualifications. He was dismissed in some circles as a non-practising obstetrician and a retired academic chosen to condemn the life saving operations carried out by Dr. Neary. As outlined elsewhere, Mr. Maresh was in fact the Lead Consultant of the Labour Ward of a large maternity Hospital in Manchester and very much a hands-on obstetrician. His advice and opinion continued to be treated with scepticism by many of the clinical staff of the Lourdes Hospital.

TWO CRITICAL REPORTS

7. When later the findings of the Lamki Review Group commissioned by the Institute of Obstetricians and Gynaecologists were circulated, the negative findings relating to many of Dr. Neary's cases in that report were made known. The criticisms made of the senior midwives for failing to recognise poor practice in Dr. Neary caused an angry reaction. A letter was written and signed by most of those sisters condemning the findings, as they believed that there had not been a sufficiently comprehensive series of interviews with the senior midwives.

8. Within six months of concerns being expressed by the small group of midwives as outlined in Term of Reference 3, three reports had been commissioned into Dr. Neary's practices regarding peripartum hysterectomy. The first had exonerated him. The second had raised very serious concerns relating to his ability to handle haemorrhage and questioned his judgement. The third, which was the most comprehensive, had looked at his practices in the context of the ethos of the hospital and the conditions under which Dr. Neary worked. The Review Group recognised that there was an acceptance of peripartum hysterectomy within the Unit that was inappropriate. Probably much more important, they noted that there was a very high number of caesarean sections in the Unit echoing the connection which the Matron of the Maternity Unit had made earlier between caesarean sections and caesarean hysterectomies.

RETRAINING FOR DR. NEARY

9. Recognising the context within which the operations had been carried out, the Lamki Review Body recommended that a 6 month retraining in The National Maternity Hospital would update Dr. Neary in modern obstetrics and remedy the defects in his judgement, especially in relation to his abnormal reaction to haemorrhage. When pressed on this point, one member of the review body was quite confident that retraining would have produced appropriate results although he admitted that Dr. Neary would have to change his belief that each hysterectomy was lifesaving and develop some insight into his propensity to exaggerate danger.

10. The Review Group believed that Dr. Neary had fault lines but was an otherwise valuable asset to medicine. He had many valuable skills that could usefully be put to work in a busy hospital but he did require serious supervised retraining.

11. The opportunity to retrain was not offered to Dr. Neary as by the time the report issued, he had already been suspended by the Medical Council and had taken early retirement from the Unit as retraining was not an option favoured by the Health Board.

12. The fact that the Lamki peer review had recommended a period of retraining circulated within the hospital, fostering the continued belief that Dr. Neary had

been unfairly treated and that management and The Health Board had engaged in a vendetta against Dr. Neary. The Review Group's main finding that most of Dr. Neary's peripartum hysterectomies were unjustified was lost on his supporters.

SUSPICION OF HEALTH BOARD MOTIVES

13. Without dwelling too much on the painful past and immediate aftermath of the disclosures relating to the Maternity Unit, it nevertheless has to be said that the need to change was only slowly recognised and change was frequently obstructed. The huge efforts by the Medical Director of the hospital, the Director of Nursing and the Assistant CEO of the North Eastern Health Board to introduce reforms and promote changes in practice took considerable personal strength of character and commitment. They were frequently vilified, condemned and isolated. There was the continued strong belief held by a significant number of consultants and other hospital personnel that Dr. Neary's suspension was contrived and formed part of a larger picture to rid the Health Board of a number of consultants who held out for complete clinical independence. Dr. Neary's troubles with management were believed to be part and parcel of the continuing move within Health funding policies of the time to measure efficiency in hospitals by increased throughput of patients, increased use of day care facilities and shorter bed stays. The impression that he was in part being penalised for his stance against Health Board policy in this regard was widespread.

14. Such was the loyalty to Dr. Neary and the suspicion with which the actions of management and the Health Board were viewed, that the doctor brought in as locum to replace Dr. Neary was not welcomed and was treated with silence and coldness for several years. The Medical Board in the hospital voted to condemn the actions of the Health Board in suspending Dr. Neary and was very critical of the Medical Director. A vote of no confidence in his leadership was passed.

RESOURCES AND INFRASTRUCTURE DEFICITS

15. Over time the internal professional conflict began to settle as more objective information became available and was disseminated. The intervention of the Medical Council contributed to the process of re-evaluation particularly among the consultants and midwives. Their respective work pressures and

their unsatisfactory working environment over many years came under increasing scrutiny. These factors quite properly began to take centre stage.

16. Few resources were spent in updating skills and attending clinical courses until 1997 when the Health Board took over. Finance or the lack of it seemed to occupy much of the managers' time during the period before and after the takeover. A consultant's bad behaviour could be reprimanded if a complaint was made but consultants were deemed untouchable where clinical matters were concerned. Hospital managers or midwifery managers had very little influence on the consultants. Some midwives described how it was very difficult to question practice and it was unusual to articulate an opinion. There was no mandatory continuing medical education although there was some evidence that Dr. Neary at least was an active member of the Nuffield Visiting Society and did attend meetings. None of the obstetric consultants had time or made time to publish papers or engage in research.

17. Many midwives were in temporary positions and the Unit relied heavily upon student midwives. As mentioned in many places in this report, midwives and consultants frequently carried very heavy workloads. Midwives reported nervousness in seeking maternity leave because of the effect of their absence on their colleagues. There were no care attendants and there was very little clerical assistance.

18. A report on midwifery practices commissioned just before the complaints against Dr. Neary were aired found that Midwifery management in the Maternity Unit focused on *"managing individual midwives rather than managing the midwifery service and developing midwifery practice."* This report identified deficits in the managing skills of senior midwives and recommended management courses. It recommended many changes including *"The midwives must ensure that they fulfil the role for which they are trained by being assertive, questioning and proactive in ensuring that their practice is evidence based."* The midwife specialist brought in to the Unit to examine midwifery structures was not told of any concerns about obstetric practices in the Unit nor did the expert identify any such concerns.

A SEPARATE AND ISOLATED UNIT

19. There was a long and documented history of sensitivity to perceived interference from Nursing Management in the general hospital with the Maternity Unit. Relations between the two Matrons were always difficult. Information was not exchanged between the Maternity Unit and management in the general hospital and when sought, was not always forthcoming. The distance between each end of the link tube corridor that connects the two hospitals, took 20 seconds to cover by foot but years to integrate. The Maternity Unit enjoyed its history of self-containment and saw no benefit in opening up to or applying the changes being introduced in the general hospital. Almost every review of the Maternity Unit noticed and commented on the tensions between senior nursing management in the two parts of the Lourdes Hospital. Vestiges of this history of resentment were still apparent to the Inquiry in our investigations.

20. The effect of this de facto separation between the two hospitals meant that no one who had any concerns about the peripartum hysterectomy rate in 1998 or earlier considered going to the General Manager of the hospital, to the Medical Director or to the Director of Nursing. Problems were not vocalised and outside resolution was not considered. The Matron of the Maternity Unit expressed fears that she might be sued if she voiced her concerns about Dr. Neary's peripartum hysterectomy rate and was subsequently proven wrong. It was against this background that everybody had to move on and pick up the pieces.

IMMEDIATE CHANGES

21. While all these battles were being fought, babies were still being born in the Maternity Unit and life had to continue. The first effect of Dr. Neary's departure was that the force of his strong personality was removed. The other consultants and midwives with management skills but milder personalities and a little more insight began to implement effective changes. No peripartum hysterectomies were carried out in 1999. Regular meetings were set in train where midwives and obstetricians discussed the week's throughput of patients and the results. The Director of Nursing instituted a reporting procedure between the Maternity Unit and her office. Senior

midwives were encouraged to attend clinical courses and to acquire management skills.

RECOMMENDATIONS FOR IMPROVEMENT HAD PREVIOUSLY BEEN MADE

22. The Institute or Lamki Review Group recommended that an audit system should be put in place urgently with weekly meetings involving medical and midwifery staff. It recommended monthly perinatal conferences with paediatric and pathology involvement, a Journal Club and a forum for case discussion with frequent departmental meetings involving midwives, postgraduates and under-graduate trainees. It should be noted that most of these recommendations had been made following an inspection by the RCOG in late 1992.

    The Review Group advised that consideration should be given to producing an annual clinical report in addition to the returns made to the RCOG in London. It recommended that the Institute of Obstetrics and Gynaecology, the Royal College of Physicians in Ireland and the RCOG London should visit the Unit regularly. It suggested that under-graduate or post-graduate training *programmes should be formalised.*

23. The Review Group recommended that sterilisation be introduced urgently and that the Maternity Unit should be more closely integrated into the hospital. They noted the difficulties that had arisen between nursing personnel in the Maternity Unit and the general hospital and stated *"there is an urgency for confrontation to be replaced by cooperation. By achieving this, hopefully everyone will benefit, not least the patients."*

EXAMINATION OF SYSTEMS AND PRACTICE

24. While the peer review of Dr. Neary's caesarean hysterectomies was being carried out, the assistant CEO of The North Eastern Health Board engaged HRRI in a long series of analyses of current and past practices in the Unit. This exercise was an effort to determine what had gone wrong in the Unit, which had permitted a systemic acceptance of resort to hysterectomy at a fairly low threshold. HRRI were specifically engaged to identify risk factors and to recommend action to minimise risk for the future.

25. The reports identified many weaknesses and made many recommendations. Very poor nursing note keeping was identified together with deficiencies in the recording of events by all theatre staff including consultants in the maternity theatre. They advised on the necessity of clinical audit, on improving consent procedures, on improving documentation and record keeping and on the importance of formulating a risk management policy. They expressed concern at Dr. Neary's high personal rate of caesarean section. The slowness in replacing retiring consultants, midwives on maternity or sick leave or recruiting additional staff to meet current requirements was highlighted with embarrassing frequency in every report and to the Inquiry. The problem is ongoing. These measures have been fully dealt with in Term of Reference 2.

26. The tragedy for this Maternity Unit and the patients is that the visiting committee of the Royal College of Obstetricians and Gynaecologists had identified deficiencies in the system and the absence of clinical audit in the Unit as early as late 1992. These deficiencies, especially the lack of audit and poor consultant involvement in incident reporting continued to be repeated and highlighted by HRRI over the next few years without any notable recognition by the hospital paymasters that audit must be resourced and supported. The Inquiry sometimes wondered how many reports must be written before anything really changes and whether there is really a will to change in institutions, which show more enthusiasm for obtaining reports than for providing infrastructure change and support.

27. HRRI reviewed the care provided by Dr. Neary and reviewed all caesarean hysterectomy records. The extent of missing birth registers and other documents was realised. They reviewed the peripartum hysterectomies carried out by the other two obstetricians in the Unit. Mr. Michael Maresh reviewed two peripartum hysterectomies carried out by Dr. Seosamh O'Coigligh, the recently arrived obstetric consultant. He expressed no concern with those caesarean hysterectomies, which he noted were justified and appropriate. He observed that his records were a vast improvement on the previous recording of care in the Unit.

28. HRRI and Mr. Maresh reviewed the practices of Dr. Finian Lynch in relation to 15 caesarean hysterectomies carried out by him in the new Maternity Unit between 1992 -1997. Mr. Maresh's main concern in relation to those 15 cases referred to him was what he perceived to be this consultant's practice of performing caesarean hysterectomies as a method of sterilisation. He was hopeful that the practice had been discontinued. He expressed no major concerns in relation to technical competence and surgical decision-making. The Unit had a high caesarean section rate and HRRI advised that Dr. Lynch's caesarean sections should be referred for peer review, which took place in 2004 when no adverse findings were made.

29. HRRI continued reporting on practice within the Maternity Unit over the next 4 years and reviewing the progress and implementation of their recommendations. Progress in some areas was slow.

SLOW PROGRESS

30. As we outlined in Term of Reference 3, the initial stages of the Inquiry gave no impression of an acceptance that very valid criticisms were made by the many reports commissioned into the events in the Maternity Unit. We heard that the staff who had been loyal to the Unit and the consultants now wanted to "move on" and "put the past behind them". There was very little evidence of any acceptance of a collective role as enablers or for accountability although there were some notable exceptions. The former tutor who had raised concerns to the Matron of the Maternity Unit and the Cardinal in 1980 expressed deep regret that she had not done more to prevent so many women from unnecessarily losing their fertility and femininity and that whatever effort she made to raise her concerns did not have a better outcome at the time. Some of the midwives who had simply never wondered or questioned, reported that they have been asking themselves since how they were so accepting; how they had no suspicions as they now see that the signs were there. They believe that their training moulded them never to question. As detailed previously in the report, many of these midwives wept at the sadness of what happened and are full of regrets. Others wished that they had had more confidence to do something earlier.

31. The Review Group's recommendations and those of the HRRI relating to monthly perinatal conferences with paediatric and pathology involvement, a

Journal Club and a forum for case discussion with frequent departmental meetings involving midwives, postgraduates and under-graduate trainees were put into effect. While much suspicion and mistrust remained within the various factions within and outside the hospital, Dr. Neary's departure removed some fear factors and opened the way for new leadership. The doubters had eventually to be impressed by the drop in the number of caesarean hysterectomies and to realise that there were several effective ways to stop haemorrhage. This comment is not intended to mean that haemostasis is always achieved or that a woman must be moribund before a hysterectomy is carried out. We are aware that hysterectomy has a place in the clinician's armoury and that the decision to proceed to hysterectomy is a question of sound judgement and timing.

ROLE OF VISITING COMMITTEES FOR ACCREDITATION OF TRAINING

32. It has been stated by a number of witnesses that recognition of a Maternity Unit for training in obstetrics and gynaecology confers a status on that clinical unit. Although technically the remit of the Royal College of Obstetrics and Gynaecology and latterly the Institute of Obstetrics and Gynaecology of Ireland relates only to suitability for training, the Inquiry believes that the purpose of a visit to a clinical unit must or should involve some assessment of the quality and standard of care delivered to patients. Dr. Neary had taken the responsibility for filling in annual returns on obstetric and gynaecological activity, which were sent to the RCOG in London. As mentioned earlier in the report, there was no space reserved for peripartum hysterectomy. Some of the annual returns appeared to overstate the activity in the unit especially in gynaecology and presented the teaching of junior doctors in a more favourable light than witnesses confirmed to be so. No witness ever confirmed attending at a clinico-pathological conference in the Maternity Unit yet the annual returns indicated that such conferences regularly took place.

33. The Maternity Unit was assessed for suitability for training in 1987 and 1992 by the Visiting Committee of the RCOG. On both occasions, the visiting committees identified deficiencies in the training of the senior house officers and registrars. They made a number of pertinent recommendations regarding audit and training of doctors. In particular, they recommended that *"Thought should be given to constructing timetables which produce more even experience, better continuity of care and less frequent change of timetable."*

It is worth repeating what the Hospital Recognition Committee wrote in its report dated 29th March 1993.

34. *"The Council recommends that the following points are worthy of attention:*

> *There should be regular perinatal audit meetings with Consultant staff in attendance;*

> *A formal tutorial and meetings programme should be produced;*

> *There should be formal instruction in neonatal resuscitation at the beginning of each six month period;*

> *Provision should be made for instruction in family planning;*

> *SHOs should be made aware of and attend clinico-pathological meetings;*

> *A rolling weekly rota seems disruptive. Thought should be given to constructing timetables which produce more even experience, better continuity of care and less frequent change of timetable;*

> *Regular audit meetings should be introduced; and*

> *Junior staff should be circulated in writing concerning other hospital clinical meetings and clinico-pathological conferences."*

35. The recommendations suggest that when junior doctors were questioned by the Visiting Committee about their attendance at clinico-pathological conferences and meetings, they appeared unaware of their existence. The evidence heard during the Inquiry indicated that no such Conferences or meetings ever took place in spite of averrals to the contrary in the annual clinical returns.

36. Had the recommendations of the last visiting Committee been applied or had the hospital been visited again to ensure compliance, a more detailed scrutiny by the Committee might have revealed the infrequent meetings and the lack of audit. Family planning, regular perinatal audit and clinico-pathological meetings if in place could have identified the high caesarean section rate and the rising peripartum hysterectomy rate.

37. In the event no visiting committee from the British or Irish bodies or from An Bord Altranais ever identified any concerns regarding any clinical practices. No person ever availed of the opportunity to say anything to the visitors. The likelihood is that they were simply not aware that anything was amiss yet in 1991 there were 12 peripartum hysterectomies carried out, 8 in 1992 and 15 in 1993. Some witnesses who formed part of previous visiting committees reported that the Lourdes Maternity Unit was seen as something of a special case because of its strong Catholic ethos. The Inquiry inferred from this that there was a reluctance to be too inquisitive.

NO COMPUTERISED SYSTEM FOR RETRIEVING DATA

38. A number of medical witnesses postulated that if a computerised system of recording key data for audit purposes had been in place, the unusual numbers of peripartum hysterectomies would have been noted earlier and acted upon. In the context of the facts determined in this case, the inquiry was not convinced that the lack of computerisation played a major role in the failure to question practices. Even without computerised data the caesarean hysterectomies were always recorded in the periodic reports that continued until 1984. No queries were raised by any recipients of those reports about the caesarean hysterectomy rates.

39. Given the incurious mindset of the clinical staff in the Maternity Unit and of the other consultants, it is questionable that computerisation of data would have raised the level of awareness of the hysterectomy figures in the absence of a recognition of the need and purpose of audit. Clearly, computers are an essential tool for the recovery of data for statistics and audit but in this Unit the available data was ignored. Furthermore, there was no evidence that consultants or the general manager of the hospital attended to the recommendations made by the visiting committee as nothing changed following their visit. The junior doctors continued on rolling weekly rotas, being attached to wards rather than to consultants, there were no clinico-pathological conferences or perinatal audit meetings; there were no changes in family planning and there were no audit meetings. There was no evidence that there was any clamour for the installation of a computerised data collection system.

40. While many consultants attributed their lack of awareness of the extent of the peripartum hysterectomies to the lack of clinical reports, the Inquiry remains convinced that overall confidence in the competence of the obstetric consultants without any independent supportive evidence might have diluted the effectiveness of any such reports. The concept that critical analysis of adverse outcomes and near misses was a medical imperative was lacking at all levels of ownership, management and daily clinical practice and training insofar as the Maternity Unit was concerned.

41. The Inquiry had to return over and over to the fact that the preponderance of evidence from those present in theatre was that Dr. Neary was a safe pair of hands and a skilled surgeon. Even at this remove and with the benefit of hindsight, most witnesses still found it difficult to believe that objective medical opinion found that many of the hysterectomies were precipitate and unnecessary. The Inquiry concludes that the only process that could have identified the failings and institutional weaknesses of the Unit was robust and meaningful peer review and audit where clearly computerisation would have been a useful tool. However it is clear that computerisation of data without belief in the value of audit is of little use.

42. It was not recognised that Dr. Neary's abnormally low tolerance of peripartum bleeding – we avoid the word haemorrhage as it implies significant blood loss - was potentially harmful to the welfare of patients notwithstanding his other undoubted commitments to his patients. Peer review, which throughout the State has maintained standards in medical practice, failed in this Unit as there was no recognition among the consultants of the need for objective analysis of outcomes. As we have said elsewhere, there was the belief that it was inappropriate for one consultant to involve himself with the private patients of another consultant. This Maternity Unit had a relatively large number of private patients. It is very possible that if audit had occurred in the Unit, those private patients may have been excluded from audit.

43. Audit has been in place and was practised for many years in the Department of Surgery with the participation of the Pathology department. The concept was therefore not unknown in the hospital. The annual and biannual reports had been a long-standing and excellent form of audit. When the duty fell on

Dr. Finian Lynch to prepare the annual reports, he was unwilling to engage in their preparation without a computer system for collecting data. As a result the production of Maternity Annual Reports ceased. The MMMs felt that fear of litigation was the reason for their suspension and believed that they may have received legal advice on this point. Whatever the reasons, the effect of their cessation was that there was no audit of performance between 1984 and 2002. The lack of audit in the Maternity Unit had been recognised and highlighted by the Visiting Committee of the RCOG on the Maternity Unit in 1993.

RECOGNITION OF 'WHAT AUDIT MEANS' A PROBLEM

44. In the first three years following the revelations of unusually high rates of caesarean hysterectomy, all reviews of practices within the Unit noted some improvement but no real understanding of what audit meant. There was little evidence of appreciation by Health Board management that audit must be resourced and protected time must be set aside for department wide audits. Until very recently, there was no clinical audit committee or multidisciplinary audit. This is only scheduled to change in 2006. Staffing levels and slow and bureaucratic replacement and recruitment procedures continue to be a real problem. For a while it was extremely difficult to recruit suitably qualified locums for the Maternity Unit.

45. Throughout 2003 many of the highlighted deficiencies identified though HRRI and the Review Body were addressed. The deficiencies that remained were contributed to by the lack of administrative support and the lack of space, tools or manpower. These issues were out of the hands of clinical staff and should have been addressed by management and financial allocation.

THE TREATMENT OF HAEMORRHAGE AFTER DR. NEARY'S DEPARTURE

46. An unusual feature of the Maternity Unit was the lack of teamwork in relation to the treatment of severe haemorrhage. There were no written or agreed oral protocols or even a policy on what constituted severe haemorrhage. Each consultant had his own way of assessing and handling haemorrhage. The measurement of blood loss was unscientific and individualistic. There was no policy of seeking assistance or a second opinion before carrying out hysterectomy. On the other hand the reality is that for much of the 90s, one of

the consultants was in poor health and Dr. Neary had to proceed on his own. He thus developed a custom of managing without assistance. His opinion and assistance was far more likely to be sought than the other way round. There was no haematologist in the hospital to advise on blood replacement or on any developing coagulopathy.

47. The Inquiry concludes that the culture of hysterectomy was associated with a lack of understanding, knowledge or faith in methods of managing blood loss and preserving the uterus. The possible adverse psychological effects of unplanned sterilisation were not recognised. Sometimes the impression given was that hysterectomy in a woman who already had children was not deemed a serious event. In fairness, this sentiment has to be judged in the light of the frequency with which gynaecological hysterectomies as planned elective operations were performed generally in the country as a whole. Until new staff came into the Unit in the late 90s there was a ready acceptance that every peripartum hysterectomy was carried out to avoid a maternal death. It was assumed that the same procedures were carried out elsewhere and were therefore unremarkable.

48. Dr. Neary's method of staunching bleeding was for the anaesthetist to give syntocinon and ergometrine while he would pack and compress the uterus or oversew the placental site. His tendency was to proceed quickly to hysterectomy if the methods used did not have immediate effect. Prostaglandin derivatives were not routinely used. Dr. Neary was perceived by the anaesthetists to be the most experienced man in dealing with severe haemorrhage. As he did not use Haemabate or Cytotec in the treatment of haemorrhage the theatre staff was unfamiliar with the role of these drugs.

Saving a woman's uterus in the presence of severe post partum haemorrhage takes time trying many different procedures and involves many adrenalin driven moments. Some consultants felt that those assisting in theatre who were used to the previous culture had little faith in the efficacy of the efforts being made. In the short period after Dr. Neary left the Unit, some of these consultants felt isolated as the custom of hysterectomy at an early stage was almost entrenched. There was reluctance to change and an inappropriate fear of losing a mother. If a mother was very ill following severe blood loss and no hysterectomy had been carried out, comments to the effect *"that wouldn't have happened if Dr. Neary had been here"* were passed.

THE TREATMENT OF HAEMORRHAGE CHANGED

49. With the passage of time and the introduction of so many new obstetricians, there is an awareness of accepted norms, new practices and a definite change in thinking in relation to the importance of preserving a woman's uterus. All hysterectomies carried out now involve teamwork and at least two obstetricians and two anaesthetists. The possibility of hysterectomy as a consequence of placenta previa with accreta is now almost always recognised in the antenatal period and is fully discussed with the patient and her partner in advance of the operation.

50. Prostaglandins began to be routinely used in the treatment of post partum haemorrhage from 1999 as are other methods, such as the B Lynch suture, the haemostatic balloon, leaving the placenta in situ in combination with the use of methotrexate (a cancer drug) and antibiotic therapy. There are still occasions where bleeding continues and timely hysterectomy remains the appropriate and only solution.

51. In the years following Dr. Neary's departure serious communication issues with the laboratory were encountered and were the subject of heated discussion. Dr. Neary had always insisted that cross-matched blood be available for every caesarean section. For much of the time the blood was not used resulting in wastage of blood and laboratory time. A history of overreaction to blood loss in the past had created a climate of a relaxed response to "urgent" requests for blood from the maternity theatre even after Dr. Neary had left. The laboratory did not react appropriately when new consultants called for urgent blood supplies. These difficulties took several years to resolve. Strong protocols are now in place.

52. When attitudes towards caesarean hysterectomy changed the unacceptable delay in obtaining the fresh frozen plasma (FFP) was recognised. It was defrosted on a different and distant floor. There was no microwave or warming bath in the maternity theatre. It took several life threatening emergencies for the system to change and for a protocol for the ordering of urgent blood supplies to be worked out and warming baths and a microwave

to be installed in the operating theatre.

TUBAL LIGATION AND FAMILY PLANNING

53. Tubal ligations were introduced at the end of September/October 1999 without obstruction or objection from any quarter. A full range of contraceptive choice and advice is available since then. Newer consultants have introduced more modern procedures in gynaecology. Within a short time the number of hysteroscopy and other laparoscopic procedures increased dramatically with a commensurate fall in gynaecological hysterectomies in women of child-bearing age. More infertility investigation and assisted reproduction is carried out.

CHANGES TO MIDWIFERY SERVICES

54. During the past three years the new Assistant Director of Nursing in the Maternity Unit pushed forward several changes on the ground. Midwifery led changes include the introduction of updated admission forms containing more relevant data and the use of patient satisfaction surveys. Midwives are now managing low risk pregnancies. Improved training and skills-updating was made available and all line managers have attended management courses. Midwives no longer carry out non-nursing duties as care assistants have been employed. The dependence on student midwives to fill staff numbers has ceased. There is a strong association between the Lourdes Hospital, the Rotunda Hospital and the School of Nursing in Trinity College, Dublin. There is increasing emphasis on continuing midwifery education and attendance at workshops and seminars is encouraged. The strong criticism of the poor standards in documenting patient care has been heeded and continuing education on writing up of notes has been introduced. Bord Altranais guidelines for record keeping published in 2001 is in place. The format of the birth registers has changed to include far more detail on the condition and care of the baby. Mothers are given their own antenatal notes to keep and bring with them to hospital visits. A more structured appointments system has been introduced. More day care procedures are carried out and more community based antenatal care is taking place. A Clinical Governance Group within Maternity Services originally led by Dr. Lynch and then by Dr.O'Coigligh and new Assistant Director of Nursing was established and meets once every week to review weekly figures and outcomes. Junior

doctors and midwives were encouraged to attend, question and discuss events with the consultants.

55. The Condon Review recommended the closure of the obstetric units at Monaghan and Dundalk. The implementation of this recommendation in 2001, together with the opening of a large refugee reception centre in Mosney contributed to a 40% increase in the number of births at Drogheda without any commensurate increase in beds or staff. The problems associated with a foreign and frequently stressed asylum seeking population seem to have been handled with equanimity by the staff of the Maternity Unit even though many of the medical problems were new and staff numbers were very stretched. Staff recruitment in midwifery remains a problem.

MEDICAL COUNCIL REPORT

56. On 29th July 2003, the Medical Council considered the report of the Fitness to Practise Committee on the complaints made against Dr. Neary. The Committee upheld most of the complaints and found that Dr. Neary had been guilty of misconduct in carrying out peripartum hysterectomy on 10 patients who had lodged complaints and they recommended that his name be erased from the register of medical practitioners. The Medical Council took the unprecedented step of making the transcripts of the proceedings available to the general public on payment of a small fee for the CD rom version.

57. The publicity and public debate associated with the release of the information reopened many old wounds in the Maternity Unit. Two months later when HRRI/Capita Consulting returned to the Unit to report on the implementation of their previous recommendations they noted:

"the very significant emotional distress that remains in relation to historical events within the hospital and to the effects of high profile medical negligence actions… Many staff are still working in an atmosphere where they feel that past events exercise undue influence over the present working practice and professional outlook. Furthermore the idea that some patients may have been harmed by care delivered within the department is of deep concern to most staff".

58. They found then as we did during the Inquiry, a reluctance to face the past with very little discussion of historical events. The Medical Council Committee

report unequivocally condemned Dr. Neary's over reaction to what was perceived by him to be copious bleeding resulting in an over precipitous resort to hysterectomy. There could no longer be any doubt that Dr. Neary's practices were questionable and fell below the standard to be expected by patients of a consultant in the Lourdes Hospital or generally in the country. The Committee expressed criticism of a curious internal and external culture of isolation and absence of consultation within the hospital.

59. The ongoing reviews of HRRI/Capita Consulting and the Institute Review Body had highlighted the same unusual isolation as found by the Medical Council. By the time the report on Dr. Neary was publicised, there had already been major changes in practice in the Maternity Unit to minimise or entirely remove this isolation. Much credit for recognising that change was due must be attributed to Dr. McLoughlin the Assistant CEO of the North Eastern Health Board and to the former Medical Director who had the courage to follow through on the complaints made to the Health Board Solicitor and to act on their own instincts after the maternity theatre register had been scrutinised. Their actions in seeking that Dr. Neary should be suspended were vindicated. It is a great pity that both men and to a lesser extent the Director of Nursing of the Lourdes Hospital were subjected to personal vilification during the process.

MOST RECOMMENDATIONS ALREADY IN PLACE

60. By the time the Report from the Medical Council issued, many of the recommendations contained in that report had already been addressed in previous reports and had been put into effect. The importance of improving communication within a hospital service was recognised. Organised education sessions on identifying adverse events, learning from the experience and disseminating information on avoiding repetition were underway. An obstetric lead clinician was in place and the first annual report from the maternity department since 1984 had been published. For the first time, the midwives contributed a section dedicated to midwifery. The departments of anaesthesia and neonatology also contributed separate sections. The climate of isolation and its dangers had been recognised and remedied.

61. All permanent consultants were taking roles in formalised teaching of trainee doctors and MRCOG candidates. A culture of reporting was beginning to find acceptance although still meeting some reticence. Improved practices in the training and coordination of ultrasound services had been achieved. Registrars and SHOs were now attached to specific consultants instead of working to a general rota. Regular obstetric/midwifery meetings were held where open discussion of clinical practice and difficult cases was accepted as the norm. Key policies and protocols had been drafted and ratified. Procedures covering a broad range of clinical requirements were in place and were deemed by Capita/HRRI to be of good quality, evidence based and with review dates.

62. There was a developing association between Trinity College School of Nursing and Midwifery and the Maternity Unit in determining best practice in midwifery protocols. The Maternity Services Task Force set up by the Health Board included a number of external experts to assist in the implementation of recommendations made by HRRI and the Lamki Review Group. There was much new blood in the department of Obstetrics bringing experience of best practice from the major hospitals in which those clinicians and midwives had worked in Ireland and overseas. Work was still in progress in relation to policies and protocols on consent, the management of obstetric emergencies, spontaneous abortion, referral criteria, induction of labour and the management of diabetes in pregnancy. All of these improvements took place at a time when the delivery rate had almost doubled in the space of 4 years and in the presence of high midwifery stress levels associated with the takeover of the hospital, the attempts at integration of the two hospitals, the events associated with Dr. Neary and the seemingly endless reviews, inspections and reports.

63. There were however some areas which still required work. Individual appraisal and competence assurance frameworks were still absent. Specific competency and training needs remained and there was still no planned programme of clinical audit for all areas of obstetrics and gynaecology. The need for good quality clinical information enabled by a technology management information system was still not available. Dr. Lynch complained in 1982 of the lack of a computerised database. At the time of

writing the report this system is not as yet in place although yet again, it is expected shortly.

64. **ANAESTHETIC TRAINING IN OBSTETRICS**

While most of the anaesthetists had been exposed to obstetrics during part of their specialist training none had attended obstetric specific courses since taking up their appointments at the Lourdes Hospital. The limitations of their training in obstetrics were recognised and cured by the recruitment of a consultant anaesthetist with extensive experience and accreditation in obstetrical anaesthesia. She is now lead clinician in obstetric anaesthesia. The anaesthetic team had remained almost unchanged until mid 1996. All the evidence we heard suggests that for much of the time the anaesthetists were thinly spread especially after March 1993 when patient demand for epidural pain relief was finally met. Between 1998 and 2003 four new anaesthetic appointments were made. Three more consultants were appointed in late 2004. Several HRRI/Capita reports have criticised the lack of dedicated anaesthetic night cover for the Maternity Unit and this problem continues.

2004 WAS A VERY DIFFICULT YEAR

65. In late Spring the Unit was hit with an extraordinary series of tragic incidents. The lead consultant became gravely ill and required very major surgery; one of the locums suffered a tragic bereavement, another consultant's spouse became gravely ill and died and one of the newly recruited consultants went on maternity leave. Suddenly the Unit was down to one permanent consultant, no lead clinician and several urgently recruited locums. The clinical teaching programme was seriously affected.

66. During what has been described by the consultants as an *annus horribilis,* the Unit had its first visit from a Hospital Recognition Committee for suitability for Obstetrics and Gynaecology training. This was the first visit since 1992. Adverse comments were made on the inadequate permanent consultant staffing of the Unit.

67. In the rest of the hospital the acute shortage of beds and the extraordinary number of ill A&E patients occupying trolleys meant that all gynaecology

beds were taken over for A&E admissions. The lack of gynaecology beds has had a negative effect on the training of junior doctors.

68. The visiting committee warned hospital managers that the lack of major gynaecology surgery, if not rectified, would affect the approval of the hospital for registrar posts in obstetrics and gynaecology. They therefore made a number of recommendations and wished to see a progress report within one year. They recommended rotation of registrars and SHO posts between the Lourdes Hospital and the Dublin teaching hospitals; increased ward round teaching sessions and training programmes in ultrasound were recommended.

69. The Obstetric expert employed by Capita/HRRI also visited the Unit to assess progress and noted the absence of the permanent consultants but acknowledged that the Unit was fortunate in having high quality short term locums. He was complimentary of many recent improvements in the Unit. He was happy with the guidelines for managing massive haemorrhage and was impressed by the ability of the risk adviser although he observed that some consultants' understanding of the value of critical incident reporting or of risk management was deficient. In terms of adverse outcome reporting and the implementation of a risk management programme he felt that the Unit still had a way to go. Staffing levels in anaesthesia remained deficient.

70. He expressed serious concerns in relation to audit, the lack of support structures to support the risk manager's work and the lack of a risk management committee. He did not believe it appropriate that the Risk Adviser reported to Patient Liaison and not to a senior clinician. He expressed the need for the establishment of a clinical risk management committee at department level, led by a senior consultant, which should report to a central clinical risk management committee also with senior clinical leadership.

71. He commented in his report:

"There is no organised departmental system of clinical audit. The clinical governance meetings are a useful forum but discuss chiefly caesarean

sections. There have been several audit projects undertaken by individual staff members but these do not, in my view, represent a proper approach to audit which should be multidisciplinary and unit wide. It is essential that there should be a clinical audit lead to plan the programme and evolve responsibility for individual projects"

Very shortly after the review took place, the consultant numbers fell to one and later two with the arrival of a newly appointed consultant in July 2004. There were extreme difficulties in recruiting locum cover causing the midwives and remaining doctors to be very overstretched. There was no lead clinician and no possibility of setting up a clinical risk management committee or multidisciplinary unit wide audit. It is to the credit of the midwives and consultants and a tribute to their professionalism that under trying and testing conditions, a maternity service was delivered to the women of the North Eastern region. In spite of the calls on their time, these same overworked people were generous of their precious time to this Inquiry.

Plans to open a midwifery led unit on an experimental basis went ahead in spite of the acute shortage of consultant cover, the views of the remaining consultant, the views expressed by the Institute of Obstetricians and Gynaecologists and against the advice of Mr. Finbar Lennon, the Medical Adviser to the Health Board. All these parties had recommended waiting until the full complement of consultant obstetricians was in place. The Inquiry had difficulty understanding the political imperative to open the new midwifery led unit in such circumstances and contrary to the advice of the Medical Adviser. The idea was a good one but the timing was unwise and a cause of unnecessary stress for the few consultants covering the Maternity Unit. Such were the workloads on staff in the Unit that had we been presenting this report at the end of 2004, our hopes for the future direction of the Unit would not have been as sanguine. While all these events were taking place and while the consultants were involved in an industrial dispute, hospital management engaged the new Hospital Accreditation Board to engage in an accreditation of the Maternity Unit. The accreditation remains incomplete and identified "pockets of excellence".

72. By the Autumn of 2004 the Health Board, conscious of the problems created by the lack of a lead clinician, persuaded Dr. Shane Higgins who was due to join the consultant staff in January, to come a month earlier and take over the position as Lead Clinician of the Maternity Unit. He brought his valuable experience as Clinical Director of the Labour Ward of a busy University hospital in Melbourne and with a special interest in fetal medicine to the Unit. Gradually, the unusual combination of health problems and tragic events, which contributed to the absence of so many of the consultants, began to resolve and the Unit began slowly to recover from the very difficult year.

2005 AND FINALLY A FULL TEAM WITH LEADERSHIP

73. This last year has seen much progress and is a success story. It was reported that newer and younger consultants are strongly committed to clinical audit, risk management, continuing medical development and quality assurance frameworks.

74. The Maternity Unit has now undergone a long series of evaluations and reviews. As one expert advised "there is the danger of creating institutional paralysis by analysis." Management should now be aware of its strengths and should support its weaknesses, which are contributed to by lack of administrative support systems. Within the Unit, it is obvious that the tensions and despondence associated with the problems of consultant absence in 2004 have lifted. The Unit has a dynamic lead clinician. The former lead clinician is back at work and has taken charge of coordinating audit and risk management. The Unit has an almost full complement of consultants. There is only one locum. Cross cover is provided for any consultant absences. The rota is 1:7 which is a luxury never available to Dr. Milner or Dr. Akpan in 2004 or to the previous consultants. The current consultants speak through their lead clinician and have developed a strong collegiate approach to practice. There is now little doubt that the Unit is engaged in moving forward and offering care which is evaluated against known benchmarks.

75. The Maternity Unit works with a very much enhanced and impressive paediatric department with two neonatologists and three paediatricians. There have been three recent consultant appointments in anaesthesia bringing the total to eleven although a second anaesthetist with specialist obstetric experience would be desirable. A third pathologist has been

appointed. At last a haematologist had been appointed. All departments – anaesthetics, haemovigilance, pathology, paediatrics, midwifery and obstetrics have engaged in a joint consultative process in drafting and agreeing protocols which are visible, available and subject to review dates. Almost all departments now have an agreed lead clinician.

The new lead clinician very quickly made himself aware of the history of the Unit and the identified areas of strength and weakness. He is determined to lead a team dedicated to the provision of a top class obstetric and gynaecology service to the women of the North East region. He has introduced consultant cover for the labour ward on a rostered daily basis with active teaching on the ward. The Unit wishes to be in the position to offer full consultant cover for the labour ward on a 24/7 basis and thus requires more consultants.

76. The Institute expressed concerns regarding continued recognition of the Unit for training because of the lack of a full gynaecology service. The lead clinician therefore secured and ring-fenced 2 gynaecology beds per day for major operations. He has presented a plan to provide a one-stop gynaecology clinic for referrals from GPs. This would be a very positive step for women's health and would make use of the considerable expertise in gynaecology in the Unit. The nursing and consultant staff are already in place but a sonographer, colposcopic nurse and colposcopic secretary are necessary to set up the service. A very recent discussion with the lead clinician indicated a disappointing management response to the considerable effort expended in presenting this plan.

77. Under this new leadership, the consultant team now insists on support and backup to provide an effective service. For the first time, the consultants have an office in the Unit that they share. Each desk has a computer terminal. The consultants were involved in the selection of an IT system and in evaluating the software. The lead clinician is a strong supporter of clinical governance and understands the components of such governance, which include continuing audit and education. A project officer has been appointed and training is to follow. A leadership team has been appointed to oversee the introduction of the system. The software will be available for both the general

labour ward and the Midwifery led unit.

The lead clinician has extensive experience of the problems associated with repeat caesarean sections and was involved in an audit in Melbourne on a sudden surge of caesarean hysterectomies there. The investigation revealed a statistical blip. The protocol now operating in the Lourdes Maternity Unit is that a second and often third opinion is sought from a consultant obstetrician if it is thought necessary to proceed to hysterectomy, and if required, another anaesthetic colleague is called. The decision to proceed to hysterectomy is a team decision. Two caesarean hysterectomies were carried out last year. There were almost 3200 deliveries. Clinico pathological conferences (CPCs) have taken place in the last six months introducing open discussion between obstetricians and pathologists for the first time. Obstetricians regularly visit the pathology department to discuss surgical specimens.

78. The fact that the Inquiry was taking place has played a role in opening communications lines between all the various areas of clinical specialty involved with the Unit. A Policy and Procedures Committee is in place where policies and guidelines are constantly reviewed and updated with emphasis on evidence-based practice and research. Meetings have taken place with the maternity staff of Cavan Hospital and a regional forum has been set up where regional clinical midwifery guidelines are being formulated. A research Midwife with specialist training in writing clinical practice guidelines has been engaged. It is hoped that patients in both Maternity Units will thus be managed in accordance with common midwifery guidelines, which will eventually be available on the Internet.

79. The possibility of this Unit falling behind in current practice is now remote. A number of audits are planned for the department and 5 research papers have been produced and presented at scientific meetings under the tutelage of Dr. Milner who has been appointed senior lecturer with the RCSI. She is actively involved in lecturing to students at the Unit. She is on the Membership of Institute exam committee, and sets questions for the exams. It is no longer necessary for specialist trainees to sit Membership exams set by the Royal College of Obstetricians and Gynaecologists. The department of obstetrics has been instrumental in obtaining funding for a multi-centre Health Research

Board ultrasound project with 8 other participating hospitals thus putting the research capability of the department on an even more secure footing. One of the current registrars has been accepted into a Dublin based specialist registrar training programme and there are plans by the Institute to visit the Unit later this year to establish its suitability for SPR programmes. If successful, a candidate has been identified and will take up the place in July. In the same month, a senior registrar from the Women's Hospital in Melbourne will take up a twelve-month position in Drogheda. It is hoped that this will be the first of a series of visits from registrars on the specialist training programmes. There is a great deal of new blood and movement of registrars who have trained in centres of excellence. It is hoped that more Irish candidates will seek training if the Unit is recognised for SPR training.

80. The current Chair of the Medical Board of the Lourdes Hospital promotes strong inter-departmental and cross-departmental working relationships and supports the development of robust risk management to support high quality patient care. Under his chairmanship, the Medical Board and the new consultants have the motivation, the skills and the energy to move the Lourdes Hospital forward as a fully recognised teaching hospital with Specialist Registrar Training in all their departments. At the moment the departments of Obstetrics and Gynaecology and Pathology are not recognised for SPR training. It is hoped that this will change. If the Unit is recognised for SPR training, this will be the final recognition that the Unit has changed radically and has joined the rank of hospitals with full teaching status.

81. The biggest difference in the hospital at the present day is the presence of so many new consultants. Senior nursing positions have changed radically. The old hierarchy has been replaced by teamwork. Clinical team meetings take place regularly thus ensuring that communication is effective and organised. The new consultants to whom we spoke do not appear complacent; they do not accept the concept of standing still; they engage in research; they engage in and with management and they accept fully the need for meaningful audit and the concept of competence assurance. They are not prepared to be associated with a hospital with a poor reputation. They wish the Lourdes

Hospital to become a place where the best specialist trainees seek to train and practise.

82. As for the past tragic events that are the subject of this Inquiry, there is a general sense that what happened should not have been tolerated and serious questions should have been asked long before October 1998. The concerned midwives should have been fully supported and their questions investigated earlier. The obstetric hysterectomies should have been brought to the attention of the Medical Director or the Medical Board or to Management at a much earlier stage. Dr. Neary's caesarean hysterectomy rate should have been questioned by his peers in the late 1970s. The observation that he "was afraid of haemorrhage" should have been further examined to determine whether patients might be at risk as a consequence of this fear. While it is true that no patient died, the unplanned sterilisation of a young woman - as some of his patients were - was too high a price to pay for a surgeon's phobias. Dr. Neary was permitted to carry too much of the workload for safety. He was either unable or unwilling to call on his colleagues for assistance, as he perceived them as unwilling or unavailable to come in after hours. There is little doubt that junior doctors were more inclined to call on Dr. Neary rather than on his colleagues for assistance. Opportunities for peer review and assessment were thus even more limited. His praise and reward came from the gratitude of struggling junior doctors and midwives who came more and more to count on his reliability and availability.

83. The Inquiry has been reminded many times not to apply the wisdom of hindsight or the practices of 2006 to the overworked and cash strapped provincial hospitals of the past. We have tried sincerely to act on this advice but nevertheless, had difficulty understanding why so few had the courage, insight, curiosity or integrity to say, "this is not right". Had anyone had that courage after a failed attempt in 1980, there would be the satisfaction that at least they tried and they may have prevented many medically induced injuries. The former tutor who had raised concerns to the Matron of the Maternity Unit and the Cardinal in 1980 expressed deep regret that she had not done more to prevent so many women from unnecessarily losing their fertility and femininity and that whatever effort she made to raise her

concerns did not have a better outcome at the time. Some of the midwives who had simply never wondered or questioned, reported that they have been asking themselves since how they were so unquestioning; how they had no suspicions as they now see that the signs were there. They believe that their training moulded them never to question. As detailed previously in the report, many of these midwives wept at the sadness of what happened and are full of regrets. Others wished that they had had more confidence to do something earlier.

84. There have to be systems of independent safeguards in place to recognise aberrant practice soon after it occurs. Those systems have to include reviewing the practices of apparently dedicated and popular doctors in an effective and dispassionate manner to prevent their practices from falling below acceptable standards. We do not recommend a system where midwives and junior doctors openly challenge consultant decisions but recommend teamwork with appropriate discussion before and after events. We recommend much more involvement of all staff in weekly reviews and we recommend an awareness of all team members of the importance of continuous learning and competence assurance of incident reporting, follow through and audit. Regular team meetings should be attended by all staff and not left to the dedicated few. It should not be considered bad manners to discuss the outcomes of treatment of a colleague's patient. There should be no difference in the standard applied to a private or public patient. A consultant should not be engaged in so much private practice that sleep deprivation interferes with public duties.

85. The strangest finding which this Inquiry has made is that - apart from the Matron of the Maternity Unit and a tutor in 1980 - no one had any worries, concerns, apprehensions, unease or disquiet until the very late 1990s. While some of this can be explained by the belief that perhaps some hysterectomies were sterilisations, or that the consultants were intimidating, or that Dr. Neary appeared to be such a competent surgeon, they are not very convincing arguments for a brand new hospital in the 1990s. There is the suspicion that given the same set of circumstances, what happened in this hospital in Drogheda could be replicated in other hospitals where

loyalties to staff might be stronger than duty to patients and the profession of medicine.

86. *"Clinical independence" or "clinical autonomy "* was so often cited as a reason why bad practice in consultants was accepted that we wondered if perhaps this was an easy excuse to say, *"it was not my business".*

87. We do not believe that clinical independence or clinical autonomy was ever meant to provide unfettered freedom to practise medicine in accordance with personal dictates without regard to accepted standards. All consultants have a duty to practise their skills in compliance with best practice. Their position is a privileged one and their status as consultants recognises their learning and expertise in their chosen specialty. Consultants are deemed competent to lead a team of doctors, nurses and other health professionals in their field of specialty and to teach trainee doctors. Patients are referred to them for specialist advice and treatment. Patients should be able to trust consultants who owe a duty of care to provide those patients referred to them with the most appropriate and effective treatment. They do not have the right to practise outmoded medicine or to lose their competence while enjoying the status of "specialist".

88. The Inquiry has been referred several times to the aviation industry as a model for risk management and competence assessment. If a pilot is flying commercial aircraft, he/she is obliged to update his/her skills on a regular basis and to attend assessments. All incidents and accidents are fully investigated to identify root causes. If appropriate, pilot error is acknowledged and openly and fully discussed. If the pilot in error does not satisfy aviation authorities' exacting standards, he does not fly until he does. We have been told that medicine has a lot to learn from this model. It is difficult to disagree.

89. We understand that new legislation is awaited to impose statutory obligations on all doctors to attend regularly for continuing medical education and development at approved courses and to show proof at regular intervals that they have done so. Clinical competence assessment every 5 years of all specialists in practice is also planned. The legislation is long overdue and

eagerly awaited by the Medical Council and the Institute of Obstetricians and Gynaecologists.

TERM 7

To advise the Minister for Health and Children on whether additional protocols and systems of control should now be put in place to prevent a recurrence of the events that gave rise to the findings of the Report.

RECOMMENDATIONS TO PREVENT SUCH OCCURRENCES IN THE FUTURE

1. Before the Inquiry was in a position to make suggestions for the future we had to understand the past. We learned that most obstetricians carried out between two and ten peripartum hysterectomies in their lifetime. It was difficult to fathom therefore how one obstetrician could carry out nearly 130 peripartum hysterectomies over twenty five years without questions being asked. It was even more difficult to understand how more than 50 of those peripartum hysterectomies were carried out by Dr. Neary between mid 1990 and the end of 1998 in the new Maternity Unit. Other consultants or registrars carried out 38 such procedures during the same period when an average of 1800 babies a year were being delivered. Of those 91 hysterectomies carried out in the new Maternity Unit, probably no more than 20 could be statistically justified. (Some of the cases have been reviewed by external experts and found to have been necessary and justified.)

2. It had already been established by several medical review bodies that Dr. Neary, a respected and dedicated doctor had engaged in poor and even bad practices. It is evident that neither he nor his work colleagues recognised his failings. Some of those practices became systemic as is proved by the peripartum hysterectomy rate compared with other similar sized units. It took a great deal of courage and effort to question those practices and change the system. It is clear that if a repetition of the systemic acceptance of poor practice is to be prevented, safeguards must be in place to identify such questionable or outdated practices and to quickly retrain or remove such doctors to protect the public. These systems and safeguards must be capable of promptly identifying an aberrant practice soon after it occurs. Frequently the root cause of the questionable practice lies in the environment in which the consultant works and which in turn facilitates such practice. The work of all doctors including highly regarded consultants has to be reviewed in an

effective and dispassionate manner. Failure to engage in effective peer review and independent audit will ensure that history will repeat itself.

3. The Maternity Unit was unusually self-contained and isolated with a strong unvalidated belief in its excellence. Although major changes have taken place in the last few years there is still work to be done and lessons to be learned. Meaningful audit is not yet in place. The Unit was very exposed during part of 2004 when in spite of industrial action and a diminished numbers of consultants and midwives, a new midwifery led unit was introduced and management engaged in a partial accreditation process.

4. In making recommendations we are aware that our Inquiry has been uniquely confined to an examination of documents, practices and structures in the Lourdes Hospital Maternity Unit. It is therefore not clear whether this Maternity Unit was unique in its practices or whether similar practices and attitudes are found in any other peripheral hospitals in the State. The recommendations are directed to the Lourdes Maternity Unit but may have relevance for other similar sized units.

5. The changes recommended are not high tech or hungry of resources but require the attendance and involvement of rested and unstressed hospital personnel who work in a safe environment. Such personnel require effective support services so that nurses and midwives do not carry out non-nursing duties reserved for secretarial or administrative staff and doctors do not waste skills because equipment is not maintained or beds are not available. We recommend involvement of all consultants at daily labour ward handovers and at regular multidisciplinary throughput reviews and we recommend an awareness of all team members of the importance of continuous learning, competence assurance, incident reporting with follow through and audit.

6. Regular team meetings should be attended by all staff and not left to the dedicated usual few. It should not be considered bad manners to discuss the outcomes of treatment of a colleague's patient. There should be no difference in the standard of care applied to a private or public patient. A consultant should not be engaged in so much private practice that sleep deprivation or exhaustion interferes with public duties. We do not recommend a system

where midwives and junior doctors openly challenge consultant decisions but recommend a teamwork approach with appropriate discussion before and after events.

7. The Inquiry recognises the contribution made by obstetricians and midwives to the health and well being of the citizens of this State both now and during the many years when hospitals were under funded and medical staff overworked. We do not for one instant wish to decry that work by the findings we have made of the past practices in this particular hospital. Given the conditions under which so many hospitals operated in the past it is a wonder that more disasters did not occur, especially in smaller units that operated with only two consultants. We are convinced that a debt is owed to the dedication and integrity of the consultants and midwives who worked in those hospitals. However we believe that it is dangerous to rely solely on dedication, loyalty and integrity. Safe independent systems of assessment and competence assurance must be put in place.

8. Change, analysis, review and learning are the keys to best practice. All procedures must be measured against outcomes and modern literature must be considered. Medical practices must be evaluated against accepted benchmarks. Fresh ideas must circulate; education must continue and review of outcomes must take place on a regular and continuous basis. Each unit must be associated with other units and compared constantly with each other and against known standards. Leadership, training and knowledge must be recognised as key elements in every successful hospital. Support systems must be in place to enable standards to be reached and maintained. The professional bodies must play a fuller role in evaluating competence. Society needs good doctors and nurses. They deserve good working conditions and their good work should be rewarded and appreciated.

9. We have outlined that deficiencies of insight, judgement and training were the probable root to the serious limitations in some of Dr. Neary's practices. We have described the failure of peer review in this Unit and how the lack of transparency generally combined with hierarchical obedience and a narrow interpretation of clinical independence created a culture of fatalistic

acceptance where the difference between humane practice and bad practice was blurred.

10. Experience shows that small departments or institutions have a propensity to develop very close bonds of collegiate loyalty where honest peer review becomes difficult. The other direction is where small camps or cliques develop and divide staff again making honest review difficult. In both situations newcomers face difficulties in breaking in and new practices are viewed with suspicion. Objective critical analysis rarely flourishes in such a hospital. The Lourdes maternity Unit was in this position only seven years ago. In this, it probably shared features which may be present in other hospitals today. What happened in this Unit should be a lesson to those other departments elsewhere of the value of objective audit, circulation of new ideas, movement of staff and continuing education and skills assessment.

11. The enlargement of consultant numbers in the Maternity Unit with the commensurate increase in consultant appointments in pathology and anaesthesia has the potential to dilute the effect of partnerships, opposing camps and the personalisation of comment on outcomes. These enlarged departments require rotating leadership with management skills to maximise the full potential of each area of specialisation. Thus each department is integrated fully as a component of a hospital providing a good health service for the community from antenatal to geriatric care. Hospitals are not there to provide jobs but to provide services for the evolving and changing needs of the community. A good health system must surely be one of the best assets of a sophisticated democracy.

12. Many changes have taken place in the hospital and the Maternity Unit in the last seven years. It is a much busier hospital offering far more services. There are almost twice as many consultants as when the hospital was in private ownership. The practice of each consultant in the Maternity Unit operating under personal and unwritten protocols has been replaced by agreed guidelines and protocols for general application. Communication and transparency have been dramatically improved and questioning has been encouraged. Although the MMMs continue to play a pastoral role, the religious ethos has changed. A full family planning service is in place for

those who wish to avail of such advice. Tubal ligations are carried out. Many of our recommendations, drafted when the Unit was recovering from the traumas of the past and the "*annus horribilis*" of 2004, are already in place. The recommendations are nevertheless presented in their entirety to minimise the potential to repeat the same mistakes.

13. Change effected in the Maternity Unit at all levels has not been matched by commensurate changes in support for the consultants and midwives. They are still under resourced and under staffed. The extraordinary dedication of the few is still counted upon to fill gaps in services. Long-term absences are still imposing burdens on the working midwives and consultants. Lead consultants still have little say in strategic planning and good ideas are often sacrificed at the altar of annual budgetary constraints. Management structures need serious changes in training, continuity and accountability. They too need to be subject to audit and review.

GUIDE TO RECOMMENDATIONS

14. These recommendations are made following more than 18 months of hearing evidence from patients and their spouses, junior doctors, midwives, consultants, risk management experts and managers. The use of the pronoun he is intended to include she and the recommendations should be read *mutatis mutandis.*

15. The recommendations have been discussed in general terms with the lead obstetrician, Chairman of the Medical Board and lead midwives. They were largely in favour of our suggestions and have assisted with their ideas and comments. In making our recommendations, we were very conscious of the culture that existed previously at the Lourdes Maternity Unit and of the malpractices that innocently flourished within the ambit of a good service. All of these recommendations are directed specifically towards minimising the recurrence of such a culture where openness was lacking and where one doctor carried too heavy a workload and where consultants imposed too much of their personality on the Unit.

16. RECOMMENDATIONS FOR OBSTETRICIANS

16.1 LEAD CLINICIAN

➤ The unit should always have an elected lead clinician modelled on the Mastership system of the Dublin maternity hospitals. The lead clinician should be elected from the team of consultants for a period of 5 years and have protected sessions for administrative duties.

➤ The lead clinician should be assisted by a deputy lead clinician to share the workload and to step into his shoes while he is absent. The lead and deputy should strive not to be absent for extended periods at the same time.

➤ The lead clinician should have input and take responsibility for obstetric and gynaecology budgetary planning and management and should be part of the management team.

➤ The lead clinician should be responsible for organising regular clinical audit meetings, clinical pathological conferences, clinical governance and continuing education. It is recommended that the duty to ensure that regular and effective audit takes place is delegated to a specific consultant in charge of audit and that audit consultant should have a deputy.

➤ The lead clinician should be responsible for educating all medical staff on the value and importance of clinical incident reporting and should work with the Institute of Obstetricians and Gynaecologists, the Royal Colleges and the Medical Council to establish an agreed trigger list of reportable clinical events.

➤ Back up and support by way of a separate office, full time secretarial and IT services and a meeting room for discussion and presentations should be available to the lead clinician.

➤ The two consultants delegated to work on audit should have dedicated secretarial assistance with training and experience of audit procedures and specific IT programming.

➢ There should be regular liaison between the lead clinicians in the midwifery, anaesthetic, radiology, paediatric and pathology departments.

➢ The lead clinician should sit on the Hospital Medical Board with the other department lead clinicians.

➢ The lead clinician should work out a complaints or concerns procedure for all staff in the Maternity Unit. He should be made aware of all complaints received by the risk manager relating to any aspects of care in the Maternity Unit provided by receptionists and porters to cleaners and consultants.

➢ The lead clinician should liaise with the Patient Claims Office so that he is aware of the nature of all civil claims made against any practitioner in the Maternity Unit and thus be aware of what is being alleged against the service provided.

➢ The lead clinician must have authority to discuss the behaviour, practice, attendance and performance of all the Unit's consultants and medical staff with that staff and to recommend changes. The lead clinician must ensure that courtesy on the part of all medical personnel is recognised as an important component of an effective medical service.

➢ The lead clinician should have the authority to delegate duties to each consultant so that every consultant plays an active role in the department and is not solely involved in mandatory public contract sessions. He must establish guidelines of what constitutes an acceptable amount of private obstetrics practice.

➢ Consideration should be given to entering key data of sentinel events on a daily basis into a national integrated monitoring system and into an internal computer auditing system. This system will be in addition to but separate from clinical incident reporting. The purpose of this sentinel event reporting is to facilitate openness and awareness throughout the unit so that no clinician can say, *"I did not know it was happening"* again.

> The lead clinician and senior management should work out a strategy in advance to ensure relief is provided on a prompt basis when extended absence due to illness, maternity leave or family circumstances cause services to be stretched on the labour ward, in the operating theatres or the antenatal clinics.

> As retirement of a consultant or maternity leave is generally an event capable of prediction, a replacement should be recruited at least 3 months before the date of such consultant leave or retirement.

> The lead and deputy lead clinicians should be involved in the selection process of the replacement consultant.

> The duties of the lead and deputy lead clinician can be delegated.

16.2 A **deputy lead consultant** should be either elected by his/her peers or selected by the lead obstetrician.

> The deputy lead should be available to cover and take over for the lead clinician during all absences.

> The deputy lead should take charge of junior doctor training sessions and ensure that each doctor in training is attached for each six month session to a specific consultant who spends time teaching and assisting that trainee.

> The deputy lead should take charge of induction courses on changeover days for all new trainees and this course should include information of the layout of hospital, location of protocols, ID list of clinicians, rosters, meetings and lectures. Emphasis on standards of clinical and ethical behaviour and the importance of communication with patients and colleagues should be stressed and that the treatment of all patients with politeness and dignity is paramount. Guidance should be given on valid consent, communication with families and the importance of clear informative and legible discharge letters.

16.3 All registrar and consultant obstetricians should attend courses in clinical governance and risk management and understand their professional responsibilities in this regard.

16.4 Agreed, multi-disciplinary, massive obstetric haemorrhage protocols should be *clear, <u>unambiguous,</u> widely available* and practiced as a drill. Consideration should be given to the adoption of a mnemonic to aid easier application of the protocol in emergency situations. The article written by Rotunda Hospital (Rizvi et al, BJOG, May 2004) on post partum haemorrhage should be studied and similar audit carried out.

16.5 Obstetricians should keep a fair balance between private work and clinical contractual commitments. Private practice should not be so onerous that performance is affected nor should it interfere with the consultants' capacity to carry their full weight in teaching duties towards junior doctors in training, continuing professional development or clinical audit.

16.6 Research and audit projects by **all** clinicians should be actively encouraged and facilitated.

16.7 Members of Obstetric/Gynaecology staff who are given time off to attend seminars and conferences should present a short talk on what has been learned at the event so that all consultants benefit from any new research or information.

16.8 All obstetricians should be made aware of the benefits of the HIPE system and avail of that system to access data from the Unit and for audit and research.

16.9 All doctors should be reminded to introduce themselves to patients and to explain the procedures, which they are about to do and to explain the reasons for such procedures. Lack of courtesy was the complaint made most often by patients and the attribute most sought by patients of their consultants. Communication was frequently described as a skill lacking in doctors. It is not enough to say "I am Dr. X". We thought it far more helpful to say, "Mrs. A, I am John Doe the consultant gynaecologist who is dealing with your case".

16.10 All consultants must keep up their performance, skills and education and be prepared to assist other surgeons in maternity and gynaecology theatre on a regular basis so that different skills may be exchanged. Consideration should be given to assisting other surgeons at other maternity units to observe those surgeons' skills and practices. There is a role for the video recording of operations as a teaching tool.

16.11 One organised half day should be set aside each month for a full clinical audit of the previous month's work. The attendance of consultants and registrars should be compulsory except for attendance at emergency cases in the theatre or labour ward.

16.12 Each consultant must present an account of his/her personal procedures and outcomes for annual peer review. If it is apparent that skills are being lost through inadequate activity in a specialty then attendance at appropriate courses should be compulsory. The lead obstetrician should have the authority to recommend attendance at such courses where skills are revalidated. An outside assessor should attend and observe the integrity of the annual review. These guidelines are available from the RCOG and the Medical Council.

16.13 Annual clinical reports of activity and outcomes should be prepared and published within 9 months of the previous year's end. The lead and deputy lead clinicians should be responsible for ensuring the preparation of this report but all consultants should share in the burden of preparing the information.

16.14 The Unit should enter into arrangements with at least two other provincial maternity units to present their annual statistics at a joint meeting each year and to compare key outcomes. It is suggested that Cavan Hospital Maternity Unit should be one of these hospitals. An outside assessor should evaluate and comment on the reports and the lead clinician from each hospital should be given an opportunity to respond. These annual reports should be compared with outcomes from the Dublin hospitals and any major differences in outcomes discussed.

16.15 Uncomplicated procedures must be established for dealing with complaints and concerns arising from inappropriate behaviour or clinical practices where patient safety may be compromised. All clinicians in the Maternity Unit should be made aware of the procedures. Complaints must be taken seriously.

16.16 Consultants and registrars should engage in more discussion with the pathology department on unusual specimens explaining what they seek histopathology to confirm or refute. Ambiguous or unclear findings should be discussed.

17. SUGGESTED PROCEDURES RELATING TO COMPLAINTS OF CLINICAL PRACTICE

➢ The complaint or query should be sent to the lead clinician in writing. If the lead clinician is the subject of the complaint, then the complaint should be to the deputy lead clinician.

➢ If the lead clinician believes that the matter can be resolved by speaking to the parties involved then he/she should do so. If not, the complaint or concern should be considered and then forwarded for comment to the clinician against whom the complaint is made without revealing the complainant's identity.

➢ The response should be furnished in writing within 7 days. A copy of the response should be sent to the complainant.

➢ The lead clinician must then conduct an investigation of the complaint and response.

➢ The Lead Clinician Deputy determines whether to take the matter further.

➢ Either way the complainant must be made aware of response and action.

➢ If the matter is deemed too serious to resolve informally, then it must be notified to the Medical Director of the Hospital Medical Board to further investigate and take action, or refer to the Medical Council as appropriate. Complaints, which do not involve medical obstetrics/gynaecology staff, should be made to the Risk Manager who can liaise with the lead clinician and lead midwife.

18. A general complaints procedure should be in place for all users of the maternity and gynaecological services. Complaints should be assessed and **audit of complaints** of every kind whether involving clinical practice, behaviour or service carried out regularly to evaluate the nature of the complaints and the success of the remedy. The anonymous results should be published with the annual clinical report.

19. Joint measures should be taken by the RCSI and/or the Institute of Obstetricians and Gynaecologists to determine what steps are necessary to recognise the Maternity Unit for Specialist Registrar Training.

20. Consideration should be given to a system of entering key data on sentinel events on a daily basis into a national integrated monitoring system and into an internal audit system. This system will be in addition to but separate from clinical incident reporting. The purpose of this sentinel event reporting is to facilitate openness and awareness throughout the unit so that no clinician can say, *"I did not know it was happening"* again.

21. Relevant key data should be forwarded electronically to the body charged with collecting, reviewing and auditing such statistics. Consideration should be given to adapting the existing National Perinatal Reporting Scheme form returned to the ESRI (and others), and to the standard maternal discharge form being developed by the National Perinatal Epidemiological Centre at University Hospital Cork or the forms and software being developed by the Rotunda Hospital.

22. All consultants should be subjected to rigorous independent clinical competence appraisal and evaluation every 5 years and arrangements should be put in place for training and development on a needs basis in specialist centres of learning. Retraining and skills updating should be seen as the norm for all and not as a sanction for the few.

23. RECOMMENDATIONS FOR MIDWIVES

23.1 LEAD MIDWIFERY CLINICIAN

The appointment of a lead midwifery clinician, elected from the ranks of midwives on the labour ward for a period of 3 years, should be made. This is intended to ensure new ideas will be ventilated, leadership style will change regularly, and the burden of leadership on the labour ward will be shared. This position is not intended to displace the Assistant Director of Nursing in charge in the Maternity Unit or the Labour Ward Superintendent, but to be a complementary position.

➢ The lead midwifery clinician should be involved in liaison with the obstetrics lead clinician and work towards multidisciplinary **team** approaches to obstetric cases. There has to be a more constructive, complementary and fluid relationship between midwives and obstetricians, which is patient centred and not task focused, and avoids assumptions that 'natural' delivery or 'managed labour' is superior or that obstetricians or anaesthetists are interventionist.

➢ The lead midwifery clinician should be responsible for ensuring that the consultant anaesthetist on duty is apprised on a regular basis of all problem or potential problem maternity admissions. The obstetric anaesthetist should be alerted to the status of inpatients with known placenta previa, multiple pregnancy, placenta accreta, accidental haemorrhage and the possibility of caesarean section and/or blood replacement requirements.

➢ The lead midwifery clinician should have protected sessions each week to deal specifically with continuing education and discussion of adverse outcomes and near misses separately from the daily handover meetings and the weekly clinical governance obstetric meetings, to permit midwifery focused learning on evidence-based practice. Clinical governance at obstetric level may identify different issues and entirely miss midwifery concerns on the labour ward floor which could include women's comfort in birthing positions, the use of oxytocin, the length of time between delivery of the baby and the placenta, methods of rubbing up contractions, cord traction etc.

➢ The lead midwifery clinician should ensure that every member of the midwifery staff recognises and embraces clinical governance and understands clinical audit, risk management (including clinical incident reporting) and best practice, and receives appropriate training.

23.2   Continuing **medical** and skills based education should be encouraged and facilitated.

23.3   As with obstetricians, agreed, multi-disciplinary, massive obstetric haemorrhage protocols should be *clear*, _unambiguous,_ *widely available* and practiced as a drill. The article written by Rotunda Hospital (Rizvi et al, BJOG, May 2004) on post partum haemorrhage should be studied and similar audit carried out.

23.4   Information Technology

> A comprehensive, effective, user friendly IT system must be installed and become operational immediately.

> All midwifery staff must have or receive basic computer skills to input, access and transmit data electronically. The best training is 'on the job'. Information should be inputted into the system promptly as each patient is cared for on the labour ward and before she goes to the post natal ward. The use of Midwifery websites should be encouraged for increasing awareness of changing practice in the treatment of common problems.

> All patient records should be in standard format from which key data can be extracted for internal and external audit.

> As with the obstetricians, relevant key data should be forwarded electronically to the body charged with collecting, reviewing and auditing such statistics. Consideration should be given to adapting the existing National Perinatal Reporting Scheme form returned to the ESRI (and others), and also the standard maternal discharge form being developed by the National Perinatal Epidemiological Centre at University Hospital Cork or the forms and software being developed by the Rotunda Hospital.

> Until a computerised data collection system is in place, midwives engaged in audit should be apprised of the value of the HIPE system, and through the encoders obtain access to this very extensive data base for audit and research. Midwives should be encouraged to engage in meaningful clinical audit and research from a midwifery perspective.

23.5   Lecturers from other midwifery centres should be invited on a regular basis to address midwives on topical subjects to disseminate information on changing practices.

23.6   A detailed midwifery section in the annual Maternity Clinical Report should be prepared showing all activity and outcomes from a midwifery as distinct from an obstetric perspective.

23.7   Consideration should be given to regular temporary exchange of clinical midwife managers with midwives of similar rank in hospitals within the same group, or a mentor teaching hospital in Dublin or abroad.

23.8   The Assistant Director of Nursing of the Maternity Unit should meet with other directors of other maternity units regularly in order to keep in touch with new standards and benchmarks. Visits to other maternity facilities should be undertaken.

23.9   Every effort must be maintained to eliminate isolation. Awareness of best practice in the profession should be adopted. Reports of criticisms made of midwifery practice in medico-legal cases should be disseminated and discussed.

23.10   A fulltime **midwifery clinical skills facilitator** to update and evaluate all midwifery competence should be engaged. This clinical skills facilitator should meet regularly with the most senior midwives and work out training strategies.

23.11   The importance of accurate, contemporaneous and legible note taking and recording should be emphasised and regularly subject to spot random audit by the line manager or ward sister. Signatures in records should be legible.

23.12 All levels of midwifery staff should be encouraged to openly discuss concerns and complaints at regular midwife meetings.

24. ANAESTHETISTS

THIS GROUP CAUSED US CONCERN. MANY YOUNG WOMEN UNDERWENT HYSTERECTOMY OR OOPHORECTOMY WITHOUT COMMENT FROM THE ANAESTHETISTS WHO ACCEPTED WITHOUT QUESTION THAT THE SURGEON WAS THE EXPERT IN HIS FIELD. THIS GROUP SHOULD USE THE CLINICAL GOVERNANCE MEETINGS TO VOICE QUERIES OR CONCERNS. THERE HAS TO BE A WAY FOR ANAESTHETISTS TO BE AWARE OF DATA FROM THE MATERNITY UNIT.

24.1 The department should have an elected **lead and deputy lead anaesthetist** responsible for maintaining standards and updating knowledge in the department of anaesthetics. The election should be from the consultants within the anaesthetic department and be for a period of 5 years.

24.2 The lead anaesthetist should be responsible for ensuring that each member of the Department of Anaesthetics should attend a course in clinical governance in order that clinical audit, risk management are fully understood.

24.3 Training in the concept of teamwork in theatre should be mandatory.

24.4 **At least two of** the anaesthetists should have **specialist training in obstetric** anaesthesia – all the other members of the team must attend professional development courses in obstetrics related anaesthesia and haemorrhage control.

24.5 Protocols for urgent blood supplies should be agreed with the pathology department, and drills practised.

24.6 Anaesthetists must attend obstetric clinical governance meetings when cases with anaesthetic input are being discussed. Arrangements should be made to facilitate the attendance of the anaesthetists by discussing those cases as the first item on the agenda.

24.7   The numbers of consultant anaesthetists and NCHDs must rise significantly so as to be able to provide full obstetric cover on 24 hour basis 7 days a week and to provide cover for the increasing needs of the catchment area of the hospital.

24.8   Anaesthetists must be aware of advised and agreed sentinel events in obstetrics and gynaecology and must recognise their professional obligations to fill in clinical incident forms when such events occur.

24.9   The lead anaesthetist should consider and evaluate the system of partnership between certain anaesthetic consultants and obstetricians in the care of private patients and determine whether such arrangements are capable of compromising independent appraisal of clinical management of patients and if so, the arrangements should be discouraged.

24.10   There should be a high dependency unit in the Maternity Unit for patients requiring special observation following surgery. Anaesthetists should write detailed observations on such patients' charts.

25.   PATHOLOGISTS

THE INQUIRY WAS CONCERNED AT THE LACK OF AWARENESS OF THE EXTENT OF PERIPARTUM HYSTERECTOMIES IN THE MATERNITY UNIT DURING THE 1990S. AS WITH THE ANAESTHETISTS AND THE OBSTETRICIANS, THERE WAS A TENDENCY FOR EACH PATHOLOGIST TO WORK ON HIS OWN CASES WITH LITTLE TIME OR OPPORTUNITY TO ENGAGE IN TEAM DISCUSSION OR REVIEW OF CASES DEALT WITH BY COLLEAGUES. THERE WAS NO SYSTEM OF ENTERING KEY DATA INTO EXISTING COMPUTERS FOR EASY RETRIEVAL. THERE WAS NO PRACTICE OF DISCUSSION OF EVENTS IN THE MATERNITY UNIT.

25.1   A new protocol should be established requiring two consultants to view slides before histology diagnosis is made in cases where such diagnosis is critical or urgently required. The pathologists should consult with the lead obstetrician to establish such key cases but it is suggested that placenta accreta is one such case.

25.2 To facilitate Recommendation 1 there should be two histopathologists on day duty at all times.

25.3 The practice of a single pathologist reviewing pathology slides on a week on week off basis should be reviewed.

25.4 Histopathologist should attend clinical governance obstetric/gynaecology meetings where Pathology issues or histopathology results or reports are on the agenda.

25.5 Pathologists should develop the habit of telephone discussions with obstetricians and encourage obstetricians to discuss their concerns more fully than in the past.

25.6 Pathologists should engage in clinical audit and review and meet as a team on a regular basis.

25.7 All the pathologists should be able to access data of histopathology results without patient identifying names and numbers on an instant basis. For example, if information is required on the numbers of specimens received where the clinician diagnosed placenta accreta or where an obstetric hysterectomy was carried out, that information should be quickly retrievable from a computer in the pathology department. To this day, retrieving such data involves reviewing the theatre registers or labour ward hand written data.

25.8 Pathology reports should be more informative, reasoned and consideration should be given to adding digital photographs of the surgical specimen.

25.9 Pathologists and the haematologist should be aware of changing needs for blood replacement in the maternity theatres and ensure that they are involved in drafting and updating protocols with the obstetricians and anaesthetists for the treatment of massive haemorrhage.

25.10 A third pathologist, a haematologist and microbiologist should be appointed as a matter of urgency. These three additional specialists should not be required to share attendance at other hospitals.

25.11 It is recommended that formal Director of Pathology services be appointed in the pathology department and that the practice that the longest serving is automatically considered the senior consultant is discontinued. The position should revolve between the consultants in the department.

26. MEDICAL COUNCIL

26.1 The Inquiry is acutely aware of the sense of frustration felt by members of the Medical Council and the medical professional bodies at the lack of a new Statute giving the Council statutory powers to oblige doctors to engage in continuous medical education and to present for skills assessment. The Medical Council needs these powers urgently so that it can delegate those duties to those professional bodies to regulate the training and continuous assessment of their members.

26.2 The needs of the general public require that the professional bodies have the power and effective means at their disposal to monitor the competence of their members in order to ensure optimum patient care. In the past and perhaps at this present some doctors are engaging in procedures beyond their skills and some are failing to apply current practice. There is **currently no legal obligation** to keep their skills updated. This must change.

26.3 Competence assurance is not met solely by attendance at continuing professional development courses. Skills must be certified or validated. The public must have faith in an independent regulating body within the State, which should not require that review of a practitioner's practice must come from abroad as was necessary in Dr. Neary's case. The Medical Council should have the power to:

➢ Oblige all obstetricians in practice in the State - including those who have not been included on the Specialist Register - to engage in continuing professional development and independent competence appraisal at least once every 5 years. There should be a system of certification in place and a system of arranging standard courses for all specialists in practice.

➢ Oblige all obstetrician/gynaecologists, anaesthetists and pathologists to submit their practice to annual clinical audit and review. This should include private practice in both public and private hospitals.

➢ Before any consultant engages in a particular procedure ensure that he is certified to be competent in that area. The Medical Council must have the power to delegate that power to the individual recognised professional bodies.

➢ Be in a position to provide the training/support following assessment as required, with the power to impose limitations on practice in areas where requisite competence or experience is not shown on audit/review/competence assessment. If re-entering practice after significant absence then the Medical Council must have the power to adopt/adapt RCOG Guidelines for retraining/competence assurance and Recommendations in RCOG "Discussion on Further Training for Doctors in Difficulty", April 2002.

➢ Oblige all medical practitioners to attend training on clinical governance, which includes improving knowledge, engaging in clinical audit and risk management.

➢ Issue guidelines to ensure that all hospitals have an easily accessible complaints/concerns procedure in place and advise on the appropriateness of the use of such confidential procedure whenever the need arises.

➢ Set up a confidential help line for medical practitioners who have serious concerns about a colleague and feel unable to bring those concerns before their own clinical directors. There has to be a system for dealing with concerns at an early stage which does not have the stigma and ensuing upset of a complaint to the Medical Council or a high profile court action.

➢ Empower the Institute of Obstetricians to visit **all** Maternity and Gynaecology Units in the State on a continuing and regular basis. The visiting Committees should consist of **practitioners from each** of the country's maternity units so that all obstetricians eventually become aware of conditions prevailing in **all maternity units** in the jurisdiction and thus can identify standards in the services provided in each particular unit.

27.   DEPARTMENT OF HEALTH AND CHILDREN /GOVERNMENT THROUGH HSE

27.1   While much of what was discovered to be substandard in the Lourdes Hospital can best be remedied at hospital level, the Department of Health and Children and the HSE have the power to ensure that professional medical institutions have the legal authority and the financial resources to properly and effectively regulate their members. The Inquiry was unimpressed by the unwieldy bureaucracy of the Health Board in dealing with replacement and recruitment of staff, the setting up of an IT system in the Maternity Unit, the slow response to the introduction of an acceptable risk management programme, the constant turnover of hospital managers, the distance between the Health Board Chief Executive Officer and the consultants and the belief that if "Kells" did not approve of something, then it would not happen. Over and over, we were told of political interests and political motives for taking or not taking certain steps. There was the very strong impression given that hospitals were perceived first as providers of jobs in the locality rather than providers of health services.

27.2   The Medical Council and the professional regulatory bodies do not have the power to enforce compliance with continuing professional development and a system of identifying substandard doctors. Peer review works well in large university hospitals but can fail miserably in smaller personality driven units in provincial hospitals. The Inquiry was disturbed at the acceptance by many outside Obstetricians that the International Missionary Training Hospital at Drogheda was different and that different standards therefore applied. The Inquiry was equally disturbed that provincial hospitals are not expected to provide the same level of care as the Dublin training hospitals. While it is perfectly understandable that provincial hospitals cannot provide the same range of treatments as are available in nominated centres of specialisation, there is no valid reason why the standard of care in the more limited services provided in provincial hospitals should be of a lower standard. We were also disturbed that consultant posts were unfilled for extended periods; consultants were left to carry impossible workloads and there was no system for helping consultants suffering high stress levels. Only last year, in this hospital under media scrutiny, there were extended periods where one or two consultants carried the workload of the unit. It takes too long for the employing authorities to react to emergency needs and it appears that no contingency plans are in being to deal with unplanned staff shortages.

27.3 The Inquiry was concerned at the speed at which the Health Board could set up politically propelled new services while others were left to crisis manage. A midwifery led unit was funded and made operational in the Lourdes Hospital in spite of serious misgivings at the timing of such unit by the senior medical adviser to the Health Board, the one remaining consultant on duty in the Maternity Unit and the views of the Institute of Obstetricians and Gynaecologists. The concerns at the timing of the opening of the unit appear to have been misconstrued as opposition to the idea of midwifery led unit and were utterly disregarded. Had there been any serious mishap arising from the operation of the Unit at a time when only two consultants were available out of a complement of seven, this could have had unfair repercussions for the recovering reputation of the Hospital.

27.4 This Maternity Unit was inspected by various professional bodies for suitability for training of midwives and doctors but those bodies did not identify its abnormal and unusual practices. There are clearly **deficits in an approval for training process** where poor practice by professionals engaged in the very training which is being accredited is not identified. There must be a patient centred element to the approval for training process where there is an assurance of standards in the provision of care. Unusual procedures or unusual outcomes require explanation.

27.5 There is no national reporting system in place. We understand that such a system exists in Australia and Canada. We believe that **national reporting of sentinel events** would have a beneficial effect on claims and on standards in obstetrics. If every maternity unit was obliged each day to fill in key details of mother and baby into a computer programme with connections to the other maternity units in the State, and the data thus received was regularly analysed, there would be much benefit to the health system. An early warning system would operate to identify and isolate unusual practices conditions or outcomes. Poor practice must not be handed on to trainees.

27.6 The Inquiry believes that **more autonomy** should be afforded to the **management of each hospital** and particularly that the management of this Hospital should be responsible and accountable for expenditure, planning, standards of care and claims. All members of staff from porters to cleaners to assistant managers and consultants must learn that they are employed to provide a service and that they should be accountable for failure to follow best practice. Risk management training must be extended to all employees in a hospital. As the Lourdes Hospital is a major hospital in the health service, the person appointed as Manager should be highly skilled and experienced in hospital management. That person should be offered at least a five year contract and be paid a salary commensurate to skill, experience and responsibility.

27.7 The Lourdes Hospital Maternity Unit is unrecognisable since 1998. The Hospital is in lay ownership while the MMMs continue to play an important pastoral role. Last year more than 3400 babies were delivered. The increasing affluence of the nation has released funds to raise the numbers of consultants employed and improved the range of services offered but the general hospital is bursting at the seams and is often seriously overcrowded. Beds have been provided at the expense of planned operations. Highly skilled staff members are thus frequently underutilised. The A&E department is physically too small to cope with the demand on its services. The X Ray and scanning rooms are totally inadequate for the population using those services. It is impossible to park at the Hospital. For a major trauma centre the route to the Hospital is not marked nor is the appropriate exit from the motorway indicated. The services offered in the Hospital are frequently distant from the patients' homes and the time has come for the planners of the health needs of the North Eastern region to provide a centrally located new hospital with an upgraded road service to each of the major population centres in the region. It would be tragic if top quality staff begins leaking away from the hospital because of inadequate patient facilities. Perhaps the project design team will consider locating the proposed new regional hospital in a green field site equidistant from the major towns in the region but with accessibility for staff and patients in the region.

27.8 There is a well advanced draft Medical Practitioners Act in being. The Department of Health and Children and the Health Service Executive should engage in completing this process and introduce a **wide-ranging new Medical Practitioners Act** as a matter of urgency with the following key provisions:

> Give statutory powers to the Medical Council, in association with the professional bodies to set standards and enforce competence assurance. There must be an obligation on all clinicians to attend professional development courses at regular intervals **and** be assessed and certified for competence in their field.

> Empower the Medical Council to set standards for competence assurance, with input/guidance from the appropriate professional body – in this instance the Institute of Obstetricians and Gynaecologists.

> Provide adequate financial supports to enable the Medical Council and the professional bodies to carry out competence assurance, conduct inspections, issue guidelines, provide lectures and otherwise ensure professional standards. Since writing these recommendations the HSE now has taken on the responsibility for funding health projects and many of the previous of functions of the Health Boards. Obviously, the recommendations that require funding should be brought to the attention of the appropriate governmental body.

> Empower the Institute of Obstetricians and Gynaecologists to enforce standards on its members with the power to oblige practitioners whose skills are found wanting to attend for further training and the financial means to be an effective overseer of the profession. The Medical Council must have a role in censuring non-compliant practitioners.

> Provide for compulsory specialist registration with the Institute of Obstetricians and Gynaecologists in Ireland for those practising as specialist obstetricians/gynaecologists who are not on the specialist register.

➢ The HSE should consider applying the fruits of existing research into the Role of Clinicians in Management to the Lourdes Hospital. Its rapidly growing size warrants analysis of the appropriateness of the application of the concept to this Hospital.

➢ **The Department of Health and Children should introduce legislation to protect clinical governance records and risk management clinical incident report forms from the application of the Freedom of Information Act. Unless these documents are protected from FOI or discovery they are unlikely to be created and opportunities for learning from mistakes will be lost.**

➢ The Maternity Homes Act, 1934, and the regulations made thereunder have fallen into disuse and are inadequate to ensure minimum standards in maternity hospitals. There is currently no legislation regulating the setting up of a hospital. We could find no evidence of any controls over private hospitals including maternity hospitals apart from the inadequate and unused Maternity Homes Act. There must be a monitoring body for standards in all health care facilities.

28. HOSPITAL

28.1 The Medical director should be given wider powers to govern medical staff regarding clinical standards. He should play a key role shared with the hospital manager in ensuring that governance is taught, understood and practised by the entire hospital. He should attend all Medical Board meetings.

28.2 Each lead clinician and deputy should be afforded protected time for the carrying out of their specific functions.

28.3 A rolling half day for hospital wide audit should be established where all non emergency clinical work is halted and each department engages in audit processes. If the first half day set aside is the first day of the month being a Wednesday, then the next half day will be a month later on a Thursday etc. This process is up and running in Northern Ireland.

28.4 The lead clinicians should make up the Medical Board with representation from long term locums to encourage involvement in and awareness of hospital policy. There should be regular meetings between hospital administrators and lead clinicians to identify needs, planning strategies and clinical/personnel issues within hospital.

28.5 Clear effective complaints procedures should be established for dealing with all hospital matters and it should be ensured that the risk managers prepare an appendix to the annual clinical reports of all complaints received, identifying the department involved, the level of the staff member complained and whether the complaints were resolved, and compare the complaints year on year. Patients should be encouraged to identify deficits in service at every stage of their visit to the Hospital. There should be complaints forms and boxes to receive them on every floor of the Hospital. Complaints apply to every level of service from clinical complaints to cleanliness complaints.

28.6 Effective processes must be established to identify forthcoming vacancies in consultant and other staff numbers and to provide for replacements in a much shorter time.

28.7 Processes for identifying failed safety protocols in this or any unit in the Hospital should be put in place.

28.8 The hospital management which should include the General Manager, the Hospital Board, the Clinical Director, the directors of nursing, and senior nursing sisters should have autonomy in relation to budget, costs, insurance, personnel, equipment acquisition, replacement and maintenance, and claims.

28.9 There is a need for the hospital Manager to be seen less as manager of a group of hospitals, less as an administrator attached to HSE area headquarters in Kells, and more as CEO of the Lourdes Hospital, and to concentrate on giving management and leadership there.

28.10 Accommodation and secretarial requirements have been expressed, which should be dealt with as a matter of urgency by management. The Inquiry from its many visits to the Hospital is all too aware of the constraints on space (particularly evident in A & E), and problems with further developing the site, and appreciates the difficulties that this recommendation poses. It is also cognisant of the review of services in the North Eastern Area being undertaken by the H.S.E., and ideas such as the development of a new hospital on a green field site may prove to be the only answer in the long run. Any such review must take account of the need for office space for clinicians, and to facilitate necessary improvements in clinical governance, audit and risk management with a view to improving patient care.

28.11 The department of Obstetrics and Gynaecology should have a dedicated risk manager who reports in the first place to the enhanced management structures within the Lourdes Hospital. There should be continuing liaison between the lead clinicians within the department.

28.12 Risk management should apply to all levels of employment in the hospital.

28.13 The hospital must have a computerised data inputting and retrieval system in every department.

28.14 Expert opinion should be engaged to advise on secure systems of electronic storage and retrieval of hospital records. A series of security cameras should be placed where key documents are stored and security keys with memory chips should be used for access to secure areas.

29. JUNIOR DOCTORS

29.1 Comprehensive undergraduate training on the meaning and proper conduct of clinical governance with its components of learning, audit and risk management, both personal and team based, should be a compulsory module for all student doctors as should courtesy to patients. This includes introduction not merely by saying "I am Dr. A" but rather "I am John Doe, SHO/Registrar to Dr. X". It also includes explaining the procedure they are about to carry out and listening to what the patient has to say before proceeding. The complaint made repeatedly by patients was rudeness and lack of communication skills. Patients like to know who their treating doctor is and like to know what their treatment plan is.

29.2   A dedicated period of induction should be reserved at the commencement of all NCHD placements or rotations in the Hospital for introduction to layout, staff ID, rosters, clinical meetings, risk management/incident report forms and trigger lists, and management structures including complaints procedures.

29.3   Open and free discussion with consultants on clinical matters should be encouraged with an emphasis on learning and development in a non-fearful environment.

29.4   The deputy lead clinician should organise and monitor junior doctor training and study within the Unit with protected time and administrative resources made available. This function can be delegated to an appropriate consultant.

29.5   A dedicated room should be reserved for training within the Unit, and be adequately equipped with IT and internet access. A well resourced medical library with up to date texts and publications to be maintained.

29.6   Each SHO and registrar should be attached to a specific consultant and work for a specified period of training on that team. Each area of competence should be verified and logged.

29.7   Junior doctors should be encouraged to voice complaints and concerns to the lead clinician or to the consultant charged with education. A clear, structured procedure for expressing concerns or making complaints should be put in place, communicated to junior doctors at induction, and actively managed with comprehensive feedback in the case of issues raised.

29.8   While the collegiality of the link with a particular consultant should be maintained, the requirement of a formal reference prior to obtaining a further position should be removed, and replaced by a certification of competence in listed procedures and treatments and areas of expertise.

29.9   Junior doctors, SHOs or registrars should not be at risk of losing placement or continuity in training because of a bona fide complaint of a colleague or consultant.

29.10 Dedicated efforts to facilitate and integrate non-national doctors should be actively encouraged within the hospital system which should be sympathetic to their particular needs including family, work, visa and culture. They should be encouraged to engage fully in discussions on outcomes.

ADDENDUM TO THE REPORT

1. Just before the report was ready to deliver to the Tánaiste we became aware that a comparison of the numbers of files on the Morpheus database prepared in 1999 and the recheck and recording of the same files in 2003 indicated a shortfall of 165 files.

2. The Inquiry had originally been led to believe that all the so called "*missing files*" had been removed before the database was set up by Morpheus Solutions in late 1999. We had been informed that in 2003 there had been an audit of the first database and that no files were found to be missing. In fact what was meant was that none of the missing files was found in spite of taking out and examining each file. The Inquiry was anxious therefore to determine whether the numbers of files on each database were the same and it was at this stage that we were informed of the discrepancy of 165 files.

3. The report was furnished subject to this addendum. In the meanwhile, several clerical officers with experience of patient records have been engaged in an attempt to reconcile the two databases. The task was nigh impossible due to the absence of a computer disc containing the original 1999 data. A tedious and laborious hand check was carried out. This hand check was confined to the two databases: one was a print-out of Morpheus being a printed list of charts with names and personal details with box numbers where the charts were located, and the other was the computer database created in 2003 of all charts found in storage in the basement at that time and with their new box number. There was no physical examination of charts.

4. This exercise produced the following results:

   ❖ 147 patients' names appeared twice on the 1999 database. When a number of these files was removed from their stated box location, on each occasion it was apparent that information relating to the patient was placed in a different file instead of in the original file thus creating two files for the same patient. These patients did not appear at all in the 2003 database.

❖ 16 further cases of duplication were recognised, and these appeared once on the 2003 database.

❖ 287 further charts appeared on Morpheus but do not appear on the 2003 database. Further checks may locate these charts in the basement. The administrative staff remain confident that these charts are actually in the basement.

❖ 353 charts on the Morpheus print out, made up of all of the 147 and 16 referred to above, and most of the 287 referred to above have no box number, making it very difficult to locate any chart. Nevertheless, it is thought that many of these charts may be in the basement.

❖ When the charts were being checked in 2003 several dozen of them were in the Patient Liaison Office where they were stored pending requests for copy files.

5. It became clear that the only way to actually determine whether any further files were missing since 1999 was to receive a request, check the first database and locate the record of the file there, check if the same file was on the 2003 database and then look for the file in the indicated box in the basement. If the file was not recorded on the Morpheus database or the 2003 database this was an indication that the file was not in the basement when the Morpheus database was set up. If the file was on the first database and not on the second, this was an indication that it had been removed since 1999.

6. We determined that 3 of the "*missing files*" were removed between 1999 and 2003. 1 of those files was removed between 2002 and 2003. The file found in Dr. Neary's house (which did not concern a peripartum hysterectomy) was removed between 1999 and 2003.

7. Until 2003 the security system in the basement was almost non-existent. Any member of staff could task a porter to fetch files from the basement or go to the basement and search for files him/herself. There was no system of recording the use of the key or the taking of files. Files could in fact be

missing, misfiled, seriously mislaid or stolen due to lack of a signing out system or proper security. There are no cameras in the basement and no security tags to trigger alarms. In spite of all the frailties in the storage and recording systems for archived documents, all the administrative staff report that they rarely have difficulties locating files that relate to charts of patients with no connection to Dr. Neary.

8. The administrative staff in Patient Liaison or Medical Records have had no trouble locating charts for routine BCG enquiries or for any other purpose. While it is quite possible therefore that a significant number of files are missing from the archives in the basement, it is unlikely at this remove that they relate to hysterectomies. We are confident that we have established all the peripartum hysterectomies carried out in the old and new Maternity Units. We know that of the 188 identified peripartum hysterectomy patients there are charts for 144.

9. Of the missing 44 charts –

   • 3 are known to have been removed after the Morpheus database was established.

   • 3 were relatively modern cases and would not yet have been transferred to the archives but were not available to the Institute review body in late 1998. These are the cases where the records have been falsified.

   • The rest of the missing files were not available when they were sought between late 1998 and 2003 and are not recorded as being in the basement in 1999 when Morpheus were preparing a database.

10. Regretfully neither the Lourdes Hospital nor the Inquiry had the resources to check up on each file in the archives and to compare it with the contents of the 1999 database. Of the files that are known to be missing, a disproportionate number relate to Dr. Neary. The same problems cannot arise with more recent files as a computerised patient recording system is now in use and a chart tracking system is in operation. The Inquiry remains convinced that although it was not possible to reconcile the two databases

that the removal of the old maternity theatre register, the selective removal of master cards and birth registers which contain details of 40 caesarean hysterectomies and the culling of the corresponding charts is attributable to a deliberate removal of information relating to those hysterectomies. Our original conclusions are unaffected by the possibility that there is a discrepancy between the number of files on the two databases.